Hospitals in a
changing Europe

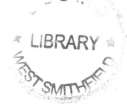

European Observatory on Health Care Systems Series

Series Editors

Josep Figueras is Head of the Secretariat and Research Director of the European Observatory on Health Care Systems and Head of the European Centre for Health Policy, World Health Organization Regional Office for Europe.

Martin McKee is Research Director of the European Observatory on Health Care Systems and Professor of European Public Health at the London School of Hygiene & Tropical Medicine as well as a co-director of the School's European Centre on Health of Societies in Transition.

Elias Mossialos is Research Director of the European Observatory on Health Care Systems and Bnan Abel-Smith Reader in Health Policy, Department of Social Policy, London School of Economics and Political Science and Co-Director of LSE Health and Social Care.

Richard B. Saltman is Research Director of the European Observatory on Health Care Systems and Professor of Health Policy and Management at the Rollins School of Public Health, Emory University in Atlanta, Georgia

The series

The volumes in this series focus on key issues for health policy-making in Europe. Each study explores the conceptual background, outcomes and lessons learned about the development of more equitable, more efficient and more effective health systems in Europe. With this focus, the series seeks to contribute to the evolution of a more evidence-based approach to policy formulation in the health sector.

These studies will be important to all those involved in formulating or evaluating national health care policies and, in particular, will be of use to health policy-makers and advisers, who are under increasing pressure to rationalize the structure and funding of their health systems. Academics and students in the field of health policy will also find this series valuable in seeking to understand better the complex choices that confront the health systems of Europe.

Current and forthcoming titles

Martin McKee and Judith Healy (eds): *Hospitals in a Changing Europe*
Martin McKee, Judith Healy and Jane Falkingham (eds): *Health Care in Central Asia*
Elias Mossialos, Anna Dixon, Josep Figueras and Joe Kutzin (eds): *Funding Health Care: Options for Europe*
Richard B. Saltman, Reinhard Busse and Elias Mossialos (eds): *Regulating Entrepreneurial Behaviour in European Health Care Systems*

The European Observatory on Health Care Systems is a unique project that builds on the commitment of all its partners to improving health care systems:

- World Health Organization Regional Office for Europe
- Government of Greece
- Government of Norway
- Government of Spain
- European Investment Bank
- Open Society Institute
- World Bank
- London School of Economics and Political Science
- London School of Hygiene & Tropical Medicine

The Observatory supports and promotes evidence-based health policy-making through comprehensive and rigorous analysis of the dynamics of health care systems in Europe.

European Observatory on Health Care Systems Series

Edited by Josep Figueras, Martin McKee, Elias Mossialos and Richard B. Saltman

    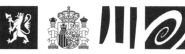

Hospitals in a changing Europe

Edited by

Martin McKee and Judith Healy

Open University Press
Buckingham · Philadelphia

Open University Press
Celtic Court
22 Ballmoor
Buckingham
MK18 1XW

email: enquiries@openup.co.uk
world wide web: www.openup.co.uk

and
325 Chestnut Street
Philadelphia, PA 19106, USA

First Published 2002

A catalogue record of this book is available from the British Library

ISBN 0 335 20928 9 (pb)   0 335 20929 7 (hb)

Library of Congress Cataloging-in-Publication Data
Hospitals in a changing Europe / edited by Martin McKee and Judith Healy.
        p.   cm. — (European Observatory on Health Care Systems series)
    Includes bibliographical references and index.
    ISBN 0-335-20929-7 (hb) — ISBN 0-335-20928-9 (pb)
        1. Hospitals—Europe. 2. Hospitals—Europe—Administration. I. McKee,
    Martin. II. Healy, Judith. III. European Observatory on Health Care
    Systems. IV. Series.
        [DNLM: 1. Hospital Administration—trends—Europe. 2. Health Care
    Reform—Europe. WX 150 H8345 2002]
    RA985 .H676 2002
    362.1′1′094—dc21
                                                                            2001032135

Typeset by Graphicraft Limited, Hong Kong
Printed in Great Britain by Biddles Limited, Guildford and Kings Lynn

Contents

List of figures, tables and boxes

List of contributors

Linda H. Aiken is the Claire M. Fagin Professor of Nursing, Professor of Sociology and Director of the Centre for Health Outcomes and Policy Research at the University of Pennsylvania, Philadelphia, USA.

James Buchan is Reader at the Faculty of Social Sciences and Health Care, Queen Margaret University College, Edinburgh, United Kingdom.

Nigel Edwards is Policy Director of the NHS Confederation, United Kingdom.

Nick Freemantle is Professor of Clinical Epidemiology and Biostatistics, Department of Primary Care and General Practice, University of Birmingham, United Kingdom.

April Harding is a senior specialist on private sector development for Health Nutrition and Population at the World Bank.

Anthony Harrison is Fellow in Health Systems at the King's Fund, London, United Kingdom.

Judith Healy is Senior Research Fellow of the European Observatory on Health Care Systems, and is an honorary senior lecturer in Public Health and Policy at the London School of Hygiene & Tropical Medicine, United Kingdom.

Martin Hensher is European Union Consultant in Health Economics for the Health Financing and Economics Directorate, Department of Health, Pretoria, South Africa.

Melitta Jakab is a health economist, Health Nutrition and Population at the World Bank.

John C. Langenbrunner is a senior economist at the World Bank.

Martin McKee is Research Director of the European Observatory on Health Care Systems and Professor of European Public Health at the London School of Hygiene & Tropical Medicine, London, United Kingdom.

Fiona O'May is Research Assistant at the Faculty of Social Sciences and Health Care, Queen Margaret University College, Edinburgh, United Kingdom.

John Posnett is Director of the York Health Economics Consortium, University of York, United Kingdom.

Alexander S. Preker is Chief Economist for Health, Nutrition and Population at the World Bank.

Rebecca Rosen is Fellow in Primary Care at the King's Fund, London, United Kingdom.

Douglas Sloane is Adjunct Associate Professor at the Center for Health Outcomes and Policy Research at the University of Pennsylvania, Philadelphia, and Associate Professor of Sociology at the Catholic University of America, Washington, DC, USA.

Miriam Wiley is Head of the Health Policy Research Centre and Senior Research Officer at the Economic and Social Research Institute, Dublin, Ireland.

Series editors' introduction

European national policy-makers broadly agree on the core objectives that their health care systems should pursue. The list is strikingly straightforward: universal access for all citizens, effective care for better health outcomes, efficient use of resources, high-quality services and responsiveness to patient concerns. It is a formula that resonates across the political spectrum and which, in various, sometimes inventive configurations, has played a role in most recent European national election campaigns.

Yet this clear consensus can only be observed at the abstract policy level. Once decision-makers seek to translate their objectives into the nuts and bolts of health system organization, common principles rapidly devolve into divergent, occasionally contradictory, approaches. This is, of course, not a new phenomenon in the health sector. Different nations, with different histories, cultures and political experiences, have long since constructed quite different institutional arrangements for funding and delivering health care services.

The diversity of health system configurations that has developed in response to broadly common objectives leads quite naturally to questions about the advantages and disadvantages inherent in different arrangements, and which approach is 'better' or even 'best' given a particular context and set of policy priorities. These concerns have intensified over the last decade as policy-makers have sought to improve health system performance through what has become a European-wide wave of health system reforms. The search for comparative advantage has triggered – in health policy as in clinical medicine – increased attention to its knowledge base, and to the possibility of overcoming at least part of existing institutional divergence through more evidence-based health policy-making.

The volumes published in the European Observatory series are intended to provide precisely this kind of cross-national health policy analysis. Drawing on an extensive network of experts and policy-makers working in a variety of academic and administrative capacities, these studies seek to synthesize the available evidence on key health sector topics using a systematic methodology. Each volume explores the conceptual background, outcomes and lessons learned about the development of more equitable, more efficient and more effective health care systems in Europe. With this focus, the series seeks to contribute to the evolution of a more evidence-based approach to policy formulation in the health sector. While remaining sensitive to cultural, social and normative differences among countries, the studies explore a range of policy alternatives available for future decision-making. By examining closely both the advantages and disadvantages of different policy approaches, these volumes fulfil a central mandate of the Observatory: to serve as a bridge between pure academic research and the needs of policy-makers, and to stimulate the development of strategic responses suited to the real political world in which health sector reform must be implemented.

The European Observatory on Health Care Systems is a partnership that brings together three international agencies, three national governments, two research institutions and an international non-governmental organization. The partners are as follows: the World Health Organization Regional Office for Europe, which provides the Observatory secretariat; the governments of Greece, Norway and Spain; the European Investment Bank; the Open Society Institute; the World Bank; the London School of Hygiene & Tropical Medicine and the London School of Economics and Political Science.

In addition to the analytical and cross-national comparative studies published in this Open University Press series, the Observatory produces Health Care Systems in Transition Profiles (HiTs) for the countries of Europe, the Observatory Summer School and the *Euro Observer* newsletter. Further information about Observatory publications and activities can be found on its web site at www.observatory.dk.

Josep Figueras, Martin McKee, Elias Mossialos and Richard B. Saltman

Foreword

The publication of the World Health Report 2000 entitled *Health Systems: Improving Performance* has stimulated policy-makers worldwide to look again at their health care systems. Advances in knowledge, technology and pharmaceuticals enable health care to make a much greater contribution to health than was possible in the past. Unfortunately, this potential is still unrealized in many countries. Health care systems often fail to provide effective care or to respond to patients' legitimate expectations.

The hospital plays a central role in the delivery of health care. Yet for too long it has received relatively little attention from academics and policy-makers. In part, this is because hospital reform is regarded as a difficult issue. Hospitals are complex institutions, often shrouded in mystique. Their distribution and configuration often owe more to the needs of previous generations than to those of today, and hospitals often appear resistant to change. But the demands they face, from changing populations, diseases and the need to respond to technological developments and popular expectations, are constantly changing. Thus both policy-makers and the hospitals themselves must respond to these pressures for change.

What, then, is the role of the hospital of the future? This book identifies the multiple goals of the hospital but also its centrality in promoting health. It stresses the need for governments, and those acting on their behalf, to invest in the prerequisites for effective care, including people, facilities and knowledge. It emphasizes the need to link together the different parts of the health care system, within a framework characterized by cooperation rather than conflict.

In producing this study, the European Observatory on Health Care Systems has drawn on the conceptual skills of senior academics as well as the practical experience of policy-makers to provide a basis for more effective health policy-making.

Marc Danzon
WHO Regional Director for Europe

Acknowledgements

This volume is one in a series of books undertaken by the European Observatory on Health Care Systems. We are very grateful to our authors, who responded promptly both in producing and later amending their chapters in the light of ongoing discussions.

We particularly appreciate the detailed and very constructive comments of our reviewers, Phillip Berman, Antonio Duran, Zsuzsanna Jakab, Charles Normand, Constantino Sakellarides, Richard B. Saltman, Igor Sheiman, Per-Gunnar Svensson and Andrew Woodhead. Additional material was provided by Ellen Nolte, Reinhard Busse, Elias Mossialos and Jeffrey Sturchio. We should also like to thank the Observatory's partners for their review of, and input to, successive versions of the manuscript.

Anne-Pierre Pickaert provided invaluable research assistance in the early stages on the book. Caroline White patiently and with good humour processed and formatted successive versions of chapters and coped with meeting deadlines.

We also thank all our colleagues in the Observatory. In particular, we are extremely grateful to Josep Figueras for commenting in detail on two drafts of the book and for his encouragement – as well as for his frequent reminders of slipping deadlines. Thanks go also to Reinhard Busse, who commented on several chapters. Special thanks are due to Suszy Lessof for coordinating the studies, to Jeffrey Lazarus, Jenn Cain and Phyllis Dahl for managing the book delivery and production, and to Myriam Andersen and Sue Gammerman for administrative support. We are also grateful to David Breuer for copy-editing the manuscript.

We wish to thank Random House for permission to reproduce an extract from *In Siberia* by Colin Thubron (publisher Chatto & Windus), to John Murray (Publishers) Ltd for permission to reproduce an extract from *Where the Indus is Young*, by Dervla Murphy.

Finally, we are grateful to our partners, Dorothy McKee and Tony McMichael, for their support and forbearance.

Martin McKee and Judith Healy

part one

The context of hospitals

one

The significance
of hospitals:
an introduction

Martin McKee and Judith Healy

Why a book on hospitals?

Hospitals are an important component of the health care system and are central to the process of reform, and yet, as institutions, they have received remarkably little attention from policy-makers and researchers. They are important within the health care system for several reasons. First, they account for a substantial proportion of the health care budget: about 50 per cent in many western European countries and 70 per cent or more in countries of the former Soviet Union. Second, their position at the apex of the health care system means that the policies they adopt, which determine access to specialist services, have a major impact on overall health care. Third, the specialists who work in hospitals provide professional leadership. Finally, technological and pharmaceutical developments, as well as more attention to evidence-based health care, mean that the services that hospitals provide can potentially contribute significantly to population health (McKee 1999). If hospitals are ineffectively organized, however, their potentially positive impact on health will be reduced or even be negative.

Attention to hospitals is timely, since hospitals throughout Europe are facing growing and rapidly changing pressures. These include the impact of changes in populations, patterns of disease, opportunities for medical intervention with new knowledge and technology, and public and political expectations. These changes have important implications for how hospital care is provided, since new types of care require new configurations of buildings, people with different skills and new ways of working. One implication is the need to shift the boundary between hospital and primary care, where hospitals are sometimes criticized for being slow to adapt and to take advantage of developments that permit community-based alternatives.

Hospitals are, however, changing. Since the early 1980s, many countries have sought to reduce their hospital capacity and to shift care to alternative settings (Saltman and Figueras 1997; Brownell *et al.* 1999; Pollock *et al.* 1999; Street and Haycock 1999). Hospitals increasingly focus on acute (short-term) care, only admitting people with conditions requiring relatively intensive medical or nursing care or sophisticated diagnosis or treatment. Hospitals must adapt internally to these new circumstances.

The people responsible for implementing change face many uncertainties about how to proceed. This book argues that an essential first step is to seek out the research evidence on the best strategies for improving hospital performance and also to draw on the experiences of other countries. There is now considerable information on what does and what does not work, although this is not always easy to locate and evaluate. We have tried to assist in this process by reviewing the evidence and, we hope, presenting it in an accessible way.

This book is aimed at people interested in health policy as it affects hospitals. They include, we believe, policy analysts and researchers and those working within governments, insurance funds and regional health authorities, but also practising hospital managers interested in the policy environment within which they work. This is not, however, a textbook on how to manage a hospital. For that, the reader must look to the many books on this topic published elsewhere.

This publication differs from much that has been written previously about hospitals, as it focuses on their role, as part of a wider health care system, in improving health and responding to the legitimate needs of people who use hospitals. Specifically, although this book recognizes that hospitals must be sustainable financially, it is not concerned with issues such as maximizing profits or market share. These are of little relevance in Europe, and people wishing to explore these issues should look to literature from the United States.

The focus of this book is on the hospital in Europe, both western and eastern Europe. We use these broad terms for convenience, although we are well aware that the borders of Europe as well as the acceptable terms are much debated. Where appropriate, reference also is made to sub-regions, such as the countries of the European Union, central and eastern Europe, the former Soviet Union, and the former Soviet republics of central Asia. Europe is, therefore, very diverse (McKee and Jacobson 2000), with each country's health care system reflecting its unique culture and history. Although much can be learned from the experience of other countries, we argue that a policy that works in one setting should not be applied uncritically in a very different setting. This can be illustrated by the frequently asked, but difficult to answer, question of what is the right number of hospital beds. For example, while there is general agreement (at least among western European experts) that Soviet-era levels of hospital capacity in eastern Europe should be reduced, comparisons with western countries must be made cautiously. First, the social context is quite different, with few support mechanisms in place, whether social services or supermarkets. Second, some argue that downsizing has gone too far in some western countries, such as the United Kingdom and the United States. In these countries, reductions in staff and facilities have not been matched by reductions in workload, so that increasing pressures on staff have led to a decline in the quality of care (Hensher *et al.* 1999; Reissman *et al.* 1999). Finally, there is the question of whether a reduction in hospital capacity on its own can achieve the intended savings, since the intensity of treatment in the remaining facilities increases (Shanahan *et al.* 1999).

What is a hospital?

At the outset, it is necessary to be clear about the subject of this book. What, precisely, is a hospital? One definition is that it is 'an institution which provides beds, meals, and constant nursing care for its patients while they undergo medical therapy at the hands of professional physicians. In carrying out these services, the hospital is striving to restore its patients to health' (Miller 1997). Although this captures its essence, a hospital can cover very diverse structures. A hospital might be a ten-bed building without running water in a Siberian village or a large specialist centre equipped with the most advanced technology in a western European city (Box 1.1). This diversity is not surprising, given

---

Box 1.1 Two hospitals

The hospital in Potalovo: In the mid-1990s, the travel writer Colin Thubron travelled through Siberia. Here is his description of a hospital in Potalovo, a small village on the River Yenisei in the northern Russian Federation.

> His hospital was a low, wooden ark. Reindeer moss caulked the gaps between its logs, and it buckled at either end from permafrost . . . Inside the building was a simple range of three-bed wards, a kitchen and a consulting room. It had no running water, and its lavatory was a hole in the ground. Between the double windows the sealing moss had fallen in faded tresses. It was almost without equipment. But the rooms were all washed white and eggshell blue, and three part-time nurses tended the five children in its narrow, iron beds, while a woman recovering from premature childbirth lay silent in another.
>
> (Thubron 1999: 131)

Johann Wolfgang Goethe University Hospital, Germany: Founded in 1884 by the City of Frankfurt, this municipal hospital was taken over by Goethe University medical faculty in 1914 and in 1967 by the State of Hessen, and now is run by a board of directors. The hospital is a large medical complex that carries out medical treatment, research and teaching, with an annual budget of €322 million. It has over 60 buildings, 4500 staff and 1443 hospital beds. The hospital annually treats 41,000 inpatients and 170,000 outpatients in 11 medical centres that include 26 specialist departments. Research is conducted through 26 research institutes, while as a university hospital it annually trains over 3500 medical and dental students, 180 nurses and 160 medical technicians. There are close links to affiliated teaching hospitals in Frankfurt and to other research institutes around the country.

Source: Johann Wolfgang Goethe University Hospital.
http://www.klinik.uni-frankfurt.de/en/patient/patinfo/p33.asp (accessed 21 January 2001)

that some countries in Europe spend less than €50 per head of population per year on hospitals, whereas others spend almost €14,000.

Second, the type of hospital can be difficult to classify. For example, how does one classify a facility that links a small acute care service to a larger long-term care facility? What is the difference between a small community hospital offering mainly nursing care and a nursing home visited daily by a physician? This dilemma was captured by the travel writer Dervla Murphy who, commenting on a hospital in northern Pakistan that closed on weekends, public holidays and religious feasts, described it as 'more a statistic than reality' (Murphy 1995).

Third, a hospital may spread across many buildings, or hospitals on different sites may merge into one organizational structure. Thus, the United Kingdom stopped counting 'hospitals' in 1992 and instead publishes statistics on hospital trusts, the latter often incorporating buildings on more than one site (Hensher and Edwards 1999). In other countries, multi-site hospitals may function as a single organization but are counted separately. Consequently, although data on hospitals and beds for different countries are available – for example, from the WHO European Health for All Database (WHO 2001) – these statistics can be difficult to interpret.

Fourth, does the definition of a hospital cover only the activities undertaken within its walls? Hospitals in the United States have embarked on vertical mergers that incorporate other service types such as rehabilitation and post-discharge care. Schemes such as 'hospital without walls' or 'hospital at home' link the hospital to a wide range of outreach services (see Hensher and Edwards, Chapter 5). Advances in short-acting anaesthetics create opportunities for free-standing minor surgical units offering day surgery. Midwives and nurse practitioners provide care in free-standing obstetric units, and units managing chronic diseases provide care that elsewhere would be provided by physicians.

Again, this exploration of diversity offers no simple answers. Perhaps the most that can be said is that any hospital policy must consider the type of hospital and its function within its environment. Chapter 2 (Healy and McKee) looks back in history to understand how and why different hospitals systems have developed. Analysing hospitals of the present requires understanding their evolution from the past and the pressures that may shape the hospitals of the future.

Researching hospitals

Despite the large share of the health budget devoted to hospitals, and in contrast to the growing body of research on primary care, there has been much less research on hospital performance (Edwards and Harrison 1999). The research that exists is rarely well known, and the reasons for success and failure remain poorly understood despite massive restructuring of hospital systems. The lack of research on systems and organizations in health care stands in stark contrast to the enormous amount of research on clinical interventions.

A new drug cannot be introduced . . . without exhaustive scientific trials, but we usually introduce new ways of delivering health services with little or no scientific evaluation. We rationalise, change and formulate new systems, often based upon economic and political imperatives, and yet rarely evaluate their impact upon patients. Significant morbidity and mortality may be associated with new models of healthcare delivery. If healthcare system changes were submitted to the same scrutiny as new drug evaluations, they would probably not even be allowed to move from the animal to the human experimentation stage.

(Hillman 1998: 239)

The scarcity of research on how to maximize the impact of hospitals on health may appear surprising until one considers the enormity of the task. First, a hospital is a complex organization and not a simple entity. The goals of a human service organization, such as a large hospital, are multiple and conflicting (Hasenfeld and English 1974; Wildavsky 1979) and may differ from those of individual departments, such as intensive care units and diagnostic laboratories. A hospital also brings together many professional groups, each with its own specialized body of knowledge and own value base. The evaluation of a complex organization is very different from narrowly focused, reductionist research; for example, assessing the outcome of a single intervention in a randomized controlled trial of a drug or the respective merits of artificial heart valve A compared with valve B.

This book draws, as far as possible, on a rigorous analysis of evaluative research to identify what is and what is not known. Inevitably, the empirical base is firm on some issues, shaky on others and depends on the context for many. We try not to seek excessive refuge in the argument that 'the jury is still out', but aim to offer carefully considered advice to policy-makers.

This extensive review of the research is combined with a comparison between countries that, although limited in its ability to attribute observed outcomes to specific policies, does challenge preconceived notions and offers scope to learn from experience (Healy 1998; McKee 1998). Cross-country comparisons enable policy alternatives to be identified, the success or failure of a particular strategy to be evaluated and the importance of context to be understood better (Rose 1993). Comparisons of data must, however, be treated with caution given differences in concepts and differences even in quite basic definitions, such as a hospital bed or a qualified nurse. As noted earlier, the term 'hospital' may have different meanings and functions in different countries. At the risk of generalization, most hospitals in western Europe now concentrate on acute care, whereas most hospitals in eastern Europe and some parts of southern Europe continue to provide social as well as health care functions.

This book also draws on international research, which is uneven in its geographical coverage, at least in a form accessible to the international community (Table 1.1). Much of the literature comes from the United States and United Kingdom. It was not possible, using standard bibliometric terms, to distinguish evaluations from reports and reviews, but inspection of the papers involved showed that primary evaluative research is even more concentrated in the United States and United Kingdom. This uneven coverage is inevitably

Table 1.1 Number of articles in a Medline search on hospital-related topics

	Hospital design or construction	Hospital administration	Hospital costs
Australia	0	20	20
Canada	3	29	23
France	4	17	26
Germany	4	38	64
Italy	4	11	15
Netherlands	4	10	18
Russian Federation	4	3	2
Spain	1	17	15
Sweden	5	11	24
United Kingdom	33	79	119
United States	57	311	380

Note: Articles published between 1991 and August 2000 were identified and indexed according to the country of the lead author as identified in Medline and medical subject headings.

reflected in this book, although strenuous efforts have been made to draw on the experience of as many countries as possible. We hope, therefore, that this book will catalyse more interest in hospital research among the European research community.

Several chapters focus on eastern Europe, drawing on internal reports by the World Bank and other agencies. These countries have been the settings for large-scale natural experiments, the results of which provide important information for policy-makers everywhere about how hospitals change (or do not) in the face of changing incentives.

We have chosen to range broadly in covering topics of interest to policy-makers across Europe. As we have noted, Europe encompasses countries that are very different and therefore have different health system priorities. The priority may be to rebuild a hospital sector that has been devastated by war, to enhance primary care and reduce hospital capacity, or to implement new systems for hospital governance. We have chosen, therefore, to review a broad range of strategies and tools for change. The unifying theme, however, is the need for mechanisms that support continuing development and change. Although the precise nature of the challenges may differ, health policy-makers everywhere cannot afford to stand still in an ever-changing environment.

Changing hospitals

Even where a particular policy is based on clear evidence, the implementation of change encounters many barriers. The structural inflexibility and long time frame of hospitals contrasts with their rapidly changing environments. Hospitals are remarkably resistant to change, both structurally and culturally. They are, quite literally, immovable structures whose designs were set in concrete, often many years previously. Their configuration often reflects the practice of health care and patient populations of bygone eras. In western Europe, some hospitals still occupy buildings that once were medieval monasteries, but even relatively new hospitals have failed to keep pace with changing patterns of disease and treatment. These range from rooms with too few sockets for the increasing range of electronic monitors to too few operating theatres to accommodate the rise in day surgery.

The culture, or ethos, of a hospital also must adapt to changing circumstances. Hospitals have been described as palaces of medical power, and prestigious hospitals staffed by the elite members of the medical profession can marshal opposition to threats to their survival and growth. Furthermore, hospitals are inhabited by a proliferation of occupational groups, so that considerable effort must be put into developing good working relationships. What levers are effective in promoting multidisciplinary working? How does one create a culture that places the needs of the patient before those of the professional? The concept of patients' rights, for example, is difficult to promote in many countries and is an utterly foreign concept in others.

Why now?

Given these barriers to change, why should policy-makers embark on hospital reform? First, some important lessons have emerged from the experience of health care reforms in Europe over the past two decades. One is that policies based on market principles, such as competition, have been less successful in containing costs than regulatory and budgetary policies (Saltman and Figueras 1997; Mossialos and Le Grand 1999). The latter include policies directed specifically at the hospital, such as capping hospital budgets and regulating the distribution of hospital beds.

Second, the environmental factors that affect the health of populations and, by extension, hospital care are now better understood. These include changing population age distributions, changing patterns of disease and rapid technological change.

Third, the steadily increasing volume of research on hospitals (although from a low baseline) provides important new evidence on issues such as the optimal configuration of hospitals and how to change the behaviour of health professionals. The experiences of countries in eastern Europe in restructuring their large hospital systems over the past decade also help to illuminate the success or otherwise of particular policies and their implementation.

Although hospitals are a key element of health system reform, they have long been regarded as a black box with regard to their effects on health. There are now good reasons, however, for researchers and policy-makers to look inside that black box and to ask how well hospitals are performing. Those responsible for planning and managing hospitals and for making decisions about investing in them need to understand why hospitals in each country are as they are and the nature of the challenges facing hospitals now and in the future. They must assess the arguments for different hospital configurations, how best to provide high-quality health care and how to ensure that expensive hospital facilities are used optimally.

A systems approach to the hospital

This book looks at the hospital from a systems perspective. Systems concepts and principles have been applied in many fields, including the study of complex organizations such as hospitals (Checkland 1981; Perrow 1986). Based on a biological analogy, general systems theory offers several concepts that help to explain the behaviour of a hospital and that have helped us to identify and to order the issues addressed in this book.

A key property of an open system is that it must interact with its environment to secure the resources necessary for survival, adaptation and growth. This means that a hospital must be considered within its environment and that this environment itself is an important focus of study. The way a hospital responds to policies and incentives depends on its role and function as well as the beliefs and experiences of those who interact with it. For these reasons, knowledge is needed about the past history and trajectories of hospitals in European health care systems (Healy and McKee, Chapter 2). The hospital is acted on continually by many external influences (the environment), and these we have considered collectively as a series of pressures for change (McKee, Healy, Edwards and Harrison, Chapter 3). These pressures include changes in the composition of the population being served, in patterns of diseases and in public expectations, all of which have implications for hospital services.

A second concept is that a system exists within a hierarchy of other systems, so that a hospital can be studied from different system levels. An individual hospital must, therefore, be considered within the wider hospital system, within a country's health care system and, ultimately, within the broader socioeconomic and political environment. We set the context for understanding individual hospitals by tracing trends in hospital systems throughout Europe (Healy and McKee, Chapter 2). Furthermore, examining the hospital from different levels leads to our main division in analysing policy strategies: the division between external and internal levers for change.

A third fundamental concept of systems theory is the interdependence of the various elements that comprise the organization. The systemic property arises from the organizing relations between the parts, and the properties of the parts can only be understood in relation to the whole. A hospital is a complex organization, since it contains a series of subsystems. These might include, for example, systems for recruiting and retaining staff, for running housekeeping and catering services and for performing diagnostic imaging services for clinicians. These subsystems can be expected to pursue their own interests, but any significant change to one part will have repercussions for others.

As described by Checkland (1981), a system consists of a pattern of organized relations: a configuration of components and relationships that are characteristic of a particular system. Furthermore, systems theory uses the concept of self-regulation; that is, an organization maintains a quasi-steady state through homeostatic mechanisms that involve information feedback. This analogy may be taken too far: a hospital is not a biological organism. However, this concept does help to explain why hospitals are resistant to radical change and why a hospital cannot change itself into an entirely new type of organization. Chapter 4 (Healy and McKee) addresses the differing roles and functions of a hospital.

The boundary or interface is a key concept in systems thinking, since the organization is seen as an open system in continual interaction with its environment, while the organization itself is made up of many subsystems. For the purposes of this book, we have defined the boundary of the hospital system to include acute care hospitals that provide secondary and tertiary health care, but we exclude long-term care hospitals, although this superficially simple definition conceals some major difficulties. A key question for modern hospitals is what types of health care should be provided within the hospital and what elsewhere. Chapter 5 (Hensher and Edwards) reviews the experience of shifting hospital boundaries in one country, the United Kingdom.

The elements of a system, in this case including individual hospitals, are in a dynamic relationship with one another and with changes in the wider environment. These relationships affect the optimal size of each element and how they should be distributed. Chapter 6 (Posnett) reviews the research on the optimal size of a hospital and, in particular, the relationship between economies and scale and between volume and outcome.

The impact of different systems on a hospital means that those seeking to bring about change must act at the appropriate level. Considering who has responsibility for which function is therefore necessary. *The World Health Report 2000* (WHO 2000) discusses the concept of stewardship, which sets out the responsibilities of governments to safeguard their health care systems. Although quasi-state or private organizations can undertake operational management, governments retain ultimate responsibility for health system performance. This implies that governments must set the overall goals for the health system, among which *The World Health Report 2000* includes ensuring high and equitable levels of health, services that are responsive to public expectations and fairness in paying for health services. Governments, or those acting on their behalf, should therefore play an active role in the direction taken by the hospital system, and they have at their disposal many potential levers for changing aspects of hospital services and performance.

External factors may be the most likely and appropriate way to change some aspects of hospitals and hospital systems. These include actions to enable hospitals to provide care, to specify what type of care they should provide and to monitor what they do. We have grouped together these activities as external levers for change (McKee and Healy, Chapter 7). Financial incentives can act as powerful levers for change, but their effects are sometimes unexpected. Chapter 8 (Langenbrunner and Wiley) reviews the evidence on the effects of different payment systems.

A systems approach requires that links be made between systems at different levels. In this case, incentives created outside the hospital must be consistent with those used inside it. Chapter 9 (Jakab, Preker and Harding) explores the challenges involved.

Change within the hospital involves assembling the resources needed for high-quality care, such as optimal use of buildings, people and equipment, and organizing them in a way that provides high-quality care (Healy and McKee, Chapter 10). This requires a new way of working. This has been termed 'clinical governance', a set of activities that bring together the often separate tasks of management and quality assurance. It is based on the premise that those responsible for using resources efficiently must also take account of the outcomes the resources achieve; those responsible for enhancing the quality of care must also be able to influence the use of resources.

People and technology will confront policy-makers with some of their toughest tests in the future. As the patients and conditions treated within hospitals change, so will the skills needed by staff. New types of staff will be needed, but this must take account of the changing workforce from which health care workers will be drawn in Europe. Chapter 11 (Buchan and O'May) reviews some of the emerging challenges. Advances in technology offer many opportunities, but they should promote the goals being pursued by the hospital rather than divert from them. Chapter 12 (Rosen) draws on a case study on the introduction of complex technology to offer guidance on how to maximize its health benefits.

Although many of the subsystems within a hospital are important, improving the clinical performance of staff is central to the hospital's role. The challenge is to assess the quality of care provided and to change clinical practice to make it better. Chapter 13 (Freemantle) reviews the evidence on how this can be done.

Systems theory emphasizes the importance of the culture within which activities take place. Chapter 14 (Aiken and Sloane) reviews emerging evidence that shows that a hospital characterized by good communication and relations between professions not only retains staff more successfully, but also obtains better outcomes for patients.

Returning to the hospital as a system, the many issues covered in this book clearly interact, and the boundaries between them also reflect the immediate concerns of the particular policy-maker. These issues can be grouped broadly under four headings. The first is the set of pressures to which the hospital system must respond in the future. The second relates to how the system should be configured and managed: the size, shape, distribution and functions of hospitals. The third and fourth are the levers for change, both external and internal. The relationship between these groups is shown in Figure 1.1. They provide the framework around which this book is organized.

Figure 1.1 The hospital as a system: opportunities for change

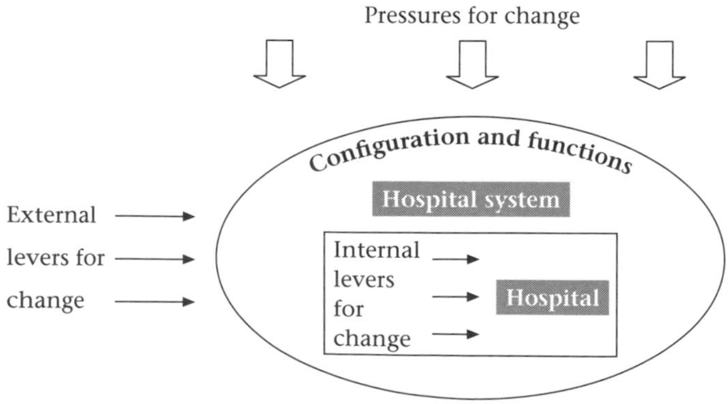

References

Brownell, M.D., Roos, N.P. and Burchill, C. (1999) Monitoring the impact of hospital downsizing on access to care and quality of care, *Medical Care*, 37(6): JS135–50.

Checkland, P. (1981) *Systems Thinking, Systems Practice*. Chichester: Wiley.

Edwards, N. and Harrison, A. (1999) The hospital of the future: planning hospitals with limited evidence. A research and policy problem, *British Medical Journal*, 319: 1361–3.

Hasenfeld, Y. and English, R. (1974) *Human Service Organizations*. Ann Arbor, MI: University of Michigan Press.

Healy, J. (1998) *Welfare Options: Delivering Social Services*. Sydney: Allen & Unwin.

Hensher, M. and Edwards, N. (1999) Hospital provision, activity, and productivity in England since the 1980s, *British Medical Journal*, 319(7214): 911–14.

Hensher, M., Edwards, N. and Stokes, R. (1999) International trends in the provision and utilisation of hospital care, *British Medical Journal*, 319(7213): 845–8.

Hillman, K. (1998) Restructuring hospital services, *Medical Journal of Australia*, 169(5): 239.

McKee, M. (1998) An agenda for public health research in Europe, *European Journal of Public Health*, 8: 3–7.

McKee, M. (1999) For debate – does health care save lives?, *Croatian Medical Journal*, 40: 123–8.

McKee, M. and Jacobson, B. (2000) Public health in Europe, *Lancet*, 356: 665–70.

Miller, T.S. (1997) *The Birth of the Hospital in the Byzantine Empire*. Baltimore, MD: Johns Hopkins University Press.

Mossialos, E. and Le Grand, J. (1999) Cost containment in the EU: an overview, in E. Mossialos and J. Le Grand (eds) *Health Care and Cost Containment in the European Union*. Aldershot: Ashgate.

Murphy, D. (1995) *Where the Indus is Young – a Winter in Baltistan*. London: John Murray.

Perrow, C. (1986) *Complex Organizations: A Critical Essay*. New York: McGraw-Hill.

Pollock, A.M., Dunnigan, M.G., Gaffney, D., Price, D. and Shaoul, J. (1999) The private finance initiative: planning the 'new' NHS. Downsizing for the 21st century, *British Medical Journal*, 319(7203): 179–84.

Reissman, D.B., Orris, P., Lacey, R. and Hartman, D.E. (1999) Downsizing, role demands and job stress, *Journal of Occupational and Environmental Medicine*, 41(4): 289–93.

Rose, R. (1993) *Lesson Drawing in Public Policy*. London: Chatham House.

Saltman, R.B. and Figueras, J. (1997) *European Health Care Reform: Analysis of Current Strategies*, WHO Regional Publications, European Series, No. 72. Copenhagen: WHO Regional Office for Europe.

Shanahan, M., Brownell, M.D. and Roos, N.P. (1999) The unintended and unexpected impact of downsizing: costly hospitals become more costly, *Medical Care*, 37(suppl. 6): JS123–34.

Street, A. and Haycock, J. (1999) The economic consequences of reorganizing hospital services in Bishkek, Kyrgyzstan, *Health Economist*, 8(1): 53–64.

Thubron, C. (1999) *In Siberia*. London: Chatto & Windus.

Wildavsky, A. (1979) *Speaking Truth to Power: The Art and Craft of Policy Analysis*. Boston, MA: Little, Brown and Company.

WHO (2000) *The World Health Report 2000. Health Systems: Improving Performance*. Geneva: World Health Organization.

WHO (2001) *WHO European Health for All Database*. Copenhagen: WHO Regional Office for Europe.

chapter two

The evolution of hospital systems

Judith Healy and Martin McKee

Introduction

Hospitals have performed many different roles and functions over the centuries: as shelters for the poor attached to monasteries in the Middle Ages; as a feared last resort for the dying in the eighteenth century; and as shining symbols of a modern health care system in the twentieth century. Considering the directions for hospitals of the future requires understanding why hospitals of the present are as they are. Present-day hospitals reflect a combination of the legacy of the past and the needs of the present. Huge advances in knowledge and technology, however, mean that a present-day state-of-the-art hospital would be unrecognizable to a physician or nurse of just five decades ago.

From a review of the past, this chapter moves on to consider contemporary trends in hospital activities. The number of acute hospital beds has fallen steadily while admissions have risen, the increasing throughput of patients being achieved by shorter hospital stays and higher bed occupancy rates. Next, these overall trends are examined in the light of experiences in countries in western and eastern Europe in restructuring their hospital systems.

From past to present

Hospitals have evolved over the centuries in response to social and political changes and changes in medical knowledge (Table 2.1). The earliest examples of institutions recognizable as hospitals were in Byzantium, no later than the seventh century (Miller 1997). By the twelfth century, many Arab towns had a small hospital, while a large hospital was built in Cairo in 1283 (Porter 1997). This concept of a building in which the sick and injured were treated was reintroduced to Christendom by the crusading orders in the eleventh

Table 2.1 Historical evolution of hospitals

Role of hospital	Time	Characteristics
Health care	7th century	Byzantine Empire, Greek and Arab theories of disease
Nursing, spiritual care	10th to 17th centuries	Hospitals attached to religious foundations
Isolation of infectious patients	11th century	Nursing of infectious diseases such as leprosy
Health care for poor people	17th century	Philanthropic and state institutions
Medical care	Late 19th century	Medical care and surgery; high mortality
Surgical centres	Early 20th century	Technological transformation of hospitals; entry of middle-class patients; expansion of outpatient departments
Hospital-centred health systems	1950s	Large hospitals; temples of technology
District general hospital	1970s	Rise of district general hospital; local, secondary and tertiary hospitals
Acute care hospital	1990s	Active short-stay care
Ambulatory surgery centres	1990s	Expansion of day admissions; expansion of minimally invasive surgery

century. Over the next few hundred years, the Knights of St John of Jerusalem (now the Knights of Malta) and the Knights Templar built hospitals across Europe (Porter 1997).

Until the twelfth century, most hospitals were small and basic and seldom offered medical care. These early hospitals were refuges for sick poor people who were admitted for shelter and basic nursing care and were also a means of isolating those with infectious diseases (Granshaw 1993). The Christian ideal of healing the sick and giving alms to the poor motivated the foundation of many early hospitals, and philanthropists (then as now) sponsored hospitals as an act of charity, in some cases to buy grace in heaven or to demonstrate their wealth and social position. By the Middle Ages, many hospitals providing medical care were attached to monasteries across Europe. St Bartholomew's was founded in London in 1123, the Hôtel Dieu in Paris in 1231 and Florence's Santa Maria Nuova in 1288 (Porter 1997).

A major era of European hospital building began in the thirteenth century. Hospitals had a recognizable medical character by the sixteenth century, although to the public they remained places of pestilence or insanity (Porter 1997). Hospitals were 'a place, not to live, but to die in' (Browne 1643), or a refuge for the elderly poor who were thrown aside 'to rust in peace, or rot in hospitals' (Southerne 1682). A second wave of hospital building in the seventeenth

---

Box 2.1 La Pitié-Salpêtrière

The Hôpital Salpêtrière illustrates the shift from asylum to tertiary care hospital. In 1656, Louis XIV ordered a group of asylums, the Hôpital Général, to care for poor and sick people, namely La Pitié, Scipion, La Savonnerie, Bicêtre and the petit arsenal de la Salpêtrière. The Hôpital Salpêtrière took its name from salt-petre, a component of canon powder, originally stored in this building on the left bank of the Seine. The Salpêtrière incarcerated prostitutes, with a resident doctor not appointed until 1783, later providing residential care for elderly women as well as the insane. During the twentieth century, it developed into a tertiary care acute general hospital with a range of medical specialties. Its buildings increasingly fell behind contemporary hospital standards, however, until the French government reformed the medical curriculum and restructured hospitals in 1958. Teaching hospitals were grouped together to create the Centre Hospitaliers Universitaires (University Hospital Centres), and the hospital consortium, Pitié-Salpêtrière, was formed in 1964. Specialist units were developed, and the standard of care was improved after substantial capital investment. La Pitié-Salpêtrière is now well known for research and teaching.

Sources: Club du Vieux Manoir (1977) and Simon (1986)

---

century, in part reflecting increasing urbanization, saw the establishment of hospitals such as La Pitié-Salpêtrière in Paris (Box 2.1). Political events in the eighteenth century following the French Revolution accelerated the secularization of hospitals. Voluntary non-religious hospitals were established, funded by private donors. As effective health care developed, some hospitals began to differentiate between 'curable' and 'incurable' patients.

In the nineteenth century, the state began to play a role, alongside the voluntary sector, in caring for poor and sick people in the rapidly growing cities. Many of today's hospitals in western European countries, therefore, had their origins in charitable institutions for the poor, while physicians treated wealthier people at home or in small private hospitals. With medical progress, hospitals became 'medicalized' in the sense that admission was determined according to medical rather than social criteria, and by physicians instead of hospital benefactors. By the end of the nineteenth century, all large European cities had both public and private general hospitals. Public hospitals became the sites for most teaching and research, typically being visited by clinicians for several hours each week (Trohler and Prull 1997).

As the role of the hospital expanded, so did the need for public support. Most European hospitals came under some form of state control in the twentieth century, since philanthropy and patient fees were no longer sufficient to cover the huge rise in costs of treatment.

The rise of the hospital from the late nineteenth century to its current dominant position came with the development of aseptic and antiseptic techniques, more effective anaesthesia, greater surgical knowledge and skills, and a revolution in technology (McGrew 1985). The entire character of hospitals changed. The infections endemic in hospitals were dramatically reduced, especially in surgical and obstetric wards. Surgeons were able to undertake more complex surgery with higher rates of recovery by patients. In the late nineteenth century, hospitals began to diagnose and treat ambulatory as well as bed-bound patients, and outpatient treatment gradually came to account for a large proportion of hospital activity. Also, the middle classes began to attend, changing the character of hospitals, which had to become more responsive to their clientele and to function in a more business-like manner.

The latter half of the nineteenth century saw the growth of medicine as a profession, the rise of professional specialties and the establishment of specialist hospitals. Some professional groups and hospitals 'focused on body parts, some on diseases; some on life events, some on age groups' (Porter 1997: 381). 'By 1900 . . . nothing could stop the scores of specialities taking root upon the balkanised medical map – involving hospital departments, research centres and distinctive career hierarchies' (Porter 1997: 388). The process of medical specialization proceeded rapidly and, together with the shift of medical care from the community to the hospital, brought about an enormous increase in the number of specialists.

By the end of the nineteenth century, infectious disease began to be understood. Pasteur had proven the germ theory and Koch had developed the practical and theoretical basis of microbiology. Semmelweis showed that washing hands before examining patients reduced the transmission of infection, a lesson that is often forgotten today (see Chapter 3). Lister's introduction of antisepsis, coupled with the discovery of safe anaesthetic agents, made elective surgery safer. In England, Florence Nightingale established a professional basis for nursing. By the twentieth century, the hospital was beginning to take on its present-day role. Advances in chemical engineering laid the basis for a pharmaceutical industry; for example, research on chemical dyes led to the invention of sulfa drugs. As the scope for clinical intervention increased, technology became more complex and expensive. Hospitals began to offer cure rather than just care.

Advances in military surgery in the Second World War had a profound impact on hospitals, with safe blood transfusion, penicillin and surgeons trained in trauma techniques. The greatest changes occurred from the 1970s onwards, however, with advances in laboratory diagnosis and the ability to treat more diseases. The massive expansion in pharmaceuticals transformed the management of diseases, such as childhood leukaemia and some solid cancers. New specialties such as oncology emerged and common conditions such as peptic ulcer, previously treated with prolonged hospitalization, were managed in ambulatory care. Whole new areas of surgery became commonplace, such as coronary artery bypasses, transplantation of kidneys and other organs, and microsurgery. Intensive care units kept many people alive who otherwise would not have survived. Physicians expanded their range of interventions, with techniques such as endoscopic and endovascular procedures and complex treatments such as chemotherapy, while investigations such as computed tomography and magnetic resonance imaging expanded their diagnostic capabilities. New technology, such as minimally invasive surgery and accelerated treatment regimens, reduced hospital stays throughout the 1990s.

During this process, the teaching hospital became the centre of modern medicine. Hospitals became 'the great power-base for the medical elite, the automated factories of the medical production-line' (Porter 1997: 647). Apart from these flagships of medical science, most hospitals before the 1950s were places where relatively simple drugs were administered, surgical procedures were limited and the time spent in hospital involved mostly bed rest. This created two tiers of acute care hospitals. Some hospitals, usually university-affiliated hospitals in the hearts of large cities, expanded into a range of medical specialties supported by complex technology and kept abreast of new developments. The other less advanced hospitals maintained a limited range of specialties and acted as district hospitals for outer-city areas, large towns and rural districts, referring more complicated cases to the tertiary care hospitals (Hillman 1999).

By the 1970s, these new technologies were diffusing out of teaching hospitals and subspecialization was increasingly emerging in district hospitals, which in many countries were also playing a greater role in teaching and research, thus blurring the boundary between secondary and tertiary care.

In many respects, this is a story of success. Hospital medicine has been responsible for major medical achievements in the past decades. The extent of its dominance in the health care system, however, has prompted a reassessment of the wider social and economic implications. In that sense, hospitals may be a victim of their own success.

Trends in hospital activity

Any review of trends in hospital activities in Europe must recognize the limitations of international comparisons. The nature of a hospital differs among countries, as noted in Chapter 1, but there are even problems with the concept of a 'bed'. Does it include all beds regardless of whether they are used? A staffed bed may be one of twenty covered by a single nurse or it may be in an intensive care unit with one-to-one care. It is often forgotten that the term 'bed' is shorthand for an entire package that includes nurses, supporting staff and, perhaps, advanced monitoring equipment. Furthermore, the widely used measure of average length of stay is sensitive to changes in admission procedures. For example, a policy of managing patients as day cases who previously were admitted overnight may, paradoxically, increase the average length of stay, since the calculation now excludes those formerly staying only one night. There are problems also in gathering valid and representative data; for example, some countries exclude the private sector or other sectors such as military hospitals (McKee *et al.* 1993). There may be funding incentives within the hospital system to distort the figures, such as exaggerated counts of patients and beds. Given these limitations, we confine this analysis to drawing conclusions about broad trends. Those who wish to pursue more detailed analysis can obtain the data for individual countries from the WHO European Health for All Database (WHO 2001).

Three broad patterns of hospital configuration across Europe can be discerned (Figure 2.1). This graph, which includes both acute and long-stay hospitals

Figure 2.1   Number of hospitals per 100,000 population in the European Union (♦), countries of central and eastern Europe (■) and countries of the former Soviet Union (▲)

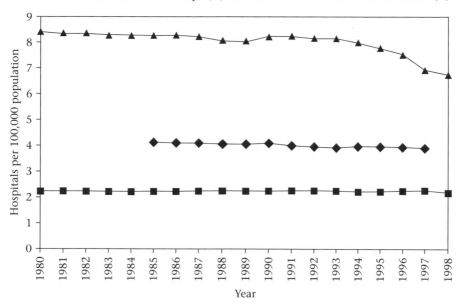

Source: WHO (2001)

(since these cannot be distinguished in all countries), indicates considerable differences across Europe. The 15 countries of the former Soviet Union have by far the most hospitals, with some very large but also many small hospitals. The 12 countries of central and eastern Europe have fewer, although many are very large (hospitals with more than 1000 beds are not uncommon), while the now 15 European Union countries have half as many hospitals for their populations. The countries of the former Soviet Union stand out as having reduced their numbers of hospitals during the 1990s from a very high level.

Turning to the slightly less problematic measure of hospital beds, western Europe has experienced a gradual but steady decline in numbers of acute beds since before 1980 (Figure 2.2). The former socialist countries of central and eastern Europe had about 20 per cent more beds than countries in western Europe in 1980, remained steady at this level through the 1980s, but started to fall in the 1990s. Their level remains about twice that in western Europe. The countries of the former Soviet Union display a quite different pattern, with levels about twice those in western Europe in 1980, actually increasing in the 1980s, but then declining dramatically in the 1990s.

Although these regional groupings are helpful as a means of summarizing trends, there is considerable national diversity. In the European Union, for example, although all countries have reduced hospital beds, they started from very different levels (Figure 2.3). Germany has nearly twice the European Union average and, despite a steep decline, Italy still has more than twice as many acute beds as the United Kingdom. There is, however, some evidence

Figure 2.2 Hospital beds in acute hospitals per 100,000 population in the European Union (◆), countries of central and eastern Europe (■) and countries of the former Soviet Union (▲)

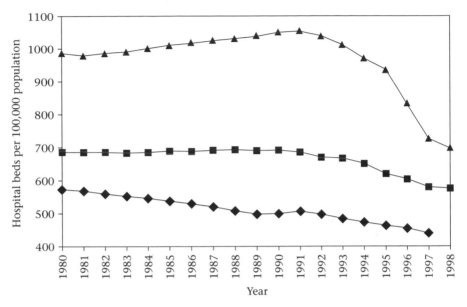

Source: WHO (2001)

Figure 2.3 Hospital beds in acute hospitals per 100,000 population, selected western European countries; ◆ France; ■ Germany; ▲ Italy; × Sweden; ✳ United Kingdom

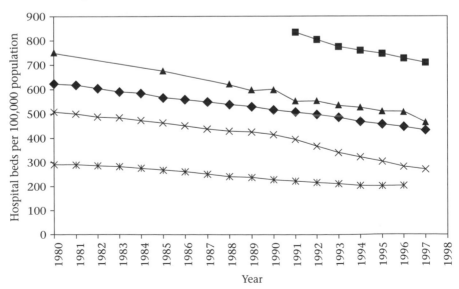

Source: WHO (2001)

Figure 2.4 Acute hospital admissions per 100 population in the European Union
(◆), countries of central and eastern Europe (■) and countries of the former Soviet
Union (▲)

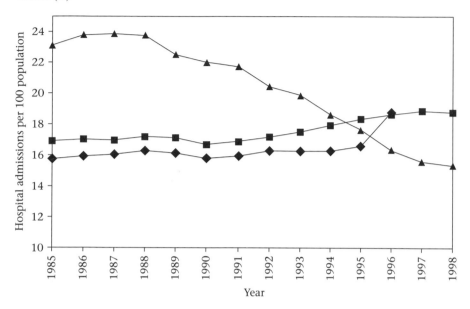

Source: WHO (2001)

that the bed stock in the United Kingdom may now be too low for current
demands (Department of Health 2000).

Information about numbers of beds provides only a partial picture. A more
comprehensive assessment requires knowledge of how many patients are
admitted to hospital, how long they stay and how intensively the bed stock is
used. Turning to admissions, responses to the falling numbers of beds have
varied across Europe (Figure 2.4). The countries of the former Soviet Union
show a spectacular fall from their high level of recorded admissions since the
late 1980s. The reasons for this are discussed later in this chapter. In contrast,
admissions in other parts of Europe began to increase in the 1990s. The
volume of ambulatory care also rose, indicating an even greater increase in
overall hospital activity in western Europe, for reasons that are still inadequately
understood. Some of the change may, however, be attributable to patients
who previously would have stayed for a prolonged period now having repeated
admissions and discharges, so that the increase in people treated may be less
than the trend lines suggest.

The second perspective is how long patients remain in these beds (Figure 2.5).
Many western European countries have moved patients who would formerly
have remained in hospital for long periods into specialized facilities providing
nursing care (such as nursing homes) or have discharged them back to their
own homes with help from community-based health and social care services.
Second, the length of stay for many acute conditions has been reduced

Figure 2.5 Average length of stay in acute care hospitals in the European Union (◆), countries of central and eastern Europe (■) and countries of the former Soviet Union (▲)

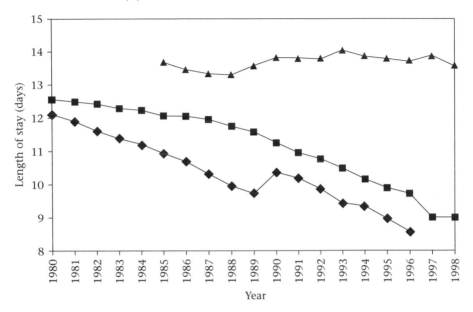

Source: WHO (2001)

substantially, reflecting policies such as earlier mobilization after surgery. Third, more cases are being handled as one-day admissions. This shift to shorter stays requires major changes in how patients are managed and how staff are deployed. In contrast, the very high lengths of stay (around 14 days) in the countries of the former Soviet Union have changed little.

Such regional comparisons are problematic, since the analysis must take into account differences in social conditions and alternative models of care as well as differences in diseases and the means available to treat them. Nevertheless, some defined conditions can be compared. Thus, women with uncomplicated normal deliveries in many countries of the former Soviet Union are kept in hospital for 7 days whereas, in western European countries, women may stay less than 24 hours. In many countries of the former Soviet Union, tuberculosis is treated primarily by prolonged inpatient chemotherapy during stays of several months, whereas similar patients in western Europe would be managed as outpatients. A better understanding of the reasons for these differences, and thus the appropriate responses, requires more information than is currently available on the precise package of care provided for specific conditions in different settings. Obtaining such information should be a high priority for health policy-makers.

The pressures on hospitals in western Europe to reduce the average length of stay has stimulated research on the reasons for delayed discharge of patients from hospital, many of whom are older people (Victor *et al.* 2000). A formal

Figure 2.6 Bed occupancy rate (%) in acute care hospitals in the European Union (♦), countries of central and eastern Europe (■) and countries of the former Soviet Union (▲)

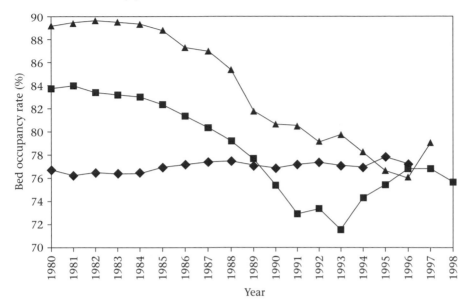

Source: WHO (2001)

utilization review, using instruments to identify patients who are inappropriately occupying a hospital bed, is part of a well-developed management system and can identify obstacles to timely discharge (Restuccia 1995). Although widely used in the United States, utilization review has only been used within Europe for local initiatives, with the possible exception of Portugal, which has a system based on monitoring length of stay by diagnosis-related groups. Research is underway to validate an instrument that could be used across western Europe (Lorenzo *et al.* 1999).

Turning to the intensity of bed use, occupancy rates have remained stable at just above 75 per cent in the European Union but declined very steeply before recovering in central and eastern Europe in the mid-1990s (Figure 2.6). In the countries of the former Soviet Union, average bed occupancy has fallen sharply from 90 to 75 per cent. The former high occupancy in part reflected the hospital funding system, with its financial incentives to maintain the maximum number of patients (at least on paper). The falls in bed occupancy and hospital admissions indicate severe crises in the post-Soviet hospital systems, as hospital budgets eroded and with them the means of treatment, so that fewer people attended hospitals (discussed further later in this chapter).

These data can be brought together to assess the amount of inpatient care provided for the overall population (Figure 2.7). Despite considerable changes in individual parameters, with the exception of the countries of the former Soviet Union where overall bed use has fallen by over a third, and a slight decline in central and eastern Europe, there has been little overall change in

Figure 2.7   Bed-days per 100 population in acute hospitals in the European Union (◆), countries of central and eastern Europe (■) and countries of the former Soviet Union (▲)

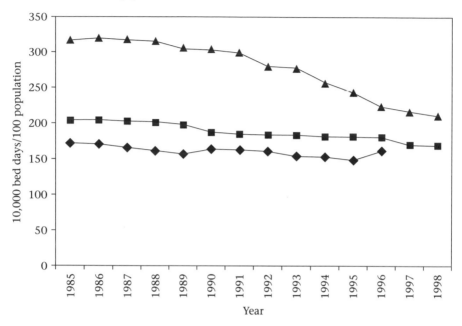

Source: WHO (2001)

western Europe. This confirms the conclusion that lower lengths of stay largely have been compensated for by increasing numbers of patient admissions.

What has happened to expenditure on hospitals? Hospitals continue to account for the largest share of overall health expenditure. Although their share has not dropped significantly over the last few decades in western European countries, expenditure growth has been contained (Mossialos and Le Grand 1999). Time-series statistics are not available for all countries, but Figure 2.8 illustrates trends for selected countries, showing Denmark with a high level of hospital expenditure and France with lower levels. Hospitals in eastern Europe take a much larger share (generally more than 70 per cent) of the (small) identifiable health budgets compared with western Europe, where hospitals take about one-third to one-half of the (larger) health budget (WHO 2001). This is, however, influenced by the uncertain scale of informal payments, particularly in eastern Europe, in the overall cost of health care.

Understanding past trends

Although regional groupings of quite diverse countries do present limitations, some general patterns can be discerned within the trends discussed above. Western European countries, many of which have sought to reduce hospital capacity, have had mixed success in closing hospitals. Bed numbers have fallen, however, and the beds are being used to treat more people, each staying

Figure 2.8   Hospital inpatient expenditure as a percentage of total health expenditure, selected western European countries: ◆ Denmark; ■ France; ▲ Hungary; × Netherlands; ✱ Spain

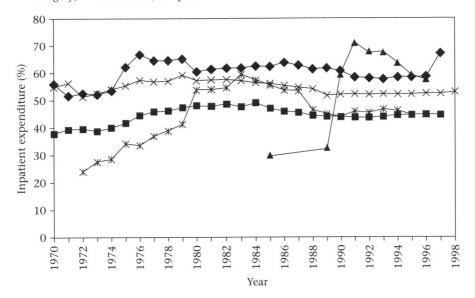

Source: WHO (2001)

in hospital for a shorter period. Central and eastern European countries reduced hospital beds after 1990 but, as in the west, did not close hospitals. Admissions to the remaining beds have increased, with patients staying for shorter periods of time, and bed occupancy rates fell in the aftermath of transition but have now recovered. The countries of the former Soviet Union exhibit a quite different pattern. They have experienced large-scale closures of hospitals, mostly small hospitals, and large reductions in beds from a very high level. Fewer patients are being admitted, but the ones admitted continue to remain in hospital for much longer than in the rest of Europe.

What are the reasons for these changes? In western Europe, the fall in hospital beds can largely be attributed to three major movements dating from the 1960s onwards, in response to cost pressures as well as changes in treatment and care options. These were the shift out of hospitals, first, of long-stay psychiatric patients, and second, of dependent older people. The third factor has been the restructuring of acute care, involving closures of very large and very small hospitals but, more often, incremental reductions in beds, accompanied by more ambulatory treatment and rehabilitation outside the hospital.

Transfer of long-stay patients out of hospital

The changing pattern of care in many high-income countries for elderly people and people with severe disabilities or mental disorders can be illustrated by statistics from the United Kingdom. There, the number of acute care and

Figure 2.9 Trends in beds (per 1000 population), United Kingdom 1977–96: ◆ acute care; ■ psychiatric care; ▲ nursing home

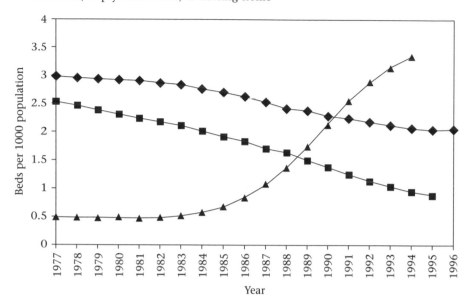

Source: OECD (1999)

psychiatric beds has dropped steadily, whereas the number of nursing home beds has risen steeply (Figure 2.9). Several factors underlie this, but their combined effects have been in the same direction. The 'normalization' movement, beginning in the 1960s, rejected a model in which medicine became a form of social control and sought ways in which people could be cared for in an environment as much like home as possible. This was facilitated by the development of new drugs that enabled patients with major psychoses to live in the community. Later, the pressures for social care of an ageing population prompted a search for alternatives to hospital care. Some of the issues that drove deinstitutionalization in the past have reappeared today: rising costs, new treatment options and changing public opinion.

Long-term psychiatric care

The number of patients in psychiatric hospitals more than halved between the late 1950s and late 1980s in most industrialized countries (Mechanic and Rochefort 1990). This was possible because psychotropic drugs reduced the need for high-security psychiatric hospitals at a time when health systems faced upward pressure on costs and when the inhumane and depersonalizing environments of institutions had become apparent (Goffman 1969). The shift began in the United States, when psychiatric hospitals the size of small towns were scaled down or closed. Psychiatric inpatient beds declined from 2.1 per 1000 population in 1970 to 0.4 in 1990 (Turner-Crowson 1993). The 1950s and 1960s are described as a 'benign' phase when the 'back doors' of mental hospitals were opened and long-stay patients were released and resettled. The 'radical' phase since the 1970s has seen hospitals close their 'front doors' and divert people to community-based services, in response both to fiscal constraints and the search for better treatment options (Turner-Crowson 1993).

Criticisms of this movement resemble current concerns about the effects of reductions in acute hospital beds. Hospitals became 'revolving doors', discharging people prematurely who later were readmitted; hospitals refused to admit many very ill people; there were long waits before admission for inpatient treatment; and the functional divisions between inpatient and ambulatory health care were unclear. Furthermore, the money failed to follow people from institutions into the community (Mechanic and Rochefort 1990).

Several lessons can be drawn from this experience. First, attempts to use old psychiatric hospitals for other health care purposes met with little success, since a large institution cannot be transformed easily into something else, such as a base for community services. Second, retraining hospital staff for roles in the community was difficult. Third, money saved in closing hospitals was not transferred to community-based services. Fourth, closing hospitals without ensuring that appropriate alternative care was available posed real risks to patients, families and the public.

The growth of nursing facilities for older people

A nursing home is a facility that provides long-term care involving regular basic nursing but not specialist medical treatment. The use of nursing homes to care for dependent older people varies between countries. For example, in a study of ten high-income countries, between 2 and 5 per cent of elderly people were cared for in nursing homes (Ribbe *et al.* 1997). These differences are due more to policy decisions (with intended or unintended consequences) than to the characteristics of older populations. Some governments have actively promoted the use of nursing homes through subsidies as a means of transferring older people out of hospitals (Hensher and Edwards 1999). This policy succeeded in its immediate aim, although, in the United Kingdom, the unexpected outcome was an enormous and unanticipated growth in private nursing homes. Paradoxically, this policy was introduced in the United Kingdom at the same time that Australia was trying to reverse a similar policy set in motion two decades earlier (Gibson 1998). The Australian government had offered a 'head in a bed' subsidy to the non-governmental sector, resulting in a 70 per cent increase in nursing home beds as a population ratio between 1963 and 1980. In the early 1980s, the United Kingdom government similarly offered a subsidy towards the cost of care of people in non-governmental homes, resulting in a 60 per cent increase in beds between 1980 and 1993. Many countries are now seeking alternatives to nursing home care by strengthening community-based services that maintain older people in their own homes for as long as possible (Tester 1996; Walker and Maltby 1997). Chapter 5 discusses the relationship between hospitals and nursing homes in the United Kingdom.

The policy of encouraging other forms of long-term care had several implications for hospitals. The most obvious is that it facilitated reductions in hospital capacity and enabled older people to be placed in settings more appropriate to their needs. A less well recognized consequence is that older people who remain in hospital are more ill and dependent than previously (Aro *et al.* 1997), with important implications for levels of nursing and support staff.

Reconfiguring acute hospital care

The transfer of long-stay hospital patients to separate nursing facilities, as well as reductions in length of stay for acute care, have provided opportunities to reduce hospital capacity. This is not to argue that radical downsizing is appropriate for all countries, since those with dispersed rural populations such as Norway may require many small hospitals (Furnholmen and Magnussen 2000).

As most western European countries are, however, trying to reduce hospital capacity, why are some more successful than others? A few themes emerge. In general, beds have been removed rather than hospitals closed. Many European countries have found it extremely difficult to close whole hospitals. For example, Germany closed 7 per cent of hospital beds between 1991 and 1997 but almost no hospitals. Closing beds alone has not, in general, released significant savings, since a considerable proportion of hospital costs is associated with buildings and other fixed costs (Mossialos and Le Grand 1999). Only a few countries have closed significant numbers of hospitals. Examples include the United Kingdom and Ireland, both of which reduced their hospitals by about one-third in the 1980s and early 1990s, although some change in the United Kingdom resulted from changing definitions.

A few countries have managed to close hospitals through regulatory approaches. Belgium implemented the following series of strategies. A 1982 decree instituted a cap on the total number of hospital beds and enabled the health insurance funds to reclassify some beds for 'nursing', which then were reimbursed at a lower rate than care in 'acute' beds. A subsequent 1989 decree, stating that an accredited 'hospital' must have at least 150 beds, led to the closing of many small hospitals (Kerr and Siebrand 2000). In Denmark, change was stimulated by development of a market between the counties but, importantly, these negotiations involved counties rather than individual hospitals and resulted in the replacement of two or more small hospitals by single larger facilities (Christiansen *et al.* 1999; van Mosseveld and van Son 1999).

Planning approaches have achieved some success. France has created 26 regional boards that seek to cut acute care beds by a further 24,000 (a 4.7 per cent reduction). During 1994–98, 17,000 beds were closed in both public and private hospitals. This enabled the development of other facilities more appropriate to changing health care needs. Thus the regional hospital agencies have opened 15 new hospitals, seven dialysis units, 20 centres for people with Alzheimer's disease and 60 new cancer units (EU News in Brief 2000; Swingedau 2000).

In contrast, change has been slower when left to the market, involving such strategies as separating purchasing and provision and giving hospitals some autonomy. This reflects several factors. First, while market forces can destabilize the system, which may help identify structural problems, they are less good at identifying what should replace the system. In particular, markets pay less attention to the health needs of the population than to managerial, corporate and professional interests. Second, giving autonomy to hospital managers also empowers them to resist closure, often by assembling powerful alliances among health professionals and local government. Third, a gradual, or even abrupt, withdrawal of resources can often be met by strategies other than closure, such as failure to maintain buildings and equipment or simply accumulating a deficit. Finally, the political visibility of major hospital closures makes it very difficult for politicians to distance themselves from unpopular change, even when they seek to transfer responsibility to 'the market'.

Change has been especially difficult where ownership is diffuse and incentives are mixed. In Switzerland, for example, there has been little reduction in capacity. There, funding is divided between taxation and health insurance, and ownership is decentralized, involving cantons, municipalities and the private sector (Minder *et al.* 2000). Although both beds and hospitals have been reduced overall in Italy, this has varied among regions. In some regions, difficulty in implementing change has been attributed to the persistence of competing incentives, with many physicians working in both the public and private sectors (Taroni 2000).

Policies based on promoting service substitution have contributed to reductions in bed numbers but have not, on their own, led to hospital closures. Such strategies include increases in ambulatory care, as in Norway, or in rehabilitation facilities, as in Germany (Busse 2000). Germany has now abolished its previous rigid separation of inpatient and ambulatory care, which had made substitution of care difficult (Busse 2000).

Closure seems more likely where two or more hospitals are replaced by a new facility, often on a different site. This avoids the impression that one site has 'won' and also provides visible benefits for staff who benefit from enhanced, modern facilities. This may also be necessary if facilities built years (or even centuries) before cannot be adapted to the needs of modern health care (see Chapter 3). In Spain, for example, it was possible to close some old and very large hospitals by building new facilities that were smaller and more accessible (Rico *et al.* 2000).

In contrast, hospitals have seen enormous structural changes over the last two decades in the United States, mainly through mergers of smaller not-for-profit tax-exempt hospitals (Arnould *et al.* 1997). Although highly regulated, greater competition from the early 1980s reduced costs and prices in hospitals, partly because insurance funds and health maintenance organizations steered patients to more efficient providers (Ferguson and Goddard 1997). Mergers between hospitals continued into the late 1990s, with an estimated 250 per year (see Chapter 14). Managed care is credited with reducing the very high health care and hospital costs in the United States, although a backlash is now developing among various groups, including patients and physicians (Enthoven and Singer 1996, 1998). Chapter 6 discusses the arguments for vertical and horizontal mergers in the European public sector, concluding that hospital mergers only produce benefits when excess capacity is eliminated or when there are clinical reasons for greater scope and scale.

Several lessons emerge from the experience of the United Kingdom, where many hospitals have been merged and closed (Robinson and Dixon 1999). As in France, a clear plan for change has been essential. Closures were often preceded by mergers of independent hospitals; for example, all the hospitals in a city were brought together into one 'hospital trust'. Given the difficulties of closing autonomous hospitals, it was much easier to close what had become one site within a large hospital grouping than to close what was previously an entire hospital. It was also important to secure support from the senior medical staff, given their influence over their colleagues and also over local public opinion. This also was the strategy pursued in Melbourne, Australia in 1995, where 32 separate public-sector hospitals were grouped into seven networks, resulting in the closure of nine hospitals and further mergers and reconfigurations across the networks (Corden 2001).

Hospital systems in eastern Europe

The countries of central and eastern Europe and the countries of the former Soviet Union are considered together here because, despite considerable individual differences, they share the legacy of the Soviet-model health care system. An understanding of changes since 1990 requires some historical background to place these changes in context. The inherited Soviet model is outlined here, therefore, followed by an overview of some factors that have contributed to change.

The Soviet model of the health care system

The countries of the former Soviet Union inherited a hospital-dominated health care system, in which hospitals were divided according to the administrative levels of the country, by the diseases they treated, the level of care they provided and the occupations and backgrounds of the patients they admitted. They are now diverging from this model, but the extent of change varies. The main characteristics of the Soviet hospital system, which also applied to some extent in the countries of central and eastern Europe, are as follows.

The first characteristic, a plentiful supply of hospitals, was (and still is) regarded as the main measure of a good health care system. The Semashko All-Union Research Institute of Social Hygiene and Public Administration in Moscow drew up normative planning standards (such as the number of hospital beds per 10,000 population) that were applied across the USSR. This emphasis on hospitals continues to starve the rest of the health care system of funds. Hospitals are funded and medicine is practised in such as way as to keep beds full. These hospitals include many small rural hospitals for the scattered population.

The second characteristic, specialization among hospitals, also is regarded as a hallmark of a good health care system. Eastern Europe is strikingly different from western Europe in its extensive network of specialist hospitals at the national, regional and district levels, including maternity, paediatrics, psychiatry, tuberculosis, cancer, dermatology, sexually transmitted diseases and ophthalmology.

The third characteristic is vertical fragmentation into tiers of hospitals according to the level of public administration: district (rayon), city, region (oblast) and national (republic). At the bottom are the rural district (village) hospitals, next the central (town) district hospitals, the city hospitals, the regional hospitals and the national tertiary care hospitals. In practice, there is little functional distinction between hospital care at the city and national level, since most patients attending national hospitals live in the capital and are treated for basic secondary care conditions. In parallel, at the district, regional and national levels, are specialist hospitals, as well as dispensaries (long-term care hospitals) for conditions such as tuberculosis.

The fourth characteristic is the existence of parallel health services. These include separate hospitals for senior party members and for the main government departments: the ministries of internal affairs, railways, and defence forces as well as large industries. These separate services for ministries mostly remain in place. For example, in Kazakhstan in 1996, they accounted for about 9 per cent of hospital beds (Kulzhanov and Healy 1999).

A fifth characteristic, a strong upward referral flow of patients to hospital, reflects several factors. Central hospitals have larger budgets, the most skilled physicians and a better supply of equipment and drugs. Primary care is poorly developed and physicians have a limited capacity (knowledge, skills and resources) to manage even minor illnesses. General physicians undertake much less diagnosis and treatment than general physicians in western Europe. Community-based physicians, therefore, perform only a minimal gatekeeping role, especially since many patients bypass them and go straight to hospital.

Finally, as shown earlier, lengths of stay in hospital are much longer than in western Europe. Much treatment is determined by centrally devised clinical protocols that typically require long stays. Also, financial incentives within the health care system (including informal payments to physicians) reward hospitals and staff for lengthy patient stays, while adequate substitutes for hospital care are generally unavailable.

In summary, most countries in eastern Europe are over-supplied with hospitals and hospital beds, at least by western European standards. Some further evidence for this excess capacity is the dramatic recent reduction in hospital admissions and occupancy rates in some countries. Hospitals in eastern Europe serve rather different functions to those in western Europe, however. They are the dominant providers of health services as well as formal social care services. The longer lengths of stay are influenced not only by financial incentives, but also by fewer resources such as technology and up-to-date knowledge and skills.

The experience of change

As in western Europe, there is considerable diversity between eastern European countries in the extent of change but, unlike the west, change more often has been a response to external circumstances. In a few countries, war or other civil disorders have been important factors (such as in Albania, Bosnia and Herzegovina, Georgia and Tajikistan). This has led to large reductions in hospital capacity, partly because of the hostilities and partly because of a lack of resources to keep hospitals running. For example, hospital beds declined by over 20 per cent between 1990 and 1998 in both Albania and Tajikistan.

The major contributor to the very large fall in hospital capacity in the countries of the former Soviet Union has, however, been the impact of economic crisis, which forced the closure of many small hospitals in rural areas. These typically had extremely limited facilities, often lacking running water, and one reason they closed was abandonment in the face of lack of funds. For example, hospital beds in Kazakhstan declined by 40 per cent between 1990 and 1997, with the number of hospitals falling by nearly half, mostly from the closure of village hospitals, down from 684 in 1994 to 208 in 1997 (Kulzhanov and Healy 1999). Planning strategies also produced closures in some countries, being called for in national health plans backed by presidential decrees, as in Kyrgyzstan (Sargaldakova et al. 2000).

The funding problems that accompanied the liberalization of the Czech Republic's health care system in the mid-1990s also led to large-scale closures. The adoption of fee-for-service payments for physicians and the failure to cap hospital payments resulted in rising hospital costs and insolvency of insurance funds. By 1998, only nine of the original 27 sickness funds remained and acute hospital beds had fallen by 23 per cent.

Elsewhere, change has been slower, although often no better planned. Many of the lessons echo those learned in western Europe. An early change, in many countries, was to make hospitals independent from central government, usually by transferring them to local government. These hospitals have continued to guard their independence jealously, making the creation of regional authorities (as in France) or mergers between hospitals (as in the United Kingdom) difficult. Thus, the government of Hungary has faced strong opposition to its repeated attempts to reduce hospital capacity (Orosz and Hollo, in press). Neither the creation of county-level committees (with limited powers) nor the introduction of payment based on diagnosis-related groups has had much impact. Acute hospital beds were reduced by only 7 per cent between 1990 and 1997, while state expenditures on hospitals rose (Gaal et al. 1999).

Expectations that changes in formal payment mechanisms would lead to significant hospital closures and cost containment have not been fulfilled in this region (Chapter 8). For example, in some countries of the former Soviet Union, formal payments are a minor element of overall fiscal flows. Thus, while Georgia's state health insurance agency has introduced case-based hospital payments, hospitals recently transformed into joint stock enterprises obtain over 80 per cent of their funding from direct patient payments, either official or unofficial.

Lessons and implications

A lesson emerging from this historical review is that hospitals must continue to adapt to changes in their internal and external environments. This chapter has described how the hospital has evolved throughout history, noting how this evolution has moved at different speeds in different places. Traditional measures of hospital activity, such as numbers of beds and length of stay, suggest that the importance of the hospital in the health care system is diminishing, but other indicators such as patient admissions suggest that hospitals are busier than ever. As the functions of the hospital change, better information is needed on the ambulatory care services and day surgery now provided by hospitals.

There are several implications for policy-makers. First, international comparative data offer no simple answer to how many hospital beds a country needs. Many countries have considerable scope for reducing existing hospital capacity by moving long-stay patients into more appropriate facilities. This does not, however, mean that all countries should emulate those with low levels of hospital capacity, since there is some concern that such low levels may be inadequate given current needs (Department of Health 2000). As one commentator has noted, no model will fit everywhere, and the policy-maker must be prepared to 'think different' (Smith 1999).

Second, where hospital capacity is regarded as excessive, planning strategies appear to work better than leaving the reconfiguration process to market forces. In particular, independent single hospitals are especially resistant to closure, while change may need to be accompanied by the creation of new organizational entities and even new facilities. Thus, it might be better for the term 'downsizing' to be replaced by 'reconfiguration'. Specifically, it should not be assumed that the problem of excess capacity can be addressed simply by closing some existing facilities and leaving others that are equally ill-equipped to address future challenges.

Finally, the largest reductions in hospital capacity in eastern Europe have arisen not from carefully planned processes but rather because of war or economic collapse. In other words, systems have been forced to react to external circumstances rather than anticipating them.

References

Arnould, R.J., DeBrock, L.M. and Radach, H.L. (1997) The nature and consequences of provider consolidations in the US, in B. Ferguson, T. Sheldon and J. Posnett (eds) *Concentration and Choice in Healthcare*. London: Royal Society of Medicine Press.

Aro, S., Noro, A. and Salinto, M. (1997) Deinstitutionalization of the elderly in Finland 1981–91, *Scandinavian Journal of Social Medicine*, 25(2): 136–43.

Browne, T. (1643/1986) Religio Medici, in *The Oxford Dictionary of Quotations*, 3rd edn. Oxford: Oxford University Press.

Busse, R. (2000) *Health Care Systems in Transition: Germany*. Copenhagen: European Observatory on Health Care Systems.

Christiansen, T., Enemark, U., Clausen, J. and Poulsen, P. (1999) Health care and cost containment in Denmark, in E. Mossialos and J. Le Grand (eds) *Health Care and Cost Containment in the European Union*. Aldershot: Ashgate.

Club du Vieux Manoir (1977) *Saint-Louis de la Salpêtrière*. Paris: Nouvelles Éditions Latines.

Corden, S. (2001) Case study: Australia, in A.S. Preker and A. Harding (eds) *Innovations in Health Care Delivery: The Corporatization of Public Hospitals*. Baltimore, MD: Johns Hopkins University Press.

Department of Health (2000) *Shaping the Future NHS: Long Term Planning for Hospitals and Related Services*. London: Department of Health.

Enthoven, A.C. and Singer, S.J. (1996) Managed competition and California's health care economy, *Health Affairs (Millwood)*, 15(1): 39–57.

Enthoven, A.C. and Singer, S.J. (1998) The managed care backlash and the task force in California, *Health Affairs (Millwood)*, 17(4): 95–110.

EU News in Brief (2000) France: 24,000 fewer beds by 2004, *Official Journal of the European Association of Hospital Managers*, 2(4): 9.

Ferguson, B. and Goddard, M. (1997) The case for and against mergers, in B. Ferguson, T. Sheldon and J. Posnett (eds) *Concentration and Choice in Healthcare*. Glasgow: Royal Society of Medicine Press.

Furnholmen, C. and Magnussen, J. (2000) *Health Care Systems in Transition: Norway*. Copenhagen: European Observatory on Health Care Systems.

Gaal, P., Rekassy, B. and Healy, J. (1999) *Health Care Systems in Transition: Hungary*. Copenhagen: European Observatory on Health Care Systems.

Gibson, D. (1998) *Aged Care: Old Policies, New Problems*. Cambridge: Cambridge University Press.

Goffman, E. (1969) The insanity of place, *Psychiatry*, 32: 357–88.

Granshaw, L. (1993) The hospital, in W.F. Bynum and R. Porter (eds) *Companion Encyclopaedia of the History of Medicine*. London: Routledge.

Hensher, M. and Edwards, N. (1999) Hospital provision, activity, and productivity in England since the 1980s, *British Medical Journal*, 319(7214): 911–14.

Hillman, K. (1999) The changing role for acute care hospitals, *Medical Journal of Australia*, 170(7): 325–9.

Kerr, E. and Siebrand, V. (2000) *Health Care Systems in Transition: Belgium*. Copenhagen: European Observatory on Health Care Systems.

Kulzhanov, M. and Healy, J. (1999) *Health Care Systems in Transition: Kazakhstan*. Copenhagen: European Observatory on Health Care Systems.

Lorenzo, S., Beech, R., Lang, T. and Santos-Eggimann, B. (1999) An experience of utilization review in Europe: sequel to a BIOMED project, *International Journal of Quality Health Care*, 11: 13–19.

McGrew, R.E. (1985) *Encyclopaedia of Medical History*. London: Macmillan.

McKee, M., Clarke, A. and Tennison, B. (1993) Meeting local needs, *British Medical Journal*, 306: 602.

Mechanic, D. and Rochefort, D.A. (1990) Deinstitutionalization: an appraisal of reform, *Annual Review of Sociology*, 16: 301–27.

Miller, T.S. (1997) *The Birth of the Hospital in the Byzantine Empire*. Baltimore, MD: Johns Hopkins University Press.

Minder, A., Schienholzer, H. and Amiet, M. (2000) *Health Care Systems in Transition: Switzerland*. Copenhagen: European Observatory on Health Care Systems.

Mossialos, E. and Le Grand, J. (1999) Cost containment in the EU: an overview, in E. Mossialos and J. Le Grand (eds) *Health Care and Cost Containment in the European Union*. Aldershot: Ashgate.

OECD (1999) *OECD Health Data 99: A Comparative Analysis of 29 Countries*. Paris: Organisation for Economic Co-operation and Development.

Orosz, E. and Hollo, I. (in press) Hospitals in Hungary: the story of stalled reforms, *Eurohealth*.

Porter, R. (1997) *The Greatest Benefit to Mankind: A Medical History of Humanity from Antiquity to the Present*. London: HarperCollins.

Restuccia, J.D. (1995) The evolution of hospital utilization review methods in the United States, *International Journal of Quality Health Care*, 7: 253–60.

Ribbe, M.W., Ljunggren, G., Steel, K. *et al.* (1997) Nursing homes in 10 nations: a comparison between countries and settings, *Age and Ageing*, 26(suppl. 2): 3–12.

Rico, A., Sabos, R., Wisbaum, W. and Jann, A. (2000) *Health Care Systems in Transition: Spain*. Copenhagen: European Observatory on Health Care Systems.

Robinson, R. and Dixon, A. (1999) *Health Care Systems in Transition: United Kingdom.* Copenhagen: European Observatory on Health Care Systems.

Sargaldakova, A., Healy, J., Kutzin, J. and Gedik, G. (2000) *Health Care Systems in Transition: Kyrgyzstan.* Copenhagen: European Observatory on Health Care Systems.

Simon, N. (1986) *La Pitié-Salpêtrière.* Paris: Editions de l'Arbre a images.

Smith, R. (1999) Editorial. Reconfiguring acute hospital services: no easy answers, but there are principles we should follow, *British Medical Journal,* 319: 797–8.

Southerne, T. (1682/1986) The Loyal Brother, in *The Oxford Dictionary of Quotations,* 3rd edn. Oxford: Oxford University Press.

Swingedau, O. (2000) The French health care system: a report, *Official Journal of the European Association of Hospital Managers,* 2(1): 30–4.

Taroni, F. (2000) Devolving responsibility for funding and delivering health care in Italy, *Euro Observer,* 2(1): 1–2.

Tester, S. (1996) *Community Care for Older People: A Comparative Perspective.* Basingstoke: Macmillan.

Trohler, U. and Prull, C.R. (1997) The rise of the modern hospital, in I. Loudon (ed.) *Western Medicine.* Oxford: Oxford University Press.

Turner-Crowson, J. (1993) *Re-shaping Mental Health Services: Implications for Britain of US Experience.* London: King's Fund.

van Mosseveld, C.J.P.M. and van Son, P. (1999) *International Comparison of Health Care Data.* Dordrecht: Kluwer Academic.

Victor, C.R., Healy, J., Thomas, A. and Seargeant, J. (2000) Older patients and delayed discharge from hospital, *Health and Community Care,* 8(6): 443–52.

Walker, A. and Maltby, T. (1997) *Ageing Europe.* Buckingham: Open University Press.

WHO (2001) *WHO European Health for All Database.* Copenhagen: WHO Regional Office for Europe.

three

Pressures for change

Martin McKee, Judith Healy, Nigel Edwards and Anthony Harrison

Introduction

The previous chapter showed how hospitals have changed throughout history. They will continue to do so, shaped by their patients, staff and technology. Diseases come and go, and the expectations of the public change. Health professionals acquire new knowledge and skills. The technology now exists to do things that were undreamed of even a decade ago. Predicting the future is an uncertain science (McKee 1995), but one can be certain that the pace of change in the twenty-first century will be faster than ever.

This chapter explores factors driving change in the hospital system and the extent to which their effects can be predicted. Many of these factors are, of course, interrelated. For example, an ageing population influences both patterns of disease and the composition of the health care workforce. These factors are discussed under three headings: demand- and supply-side changes and wider changes in society (Figure 3.1).

Demand-side changes

Changes in demography

The commercial sector puts enormous effort into tracking population trends, recognizing that this will influence demand for their products. For example, the pattern of global advertising changed markedly in 1992, shifting its target to younger people in response to increasing numbers of teenagers in the United States (Klein 2000). Much advertising results from a careful study of demographics, but this type of analysis is much less apparent in the health care sector. The composition of a population is determined by three factors:

Figure 3.1   Pressures for change in hospitals

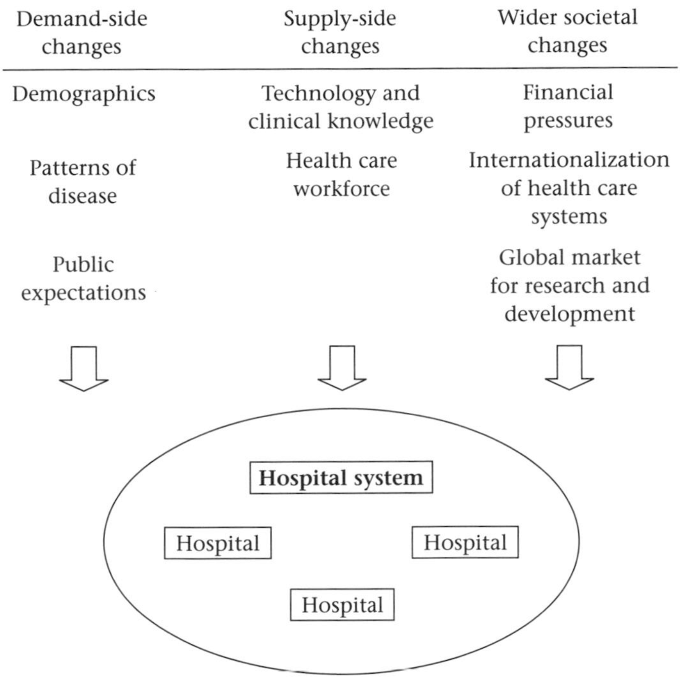

Demand-side changes	Supply-side changes	Wider societal changes
Demographics	Technology and clinical knowledge	Financial pressures
Patterns of disease	Health care workforce	Internationalization of health care systems
Public expectations		Global market for research and development

⇩   ⇩   ⇩

Hospital system

Hospital   Hospital

Hospital

births, deaths and migration. Each has implications for the health care system and, specifically, for the hospital of the future.

Fertility

Birth rates have been falling in most European countries (Figure 3.2), most markedly in the countries of southern and eastern Europe that traditionally had high birth rates. These changes have important implications for health services in the long term but, more immediately, they influence the demand for obstetric and paediatric services. In Ireland, for example, the pattern of provision that was appropriate in 1980, when a typical woman had more than three children, is no longer appropriate for a generation of women having less than two children.

Ageing

In contrast to the falling number of children, people aged 65 years and over will comprise an increasing proportion of the population in many countries in Europe (Figure 3.3). The old old population (people 80 years or older) is of particular interest, since they are the fastest growing age group, although, as with the young old, there is considerable variation among countries (United Nations Population Division 1998). It is clear, however, that Europe is experiencing both an absolute increase in older people and an increase as a proportion

Figure 3.2 Total fertility rate in selected European countries: □ 1980; ■ 1997

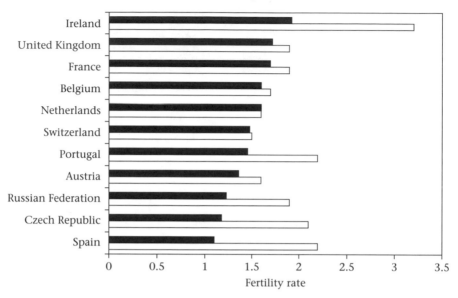

Source: WHO (2001)

Figure 3.3 Future projections of the percentage of the population aged over 65 in various regions of Europe

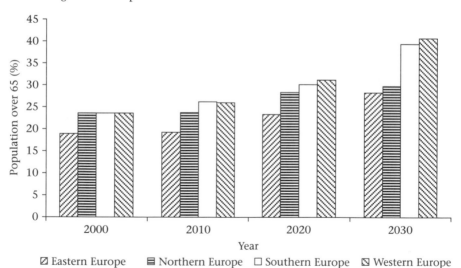

Source: United Nations Population Division (1995)

of the population. The question is whether this will mean significantly higher hospital costs.

The impact of the growth in the older population is a source of continuing concern for health policy-makers, in part because older people are the main users of hospital services. Older patients are admitted to hospitals more often than younger patients, stay longer and typically account for about half the hospital workload measured in terms of bed-days (Harrison and Prentice 1996; Walker and Maltby 1997; Victor *et al.* 2000). This has given rise to a widely held view that a future ageing population will increase the demand for hospital care and thus health care costs.

This debate has become politicized, being used by certain commentators as a device to support their view that welfare states are increasingly unaffordable (Mendelson and Schwartz 1993). The reality is rather more complex, and the conclusions depend on whether one extrapolates from current data for health services utilization or examines the determinants of health system costs. Furthermore, calculating the costs of an ageing population requires distinguishing between social and health care costs, cumulative and episodic costs, hospital and nursing home care costs, and ageing and cohort effects.

First, it cannot be assumed that the general health and hospital use of elderly people in the future will be the same as today. Future elderly people may benefit from a lifetime of better nutrition and social conditions (Evandrou 1997). For example, research from the United States predicts that the levels of chronic disability among the elderly population will decline by 1.5 per cent per year as many risk factors for chronic diseases show improvements, often linked to improved education (Singer and Manton 1998). The proportion of elderly people requiring assistance with activities of daily living halved between 1976 and 1991 (Grundy 1997). A recent projection for the United Kingdom, based on changing levels of fitness in successive generations, predicted that the total burden of disease would fall by two-thirds by 2051 (Khaw 1999).

A second point is that elderly people do not incur health care costs simply by being old (Fuchs 1984). The crucial factor is not how long one lives, but how long one takes to die. Because elderly people may be treated less intensively, the health costs associated with the last year of life may actually be less in older age groups, as seen in data from the United States Medicare programme (Lubitz *et al.* 1995). Indeed, the most costly patients are those who die young (Scitovsky 1988).

When health and social care costs are combined, the picture looks different. For example, data from the Netherlands that included the cost of social and long-term care showed that the total cost of health and social care rose exponentially with old age (Meerding *et al.* 1998). A recent study from Canada, which examined the costs of acute medical care, nursing home and social care separately, also identified the importance of proximity to death for acute care costs, which did not increase with age, although nursing home and social care costs did (McGrail *et al.* 2000). Hospitals in many industrialized countries have already transferred the long-term care of dependent older people out of hospitals and into residential care and nursing homes (discussed in Chapter 2). Thus, much of the cost has already been shifted from the health care budget to the social care budget.

Studies of the determinants of rising health system costs suggest that ageing appears to be a minor rather than a major factor leading to increased health expenditure. Health expenditure is largely driven by supply-side factors, such as technology, or by demand-side factors, such as physician and patient expectations, that have little to do with the age of populations (Fahey and Fitzgerald 1997; Zweifel *et al.* 1999).

This does not mean that the ageing of populations can be ignored. It has important implications for the type of health care that is provided. Many diseases are strongly linked to age, so, for example, an increase in the number of people aged 60 years and over will lead to more cases of cancer; on the other hand, more teenagers will lead to more accidental injuries. Many countries will have more patients with conditions such as fractured hips, strokes and Alzheimer's disease. These conditions have one feature in common: their optimal management requires coordinated multidisciplinary teamwork. This will be a major challenge in countries with a tradition of medical specialists working in isolation, and where non-medical professionals, such as nurses and social workers, play a markedly subordinate role to physicians.

Finally, hospitals of the future must take into account the specific needs of ageing populations, whether increasing provision of geriatric medicine facilities, improving access for those with impaired mobility or ensuring clearer signposting for those with impaired vision.

Migration

A third way in which populations change is migration. Many western European countries have experienced substantial migration from Africa and Asia since 1945 and, since 1990, from eastern Europe. Forced migration in the face of violence is a continuing phenomenon (Schmeidl 1997). This also involves minorities such as the Roma people of central Europe, who have been exposed to systematic discrimination in some countries (Hajioff and McKee 2000). The health needs of migrants often differ from those of the host population, for several reasons (Carballo *et al.* 1998). Some diseases may occur almost exclusively in migrant populations, such as sickle cell anaemia in Afro-Caribbean populations, and thallassaemia in migrants from the eastern Mediterranean. Other diseases may be more common among migrants, such as diabetes among South Asians (McKeigue *et al.* 1991). These chronic conditions often require specialized care, and hospitals must respond not only to medical needs but also to social needs by, for example, providing interpreting services. Those fleeing conflict, such as refugees from the Balkans in the 1990s, also have particular needs, such as for mental health services in the aftermath of trauma and torture. However, these migrants may also include health professionals who, by virtue of their linguistic ability and cultural awareness, may be able to help meet the needs of their compatriots. Finally, hospitals must ensure that they are sensitive to different cultural traditions; such responses might include dedicated prayer rooms, a choice of diets and awareness of differences in attitudes to family visiting (Mattson and Lew 1992).

Changing patterns of disease

Since the core function of the hospital is to treat illness, then it must respond appropriately as patterns of disease change. Changing patterns of diet have contributed to evolving trends in diseases such as ischaemic heart disease, which is rising among some populations as they shift to high-fat diets and falling among others moving in the opposite direction (Tunstall-Pedoe *et al.* 1999). The international marketing of tobacco has led to a global epidemic of smoking-related diseases (Peto *et al.* 1999). Other ways in which lifestyle and environment influence health are increasingly being recognized, such as the impact of fossil fuel consumption on global warming and climate change and thus on a wide range of health outcomes, such as malaria (McMichael and Haines 1997; Martens *et al.* 1999).

The interrelationship between humans and their microbial environment provides a rich source for changing patterns of disease. Throughout history, as humans have changed their habitation and lifestyles, new infectious diseases have emerged, in particular those transmitted from animals (Krause 1992). Examples include measles, influenza, tuberculosis, yellow fever and, more recently, Lyme disease. New diseases, especially those caused by infections, will continue to emerge; recent examples include the human immunodeficiency virus (HIV) and new variant Creutzfeldt-Jakob disease (Will *et al.* 1996). Although predictions can be made as to their future spread, these have wide confidence intervals and are susceptible to effective public health action, as illustrated by the wide variation in the rate of increase in cases of acquired immunodeficiency syndrome (AIDS) in Europe (Wellings 1994).

Changing risk factors

At the risk of simplification, diseases can be considered along a spectrum defined on the basis of the length of time between causation and the appearance of disease. This may be minutes, as with many injuries, or it may be many years. For example, an increase in the rate of smoking among teenagers will take up to 40 years to appear as a rise in lung cancer (Peto *et al.* 1999; Shkolnikov *et al.* 1999). It can thus be predicted with some confidence that the future need for thoracic surgical facilities will decline in Finland but increase in Portugal (Figure 3.4).

Many common diseases originate before birth or in early childhood, such as cerebrovascular disease, stomach and breast cancer. Changes during childhood, therefore, may be visible, in terms of the pattern of disease in a society, up to 60 years later (Kuh and Ben Shlomo 1997). For example, Portugal was one of the poorest countries in western Europe immediately after 1945. Thus, despite rapid economic growth since the mid-1970s, Portugal has death rates from stroke and stomach cancer in the 1990s that are far higher than other western European countries but similar to those of eastern Europe (Figure 3.5). Consequently, the optimal provision of services for rehabilitation of patients with strokes should be more closely aligned between Portugal and Poland than between the more obvious comparison of Portugal and Spain.

For other causes, the lag period is much shorter, as exemplified by changes in alcohol consumption. The dramatic reduction in alcohol consumption in the USSR in the 1980s and its subsequent reversal were associated with almost immediate changes in rates of injuries and cardiovascular disease (Leon *et al.* 1997).

Figure 3.4 Age-standardized death rate from cancer of the lung, bronchus and trachea per 100,000 population in Finland (◆) and Portugal (■), all ages, 1970–98

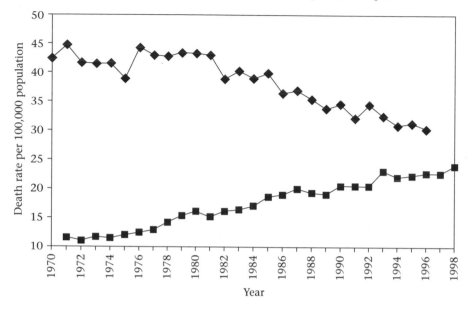

Source: WHO (2001)

Figure 3.5 Age-standardized death rate from cerebrovascular disease per 100,000 population in France (◆), Poland (■), Portugal (▲) and Spain (×), all ages, 1985–98

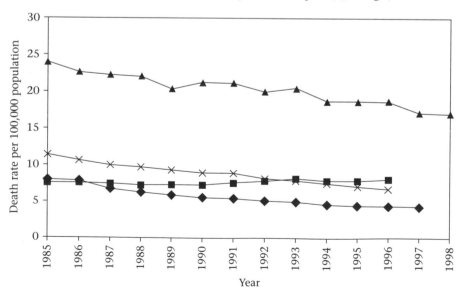

Source: WHO (2001)

Many other causes and their corresponding diseases lie between these two extremes. In central Europe, improvements in diet after 1990 led to a fall in cardiovascular disease in only a few years (Zatonski *et al.* 1998). Longstanding trends can also be modified by factors acting over shorter periods. For example, hypertension may have its origins in early life, but effective treatment can rapidly reduce the risk of cerebrovascular disease.

As this brief analysis shows, the mix of patients in a hospital will be very different two decades in the future. This has important implications for the design and configuration of hospitals.

Hospital-acquired infections

One area in which hospitals play a direct role in the changing pattern of disease is hospital-acquired (nosocomial) and, more importantly, antibiotic-resistant infection. This is an area of considerable importance to policy-makers for two reasons. First, it can directly affect the cost and viability of the hospitals; second, it is essentially avoidable. For these reasons, it is dealt with in some detail here.

By the twentieth century, for the first time in history, the risks of going into hospital were less than receiving treatment outside its walls, primarily because hospital infections were being brought under some control. The adoption of aseptic and antiseptic techniques from the late nineteenth century (Box 3.1) and the later invention of antibiotics led many to think that the battle against hospital-acquired infection had been won.

This complacency was not warranted, since rates of hospital-acquired infections are again rising. About 10 per cent of hospital patients acquire an infection (WHO 1996, 1999; Plowman *et al.* 1997; Ayliffe *et al.* 1999). Although comparative data from across Europe are limited, it is likely that rates in some countries are substantially higher. Prevalence is highest in units such as intensive care, burns, neonatal care and those treating immunosuppressed patients (Ayliffe *et al.* 1999). These infections are not only damaging to patients but also increase treatment costs for the hospital. Patients who acquire infections in hospital spend over twice as long in hospital (Plowman *et al.* 1999). The estimated annual cost to the National Health Service in England is €1.6 billion, since about 1 in 11 patients contracts an infection in hospital, with an estimated 5000 deaths per year in hospitals (National Audit Office 2000). This makes hospital-acquired infection a more common cause of deaths than road accidents, at least in the United Kingdom (Plowman *et al.* 1997). A study of surgical patients in Denmark found that those acquiring infections could expect to stay in hospital for an additional 5.7 days (Poulson *et al.* 1994).

Rates of hospital-acquired infections have been rising for several reasons (Swartz 1995). First, susceptibility to infection rises with age and patients admitted to hospital are older, reflecting ageing populations as well as the increased scope for intervention in older patients who might previously have been deemed unfit for invasive treatment. Second, procedures have become more extensive, with greater use of implants and longer operation times. Third, patients on immunosuppressive treatment are now more likely to receive invasive treatments. Fourth, the risks of blood-borne viral infections such as

---

Box 3.1 The battle against hospital-acquired infection

Surgery at the beginning of the nineteenth century was fraught with hazards. The absence of anaesthesia limited operations to those that could be performed quickly, but the skill of the surgeon counted for little if the patient died. Up to 40 per cent of operations led to death, most often due to sepsis. One surgeon noted that those undergoing surgery were 'exposed to more chances of death than was the English soldier on the field of Waterloo'. The breakthrough came at the Vienna General Hospital in 1847, where Ignaz Semmelweis became interested in why the death rate from puerperal fever was 29 per cent in one obstetric ward but only 3 per cent in another. Patients in the ward with the higher rate were tended by medical students (who had often come from attending autopsies) and the others by midwifery students. When the students exchanged wards, the death rates followed each group. Although Semmelweis was able to reduce mortality dramatically by the simple expedient of imposing hand-washing with chlorinated water, he continued to meet resistance from doubting colleagues and, in despair, left Vienna for Budapest.

Others did, however, take up his ideas. In England, Florence Nightingale revolutionized nursing and emphasized the importance of cleanliness. Joseph Lister introduced operative techniques based on removal of all clots and necrotic tissue and the liberal use of carbolic acid, showing a reduction in post-amputation mortality from 46 per cent in about 1866 to 15 per cent in 1870. Many surgeons remained unconvinced, denying that bacteria even existed. His ideas received support elsewhere in Europe. Carl Theirsch and Ernst von Bergmann in Germany, Thomas Billroth in Austria and Just Lucas-Championnère in France each adopted and disseminated aseptic and antiseptic practices. In the United States, William Halstead introduced rubber gloves.

As the nineteenth century drew to a close, the benefits of asepsis and antisepsis were becoming apparent to the most conservative of surgeons and, with the additional possibilities afforded by the development of anaesthesia, modern surgery finally became a realistic possibility. Sadly, even at the end of the twentieth century, some lessons from the early pioneers, such as the importance of washing hands when moving between patients, have yet to be applied systematically.

Source: Porter (1997)

---

hepatitis B and C and HIV are increasing. Finally, antibiotic-resistant micro-organisms have grown markedly.

The last of these factors, the rise in antibiotic-resistant bacteria, is of greatest concern. Bacteria are capable of rapid evolutionary change in response to changes in their environment, most notably the presence of antibiotics. In an infected patient, some bacteria may be resistant to the antibiotic being used, either by random genetic mutation or by transfer of genetic material from other bacteria. The appropriate antibiotic may bring the infection under sufficient control to allow the body's immune system to mop up the remaining resistant bacteria. In other cases, especially where the treatment is given intermittently or, where partial resistance exists, this may not happen. Although the bacteria susceptible to antibiotics are killed, the resistant ones multiply rapidly so that an initially antibiotic-susceptible infection becomes resistant. Inadequate hygiene facilitates the spread to other patients.

Increasing rates of antibiotic resistance are affecting many types of bacteria, but two are causing particular concern. The first is multi-resistant *Staphylococcus aureus*. *S. aureus* is common in the noses and skin of healthy people. It was initially susceptible to penicillin and other antibiotics, but new strains have evolved that are resistant to almost all antibiotics (WHO 1999). Thus, a disease that responded rapidly to a short course of penicillin five decades ago has now become effectively incurable.

The second concern is the rise in multi-resistant tuberculosis (Farmer *et al.* 1999). Tuberculosis is especially difficult to treat, as the bacteria lodge within cells, where they are protected from circulating antibiotics. Consequently, treatment must be prolonged or aggressive. Long-term administration of antibiotics provides ideal conditions for the emergence of resistance, so that multi-drug therapy is now used to reduce that risk. In some countries, especially the countries of the former Soviet Union, a substantial proportion of cases now are resistant to some or all of the first-line antibiotics used to treat tuberculosis (Kammerling and Banatvala 2001).

A key message is that these changes are not inevitable. Rates of antibiotic resistance vary greatly within Europe (Dornbusch *et al.* 1998). The lowest rates are found in hospitals that have well-designed and well-implemented antibiotic-prescribing policies and regular surveillance of patterns of resistance. Although factors driving the emergence of antibiotic resistance may reflect local practices, resistance can have consequences far afield. Infectious agents do not respect borders, and even countries that have well-designed policies in place are susceptible to imported cases. For example, the emergence of multi-resistant pneumococci in Iceland in the early 1990s has been linked to the return of a single tourist from Spain (Soares *et al.* 1993).

Increasing rates of resistant infections in hospitals pose a major threat to the progress made by health care in the twentieth century. Their control deserves to be a much higher priority among those concerned with hospital policy.

Changing public expectations

Greater health knowledge among users and higher expectations for improved quality of service may pressure hospitals, like other service providers, to do more diagnosis and treatment and to improve how they provide care (Chappel 1995; Posnett *et al.* 1998). This is manifest in myriad ways. The growth of consumerism in industrialized countries means that shared facilities, with little privacy, that might have been acceptable to patients in the past are no longer so. Patients increasingly, and legitimately, demand to be seen at times that are convenient for them rather than for health professionals. Access to clinical information via the Internet means that some patients may be better informed about their diseases than their physicians (Neuberger 2000). This does not necessarily mean that patients will demand more health care, but may be more likely to reject interventions where the evidence is equivocal (Coulter *et al.* 1994). In some parts of Europe (as discussed in Chapter 7), the concept of patients' rights is still extremely poorly developed (Platt and McKee 2000).

Supply-side changes

Changing technology and clinical knowledge

Developments in health technology (pharmaceuticals, devices, equipment and techniques) and clinical knowledge have rapidly increased the range of available interventions, and the sections of the population, especially elderly people, to whom they are applied. There is considerable variability in the introduction of new technology (Chapter 12), but the pace of change is steadily accelerating. Hip replacements have been joined by replacement of knee, shoulder and finger joints. Transplant surgeons have added the heart, liver and pancreas to their initial success with kidneys. Surgery for peptic ulcer has been largely replaced by long-term treatment with H_2 antagonists. AIDS has been transformed in affluent countries from a rapidly progressive fatal disease to one in which increasing numbers of people keep the disease under control with complex cocktails of anti-viral therapy. Improvements in anaesthetic techniques and less invasive surgery have decreased the risks of operating on elderly patients, allowing a substantial increase in per capita intervention rates across the age spectrum. Looking ahead, the implications of these changes for the hospital are considerable but complex (Wilson 1999).

New pharmaceuticals may reduce the need for hospitalization. Some drugs now tackle risk factors for chronic diseases such as atherosclerosis and allow ambulatory medical treatment instead of surgery, as with peptic ulcers (Jensen 1986). Prolonged inpatient care is being replaced by anti-viral maintenance therapy for people with AIDS (Gebo *et al.* 1999) and by the directly observed treatment short course (DOTS) strategy for people with tuberculosis (WHO 1997; Maher *et al.* 1999). Other drugs will increase hospitalization, since they extend opportunities for treatment, as with new anti-cancer agents. These drugs can expand the number of treatable individuals, either because a previously untreatable condition becomes treatable or, as side-effects or contraindications are reduced, more patients are willing to accept treatment. The potential unleashed by the rapid pace of development of genomics is enormous, with gene therapy potentially able to make many inherited diseases treatable (Morgan and Blaese 1999) or, potentially more importantly, to tailor treatment much more closely to an individual's genetic make-up, thus enhancing effectiveness and reducing side-effects.

New vaccines hold particular promise if they manage to eliminate some infectious diseases, including HIV and hepatitis C. New vaccines will also target infectious agents that cause cancer, such as human papillomavirus (a cause of cervical cancer), as well as some cancers themselves.

Advances in surgery are likely in three main areas. Minimally invasive surgery will increasingly supplant many conventional operations. Early endovascular procedures, such as coronary angioplasty, have been joined by an array of procedures directed at many different organs. Related advances in therapeutic agents, such as targeted anti-cancer drugs or those acting on blood vessel growth, will expand the possibilities further. Finally, radiosurgery, in which finely tuned beams of high-energy particles are directed at body tissues, is now used routinely to manage many intracerebral problems but, as with other techniques, is likely to extend to other parts of the body. Each of these developments has important implications for training, equipment and the configuration of facilities.

New equipment will be used to monitor the patient of the future more intensively, using sophisticated sensors providing information in real time. Taken with changes in the severity of patients admitted to hospitals, this may challenge the existing model, in many hospitals, of a single intensive care unit. Instead, current specialty-based wards may undertake much more intensive care than at present. Ward staff will need new skills, as tests that would previously have required a laboratory are undertaken using bedside kits. Improved imaging and laboratory testing will advance diagnosis and also change the boundaries of diseases, enabling what were previously thought of as single diseases to be differentiated, exemplified by the alphabetical progress of the hepatitis viruses (Zuckerman 1996). In some cases, this may lead to the emergence of entirely new specialties. Improved information technology means that the flow of information around the hospital will change. Although predictions for a 'paperless office' have proven ill-founded, medical records and X-rays are likely to be retained in digital form rather than hard copy.

This dissemination of technology will contribute to a change in the relationship between tertiary and secondary care facilities. Treatment previously restricted to highly specialized centres, such as endoscopy and kidney dialysis, can now be undertaken by other staff, and in other locations such as freestanding ambulatory care centres. The development of telemedicine is also opening up new working methods as specialists can be consulted or can carry out diagnosis 'at a distance', and health care knowledge is available from the Internet. In contrast, some new technologies, such as linear accelerators and positron emission tomography scanners, are driving even greater concentration of some facilities. Patient care within the hospital is being managed increasingly through integrated hospital information systems that, when appropriately chosen and implemented, have facilitated the sharing of patient data and contributed to the development of better coordinated patient care (van Bemmel and Musen 1997; Bakker and Leguit 1999).

Will these developments in technology dramatically increase hospital costs? The precise contribution of new technologies to rising hospital costs is arguable (Mossialos and Le Grand 1999). New technologies are not always more expensive than the ones they replace. However, even where technology is less expensive, it may lead to increased costs as other parts of the hospital are reorganized to reflect changing patterns of treatment. For example, somewhat counterintuitively, the treatment of peptic ulcers with drugs rather than surgery has increased overall hospital costs as patients undergo repeated treatments (Murphy 1998).

Some caution is also required in relation to the health benefits of new technology, which can bring threats as well as benefits. The vast growth in pharmaceutical products may have prevented millions of premature deaths, but a few have created new iatrogenic diseases. The birth of babies with limb deformities to mothers who had taken the drug thalidomide is one obvious example. In addition, many earlier predictions of vast benefits from technological advances have not been realized. Enthusiasm for the opportunities of the future must always be accompanied by a degree of caution.

Changes in the workforce

Changing population structures affect not only the demand for care but also have implications for the pool of staff that can be recruited to a hospital (Green and Owen 1995). Although different countries face different challenges, two issues stand out. One is the ageing of populations. At a time when health care needs are increasing, the pool of potential staff is shrinking, alarmingly so in some Nordic countries (Buchan and Edwards 2000). Second, an increasingly female medical workforce wishes to combine career progression with family commitments.

Chapter 11 explores the trends affecting the hospital workforce in Europe. Decentralized management and flexible employment contracts are necessary to match staff levels more closely to health care needs, offering opportunities to retain experienced individuals who might otherwise leave the workforce because of family commitments. Conversely, this concept of 'the flexible firm' brings risks that it will be used as a means of making the workforce less stable and less skilled, with adverse consequences for clinical care. As with so many policies, much depends on how 'flexibility' is implemented.

A second issue is the increasing internationalization of the health care workforce, with some countries actively recruiting health professionals from other countries. This process is likely to be accentuated by the further expansion of the European Union (McKee et al. 1996). This clearly has many important implications both for countries that are attracting skilled staff and for those that are losing them. The former must establish ways to integrate new staff with different cultural traditions and, in some cases, levels of training. The latter face adverse effects on their health care systems from the loss of skilled people (Jinks et al. 2000).

A third issue is the scope for substitution of staff by people with different skills, which reflects an emphasis on competence rather than credentials (Armstrong 1991). Physicians perform many tasks that are better undertaken by other professionals, but change may not be easy, especially where professionals such as physicians and nurses have established a statutory right to certain tasks. Substitution should not be seen simply as an opportunity to lower costs; instead, decisions should focus on the quality of care on certain tasks. Skill mix issues within the hospital are discussed in Chapter 10.

A fourth issue is the need for hospitals to ensure that their staff can respond to the rapidly changing environment. Nurses in some European countries already must prove their continuing competence to practise if they are to remain registered. This process is now extending to physicians (revalidation). Even where such policies are not implemented, it will be necessary to ensure that staff participate in continuing professional development to keep their skills up to date. This will have major implications for hospitals, such as the provision of learning time, creation of systems to monitor progress and dealing with those who are unwilling to participate. Revalidation is discussed further in Chapter 10.

Hospital workforce changes take place within a complex system of norms and values as well as within the rules and customs governing relations between professions and between employers and employees. European Union measures such as the Working Time Directive (Council of the European Union 1993) and various provisions of the Social Chapter of the Maastricht Treaty are improving working conditions in some countries, in some cases with profound implications for the delivery of health services, such as physicians' working hours (White 1996).

In summary, the health care workforce and the surrounding environmental pressures will continue to change. Key issues are flexibility and diversity. In the future, the health care workforce is likely to be more international, with fluid professional boundaries. Beyond this, however, prediction is difficult. The future will depend on a system in which employers retain sufficient flexibility to adapt to changing health care needs. Nevertheless, employees require some security, not least to continue with life-long learning, which is increasingly important in an ever more complex environment.

Political and societal changes

Financial pressures

The importance of hospitals in overall health care budgets makes them the obvious targets for governments trying to cap public expenditure or to slow the rate of growth. The sum of money allocated to health care is largely a political rather than an economic question, however, involving choices between competing priorities for public and private expenditure.

Hospitals typically consume more than half the overall health care budget. It is widely believed that they can be made to function more efficiently and that many patients can be treated more cost-effectively in other settings (Chapter 5). The result has been a vast array of measures aimed at controlling total spending, improving the technical efficiency of the hospital and raising the quality of the care delivered.

Upward pressure on health care expenditure has been a feature of most industrialized countries in the past four decades and has forced countries to find ways to constrain both demand and supply, with varying amounts of success (Mossialos and Le Grand 1999). Figure 3.6 shows the steady rise in health expenditure from the 1960s onwards as a percentage of gross domestic product (GDP) in the leading industrialized countries. The variation would be even greater if absolute values were shown, as wealthier countries tend to spend more per capita on health, although the relationship is less strong than is often assumed (Kanavos and Yfantopoulos 1999). It should be noted that there are substantial problems with the definitions involved in these comparisons (Torgerson *et al.* 1998), but some broad trends are apparent.

Figure 3.6 Total expenditure on health as a percentage of gross domestic product for the Group of Seven (G7) leading industrial countries, 1960–96

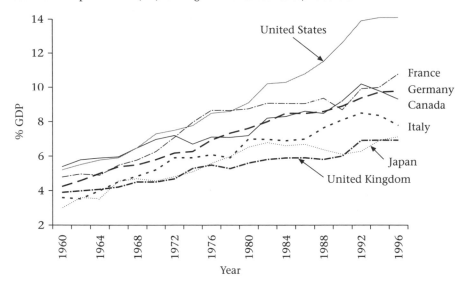

Source: OECD (1998)

Among advanced industrialized countries, the United States is the outlier, with expenditure rising steeply from the 1980s and reaching 14.1 per cent of GDP in 1996. This has clear implications for any attempt to compare experiences in the United States with those in Europe. Expenditure in the United States has slowed since then, attributed by some to the constraints imposed by the growth of 'managed care' (Enthoven and Singer 1996; Vincenzino 1998). Among the other Group of Seven (G7) leading industrial countries in 1996, the United Kingdom spent the least, at 6.9 per cent of GDP, while France and Germany each spent around 10 per cent.

In the European Union, health care expenditure has risen steadily from just above 5 per cent of GDP on average in 1970 to over 8 per cent by 1993 (Barros 1998). The issue of health care funding is covered in another book in this series (Mossialos *et al.* 2002). It is enough to note here that countries with a tax-based health financing system have contained costs more successfully since 1994 than countries with an insurance-based system (Comas-Herrera 1999). Expenditure in central and eastern European countries rose from a trough in the late 1980s to about 5 per cent of GDP in the 1990s; in the countries of the former Soviet Union, it is only around 3 per cent of GDP (WHO 2001). It must be noted, however, that GDP has dropped calamitously in many of these countries.

Hospitals in eastern Europe consume about three-quarters of identifiable health expenditure (as noted in Chapter 2), a figure underlying the strong pressure to transfer some of this shrinking health budget from hospitals to primary care. Long-term economic growth, combined with greater efficiency in collecting funds for health care, may eventually make additional resources available, but this cannot be depended on in the medium term. Simply because they are a major element in the overall health care budget, hospitals are subject to changing political decisions about the size of that budget, yet another factor to be taken into account by the health policy-maker.

Internationalization of health systems

Health services exist in an increasingly global environment (Frenk *et al.* 1997; Lee 1999). International aspects of health services include movement of patients and of providers, provision of services by organizations based in one country to patients in another one and establishment of facilities in foreign countries (Frenk and Gomez-Dantes 1995). The scale and nature of these phenomena vary greatly, influenced by such factors as tradition and language, and increasingly by economic pressures from regional trade blocs such as the European Union, the North American Free Trade Agreement and Mercosur (the Common Market of the South, including Argentina, Brazil, Paraguay and Uruguay). In an increasingly profit-driven health sector culture, United States corporations are expanding actively overseas (Gomez-Dantes and Frenk 1995).

Europe has been subject to fewer external market forces, since health care is based primarily on the concept of solidarity and private health organizations are largely not-for-profit. Health care *per se* is, formally, outside the scope of the European Commission but, in reality, is subject to many elements of European law (McKee *et al.* 1996). Health care is influenced by principles relating to the 'four freedoms' set out in the 1957 Treaty of Rome: the freedom of movement of goods, services, people and capital. In Europe, health care provided by government or under government control is, in general, not regarded as a 'service' and thus not subject to competition law. Although a detailed analysis of the impact of European law on health services is beyond the scope of this book, its importance for health policy-makers should be emphasized. One example is a recent ruling on whether individuals can be reimbursed for health care provided in another country (Kanavos *et al.* 1999). More often, however, the policies developed in relation to the internal market, and thus often not discussed by health ministers, have the most impact. An example is the transfer of ancillary staff to private contractors in hospitals in the United Kingdom; this became much less attractive to employers when it became clear that the workers' conditions of service would be protected. The extension of the European Union Working Time Directive (Council of the European Union 1993) to junior physicians will also have major implications for hospital costs (White 1996) and, potentially, for hospital configurations, as it may become impossible to provide 24-hour cover for some specialties in small hospitals.

Cross-national health care organizations (apart from pharmaceutical and insurance companies) have not so far emerged as significant players within the European Union. For-profit health care corporations, predominantly based in the United States, have not penetrated European health care systems. These organizations are exerting pressure on the World Trade Organization to gain more favourable treatment but are opposed by European countries that are concerned about the potential for destabilizing their health care systems.

Some commentators have expressed concern about World Trade Organization proposals to regulate international trade in services, arguing that this could undermine countries that have pursued policies based on solidarity (Price *et al.* 1999), although others have suggested that such fears may be exaggerated (McKee and Mossialos 2000). This is, however, an area where vigilance is required. The message for policy-makers, including those working at the local level, is that they must be aware of global developments that may have implications for what they can and cannot do.

Global changes in the market for medical research and development

Progress in basic science has created new opportunities for interdisciplinary research, which requires large research teams in multi-faculty environments and access to very large populations to recruit larger patient cohorts than are available to single hospitals. Large teams also must compete in the increasingly global market for research funds and research talent. There is intense competition between universities for publicly funded biomedical research through bodies such as the National Institutes of Health in the United States, the Medical Research Council in the United Kingdom and INSERM in France. Even more important, however, is the growth of research funded by industry (Meyer *et al.* 1998). Companies look throughout the industrialized world for the best research teams to conduct their work and do not confine their funding to universities. Claiming to deliver a research product faster and cheaper, for-profit contract research organizations now compete with academic hospitals for clinical research funding.

In some countries, research and development strategies have shifted the emphasis towards large-scale programmatic funding rather than grants for specific projects. The result of these pressures is that academic hospitals must have more capital, larger and more talented faculties, skilled research management teams and access to larger groups of patients, or they risk falling behind their competitors at home and abroad.

Many university-affiliated hospitals have traditionally subsidized their academic work from funded patient care. Judging by the experience in the United States, this may become less sustainable in an increasingly competitive health care environment (McKee and Mossialos 1998). Taken together, these developments have major implications for the future of teaching hospitals.

Responding to uncertainty

As the preceding chapter has shown, although the size of hospital systems may be shrinking (at least in terms of number of beds), the scope and scale of hospital activity has been increasing. The overall direction of the hospital of the future is hard to predict, however, and the future for particular types of hospitals still harder. Nevertheless, the immediate future of 'the hospital' does, at least, seem assured.

Some recent trends seem destined to continue, at least in industrialized countries. These include further compression of length of stay, renewed efforts to manage quality of care and greater use of options such as ambulatory care, day-only hospitalization and home care (Braithwaite 1997; Komesaroff *et al.* 1997). Further changes in hospital practice are difficult to predict, however, except that the pace of change will continue. One vision of a future hospital (at least in the immediate future) is as follows:

> The acute-care hospital will, in the future, care mainly for the sick who have a chance of recovering. Increasingly, in-hospital patients will have more complex problems and a greater number of co-morbidities. Specialised units caring for the seriously ill are increasing. Emergency departments are increasingly managing the seriously ill rather than offering primary healthcare; operating suites are performing more complex procedures for in-hospital patients. As a result, far more intensive-care and high-dependency beds are required, while the total number of acute-care hospital beds is decreasing as the more ambulant and less sick are managed elsewhere.
>
> (Hillman 1999: 326)

A key message of this chapter is the centrality of uncertainty in hospital planning, involving unintended consequences from even the best-laid plans. This creates a major challenge, since hospitals are large relatively fixed assets, built for the long term. The lead-time between drawing up the plans, obtaining the funds and completing the building can be many years. By the time the opening plaque is unveiled, the hospital might already be obsolete.

As this chapter has shown, some factors can be predicted with reasonable certainty, some can be considered as probable, but some will emerge quite unexpectedly. The challenge is to take into account those that can be predicted while allowing for the unexpected. These unpredictable areas and unforeseen consequences mean that there must be sufficient flexibility to accommodate a wide range of possible scenarios.

Future trends in population and disease are probably the most amenable to forecasting. Demographic projection methods are well established and can be used to predict both demand for care and supply of staff. Techniques such as age–period–cohort models can be used to predict, with caution, future trends in many diseases (Robertson and Boyle 1998). Such studies demonstrate that rates of ischaemic heart disease will continue to fall in many northern European countries and that rates of lung cancer among women will increase in southern Europe, with corresponding implications for health services.

Predictions of the impact of technological change or of the impact of the international economic and political environment on hospitals are more hazardous, although some trends can be foreseen. Translating these issues into a model of what a hospital might look like is, however, beset by complexity and surrounded by areas of uncertainty. This was exemplified in a model developed for the Paris University Hospital (Jolly and Gerbaud 1992).

The future is likely to lie in methods that bring together quantitative models of what can be predicted with consensus judgement about what is more uncertain (Garrett 1999). The number of examples in which these methods are being used to explore systematically potential future scenarios is growing (Box 3.2).

Box 3.2 Forecasting programmes in western Europe

The Netherlands
The Dutch Steering Committee on Future Health Scenarios established in 1984 brought together politicians, civil servants, academics and the private sector. The projects used techniques such as literature reviews, Delphi exercises and simulation to explore specific themes, which were then subjected to wide consultation. As well as detailed reports on specific topics, such as health technology and management of particular diseases, this Committee made major methodological contributions to forecasting techniques.

United Kingdom
The United Kingdom Foresight programme seeks visions of the future, looking at possible future needs and threats, and deciding what should be done now to ensure that society is ready for these challenges. It does so by building bridges between business, science and government and by bringing together the knowledge and expertise of many people. The programme was launched in 1994 following a major review of government science, engineering and technology policy. The first set of visions and recommendations for action were published in 1995, followed by 4 years of development and implementation. Work is presently underway on a new round of health care forecasting, looking at such areas as: delivering the promise of the human genome; pharmaceuticals; biotechnology and medical devices; transplantation; organization and delivery of health care; public and patients; older people; information; neuropsychiatry; and international influences on health and health care.

Sources: Schreuder (1995) and United Kingdom Foresight programme, http://www.foresight.gov.uk (accessed 21 January 2001)

References

Armstrong, M. (1991) *A Handbook of Personnel Management*. London: Kogan Page.

Ayliffe, G.A.J., Babb, J.R. and Taylor, L.J. (1999) *Hospital-acquired Infection: Principles and Prevention*. Oxford: Butterworth-Heinemann.

Bakker, A. and Leguit, F. (1999) Evolution of an integrated HIS in the Netherlands, *International Journal of Medical Informatics*, 54: 209–24.

Barros, P.P. (1998) The black box of health care expenditure growth determinants, *Health Economics*, 7(6): 533–44.

Braithwaite, J. (1997) The 21st-century hospital, *Medical Journal of Australia*, 166: 6.

Buchan, J. and Edwards, N. (2000) Nursing numbers in Britain: the argument for workforce planning, *British Medical Journal*, 320: 1067–70.

Carballo, M., Divino, J.J. and Zeric, D. (1998) Migration and health in the European Union, *Tropical Medicine and International Health*, 3(12): 936–44.

Chappel, A.G. (1995) Patients have rising expectations, *British Medical Journal*, 310: 867–8.

Comas-Herrera, A. (1999) Is there convergence in the health expenditures of the EU Member States?, in E. Mossialos and J. Le Grand (eds) *Health Care and Cost Containment in the European Union*. Aldershot: Ashgate.

Council of the European Union (1993) Council Directive 93/104/EC of 23 November 1993 concerning certain aspects of the organization of working time, *Official Journal of the European Communities*, L307(13/12/1993): 18–24.

Coulter, A., Peto, V. and Doll, H. (1994) Patients' preferences and general practitioners' decisions in the treatment of menstrual disorders, *Family Practice*, 11: 67–74.

Dornbusch, K., King, A. and Legakis, N. (1998) Incidence of antibiotic resistance in blood and urine isolates from hospitalized patients. Report from a European collaborative study. European Study Group on Antibiotic Resistance (ESGAR), *Scandinavian Journal of Infectious Diseases*, 30: 281–8.

Enthoven, A.C. and Singer, S.J. (1996) Managed competition and California's health care economy, *Health Affairs (Millwood)*, 15(1): 39–57.

Evandrou, M. (1997) *Baby Boomers: Ageing in the 21st Century*. London: Age Concern England.

Fahey, T. and Fitzgerald, J. (1997) *Welfare Implications of Demographic Trends*. Dublin: Oak Tree Press in association with Combat Poverty Agency.

Farmer, P.E., Reichman, L.B. and Iseman, M.D. (1999) *The Global Impact of Drug Resistant Tuberculosis*. Boston, MA: Harvard Medical School/Open Society Institute.

Frenk, K. and Gomez-Dantes, O. (1995) Global integration and health, in P. Freeman, O. Gomez-Dantes and J. Frenk (eds) *Health Systems in an Era of Globalization: Challenges and Opportunities for North America*. Mexico City: Institute of Medicine (USA)/ National Academy of Medicine (Mexico).

Frenk, J., Sepulveda, J., Gomez-Dantes, O., McGuinness, M.J. and Knaul, F. (1997) The future of world health: the new world order and international health, *British Medical Journal*, 314: 1404.

Fuchs, V.R. (1984) Though much is taken: reflections on aging, health, and medical care, *Millbank Memorial Fund Quarterly: Health and Society*, 62: 143–66.

Garrett, M.J. (1999) *Health Futures: A Handbook for Health Professionals*. Geneva: World Health Organization.

Gebo, K.A., Chaisson, R.E., Folkemer, J.G., Bartlett, J.G. and Moore, R.D. (1999) Costs of HIV medical care in the era of highly active antiretroviral therapy, *AIDS*, 13(8): 963–9.

Gomez-Dantes, O. and Frenk, J. (1995) NAFT and health services: initial data, in P. Freeman, O. Gomez-Dantes and J. Frenk (eds) *Health Systems in an Era of Globalization: Challenges and Opportunities for North America*. Mexico City: Institute of Medicine (USA)/National Academy of Medicine (Mexico).

Green, A. and Owen, D. (1995) The labour market aspects of population change in the 1990s, in R. Hall and P. White (eds) *Europe's Population: Towards the Next Century*. London: UCL Press.

Grundy, E. (1997) The health and health care of older adults in England and Wales 1841–1994, in J. Charlton and M. Murphy (eds) *The Health of Adult Britain 1841– 1994*. London: The Stationery Office.

Hajioff, S. and McKee, M. (2000) The health of the Roma people: a review of the published literature, *Journal of Epidemiology and Community Health*, 54(11): 864–9.

Harrison, A. and Prentice, S. (1996) *Acute Futures*. London: King's Fund.

Hillman, K. (1999) The changing role for acute care hospitals, *Medical Journal of Australia*, 170(7): 325–9.

Jensen, D.M. (1986) Economic and health aspects of peptic ulcer disease and H_2-receptor antagonists, *American Journal of Medicine*, 81: 42–8.

Jinks, C., Ong, B.N. and Paton, C. (2000) Mobile medics? The mobility of doctors in the European Economic Area, *Health Policy 2000*, 54: 45–64.

Jolly, D. and Gerbaud, L. (1992) *The Hospital of Tomorrow: Current Concerns*, SHS Paper No. 5, Division of Strengthening Health Services. Geneva: World Health Organization.

Kammerling, M. and Banatvala, N. (2001) Tuberculosis hospitals in the Russian Federation, in M. McKee and J. Healy (eds) *Implementing Hospital Reforms in Eastern Europe*. Copenhagen: European Observatory on Health Care Systems.

Kanavos, P. and Yfantopoulos, J. (1999) Cost containment and health expenditure in the EU: a macroeconomic perspective, in E. Mossialos and J. Le Grand (eds) *Health Care and Cost Containment in the European Union*. Aldershot: Ashgate.

Kanavos, P.G., McKee, M. and Richards, T. (1999) Cross border health care in Europe: European court rulings have made governments worried, *British Medical Journal*, 318: 1157–8.

Khaw, K.T. (1999) How many, how old, how soon?, *British Medical Journal*, 319: 1350–2.

Klein, N. (2000) *No Logo*. London: Flamingo.

Komesaroff, P.A., Clunie, G.J. and Duckett, S.J. (1997) What is the future of the hospital system?, *Medical Journal of Australia*, 166: 17–23.

Krause, R.M. (1992) The origin of plagues: old and new, *Science*, 257: 1073–8.

Kuh, D. and Ben Shlomo, Y. (1997) *A Life Course Approach to Chronic Disease Epidemiology Tracing the Origins of Ill-health from Early to Adult Life*. Oxford: Oxford University Press.

Lee, K. (1999) Globalisation and the need for a strong public health response, *European Journal of Public Health*, 9: 249–50.

Leon, D., Chenet, L., Shkolnikov, V.M. *et al.* (1997) Huge variation in Russian mortality rates 1984–1994: artefact, alcohol, or what?, *Lancet*, 350: 383–8.

Lubitz, J., Beebe, J. and Baker, C. (1995) Longevity and medical care expenditures, *New England Journal of Medicine*, 332: 999–1003.

Maher, D., van-Gorkom, J.L., Gondrie, P.C. and Raviglione, M. (1999) Community contribution to tuberculosis care in countries with high tuberculosis prevalence: past, present and future, *International Journal of Tuberculosis and Lung Disease*, 3: 762–8.

Martens, W., Kovats, R., Nijhof, S. *et al.* (1999) Climate change and future populations at risk of malaria, *Global Environmental Change*, 9: S89–S107.

Mattson, S. and Lew, L. (1992) Culturally sensitive prenatal care for Southeast Asians, *Journal of Obstetric, Gynecologic and Neonatal Nursing*, 21(1): 48–54.

McGrail, K., Green, B., Barer, M.L. *et al.* (2000) Age, costs of acute and long-term care and proximity to death: evidence for 1987/88 and 1994/95 in British Columbia, *Age and Ageing*, 29: 249–53.

McKee, M. (1995) 2020 vision, *Journal of Public Health Medicine*, 17: 127–31.

McKee, M. and Mossialos, E. (1998) The impact of managed care on clinical research, *Pharmacoeconomics*, 14: 19–25.

McKee, M. and Mossialos, E. (2000) Seattle and the World Trade Organization: potential implications for the NHS, *Journal of the Royal Society of Medicine*, 93: 109–10.

McKee, M., Mossialos, E. and Belcher, P. (1996) The impact of European Union law on national health policy, *Journal of European Social Policy*, 6: 263–86.

McKeigue, P.M., Shah, B. and Marmot, M.G. (1991) Relation of central obesity and insulin resistance with high diabetes prevalence and cardiovascular risk in South Asians, *Lancet*, 337(8738): 382–6.

McMichael, A. and Haines, A. (1997) Climate change and potential impacts on human health, *British Medical Journal*, 315: 805–9.

Meerding, W.J., Bonneaux, L., Polder, J. *et al.* (1998) Demographic and epidemiological determinants of healthcare costs in Netherlands: cost of illness study, *British Medical Journal*, 317: 111–15.

Mendelson, D.N. and Schwartz, W.B. (1993) Effects of aging and population growth on health care costs, *Health Affairs (Millwood)*, 12: 119–25.

Meyer, M., Genel, M., Altman, R.D., Williams, M.A. and Allen, J.R. (1998) Clinical research: assessing the future in a changing environment. Summary report of conference sponsored by the American Medical Association Council on Scientific Affairs, Washington, DC, March 1996, *American Journal of Medicine*, 104: 264–71.

Morgan, R.A. and Blaese, M.R. (1999) Gene therapy: lessons learnt from the past decade, *British Medical Journal*, 319: 1310.

Mossialos, E. and Le Grand, J. (eds) (1999) *Health Care and Cost Containment in the European Union*. Aldershot: Ashgate.

Mossialos, E., Dixon, A., Figueras, J.E. and Kutzin, J. (2002) *Funding Health Care: Options for Europe*. Buckingham: Open University Press.

Murphy, S. (1998) Does new technology increase or decrease health care costs? The treatment of peptic ulceration, *Journal of Health Services Research and Policy*, 3: 215–18.

National Audit Office (2000) *The Management and Control of Hospital Acquired Infection in Acute NHS Trusts in England*. London: The Stationery Office.

Neuberger, J. (2000) The educated patient: new challenges for the medical profession, *Journal of Internal Medicine*, 247: 6–10.

OECD (1998) *OECD Health Data 98: A Comparative Analysis of 29 Countries*. Paris: Organisation for Economic Co-operation and Development.

Peto, R., Chen, Z.M. and Boreham, J. (1999) Tobacco – the growing epidemic, *Nature Medicine*, 5: 15–17.

Platt, L. and McKee, M. (2000) Observations on the management of sexually transmitted diseases in the Russian Federation: a challenge of confidentiality, *International Journal of STD and AIDS*, 11: 563–7.

Plowman, R.M., Graves, N. and Roberts, J.A. (1997) *Hospital Acquired Infection*. London: Office of Health Economics.

Plowman, R., Graves, N., Griggin, M. *et al.* (1999) *The Socioeconomic Burden of Hospital Acquired Infection*. London: Central Public Health Laboratory.

Porter, R. (1997) *The Greatest Benefit to Mankind: A Medical History of Humanity from Antiquity to the Present*. London: HarperCollins.

Posnett, J., Baghurst, A. and Place, M. (1998) *The Rise in Emergency Admission Project: Final Report*. York: University of York, Coventry Business School, Plymouth University.

Poulson, K.B., Bremmelgaard, A., Sørensen, A.I. and Raahave, J.V. (1994) Estimated costs of postoperative wound infections: A case-control study of marginal hospital and social security costs, *Epidemiological Infection*, 113(2): 283–95.

Price, D., Pollock, A.M. and Shaoul, J. (1999) How the World Trade Organization is shaping domestic policies in health care, *Lancet*, 354: 1889–92.

Robertson, C. and Boyle, P. (1998) Age-period-cohort analysis of chronic disease rates. I: Modelling approach, *Statistics in Medicine*, 17: 1305–23.

Schmeidl, S. (1997) Exploring the causes of forced migration: a pooled time-series analysis, 1971–1990, *Social Science Quarterly*, 78: 284–308.

Schreuder, R. (1995) Health scenarios and policy-making: lessons from the Netherlands, *Futures*, 27: 959–66.

Scitovsky, A.A. (1988) Medical care in the last twelve months of life: the relation between age, functional status, and medical care expenditures, *Millbank Memorial Fund Quarterly: Health and Society*, 66: 640–60.

Shkolnikov, V., McKee, M., Leon, D. and Chenet, L. (1999) Why is the death rate from lung cancer falling in the Russian Federation?, *European Journal of Epidemiology*, 15: 203–6.

Singer, B.H. and Manton, K.G. (1998) The effects of health changes on projections of health service needs for the elderly population of the United States, *Proceedings of the National Academy of Sciences*, 95(26): 15618–22.

Soares, S., Kristinsson, K.G., Musser, J.M. and Tomasz, A. (1993) Evidence for the introduction of a multiresistant clone of serotype 6B *Streptococcus pneumoniae* from Spain to Iceland in the late 1980s, *Journal of Infectious Diseases*, 168: 158–63.

Swartz, M.N. (1995) Hospital-acquired infections: diseases with increasingly limited therapies, in B. Roizman (ed.) *Infectious Diseases in an Age of Change: The Impact of Human Ecology and Behaviour on Disease Transmission*. Washington, DC: National Academy Press.

Torgerson, D.J., Maynard, A.K. and Gosden, T. (1998) International comparisons of health-care expenditure: a dismal science?, *QJM: Monthly Journal of the Association of Physicians*, 91: 69–70.

Tunstall-Pedoe, H., Kuulasmaa, K., Mahonen, M. *et al.* (1999) Contribution of trends in survival and coronary event rates to changes in coronary heart disease mortality: 10 year results from 27 WHO MONICA project populations. Monitoring trends and determinants in cardiovascular disease, *Lancet*, 353: 1547–57.

United Nations Population Division (1995) *World Population Prospects: The 1994 Revision*. New York: United Nations.

United Nations Population Division (1998) *World Population Prospects: The 1998 Revision*. New York: United Nations.

Van Bemmel, J. and Musen, M.E. (1997) *Handbook of Medical Informatics*. Heidelberg: Springer-Verlag.

Victor, C.R., Healy, J., Thomas, A. and Seargeant, J. (2000) Older patients and delayed discharge from hospital, *Health and Community Care*, 8(6): 443–52.

Vincenzino, J.V. (1998) Trends in medical care costs – evolving market forces, *Statistical Bulletin of the Metropolitan Insurance Company*, 79: 8–15.

Walker, A. and Maltby, T. (1997) *Ageing Europe*. Buckingham: Open University Press.

Wellings, K. (1994) Assessing AIDS/HIV prevention: what do we know in Europe? General population, *Sozial- und Präventivmedizin*, 39: S14–S46.

White, C. (1996) Britain fails to stop 48 hour week limit, *British Medical Journal*, 313: 1283.

Will, R.G., Ironside, J.W., Zeidler, M. *et al.* (1996) A new variant of Creutzfeldt-Jakob disease in the UK, *Lancet*, 347: 921–5.

Wilson, C.B. (1999) The impact of medical technologies on the future of hospitals, *British Medical Journal*, 319: 1287.

WHO (1996) Methicillin-resistant *Staphylococcus aureus* (MRSA), *Weekly Epidemiological Record*, 71(10): 73–80.

WHO (1997) *Treatment of Tuberculosis: Guidelines for National Programmes*, document WHO/TB/97.220. Geneva: World Health Organization.

WHO (1999) *Removing Obstacles to Healthy Development*, document WHO/CDS/99.1. Geneva: World Health Organization.

WHO (2001) *WHO European Health for All Database*. Copenhagen: WHO Regional Office for Europe.

Zatonski, W.A., McMichael, A.J. and Powles, J.W. (1998) Ecological study of reasons for sharp decline in mortality from ischaemic heart disease in Poland since 1991, *British Medical Journal*, 316: 1047–51.

Zuckerman, A.J. (1996) Alphabet of hepatitis viruses, *Lancet*, 347: 558–9.

Zweifel, P., Felder, S. and Meiers, M. (1999) Ageing of population and health care expenditure: a red herring?, *Health Economics*, 8(6): 485–96.

chapter four

The role and function of hospitals

Judith Healy and Martin McKee

Introduction

This chapter explores the different roles and functions that a hospital might be expected to perform and how these are changing as the internal and external environments of the hospital change. A hospital may undertake several functions, depending on the type of hospital, its role in the health care system and its relationship with other health care services. The questions commonly asked by policy-makers include: What size population should the hospital serve? How many patients, beds and specialties should it contain? Where should the boundary lie between the hospital and other health services? The answers will depend on the values and objectives of the individual or organization asking the questions. In many cases, competing objectives must be balanced. For example, surgeons may want large hospitals that can support large clinical teams and complex equipment, whereas the public may want 'their' hospital close to where they live. This chapter compiles the evidence that can inform these decisions.

Functions of an acute care hospital

The core function of a hospital is to treat patients who are ill, but an analysis confined to this function would be misleading (Figure 4.1). The hospital may also be an important setting for teaching and research and may actively support its surrounding health care system. Furthermore, the hospital may be an important source of local employment and may play several societal roles. The expectations that accompany each of these roles have important implications for the organization of the hospital and its relationship with its wider environment.

Figure 4.1 Functions of an acute care hospital

Patient care

Inpatient, outpatient and day patient
Emergency and elective
Rehabilitation

Teaching

Vocational
Undergraduate
Postgraduate
Continuing education

Research

Basic research
Clinical research
Health services research
Educational research

Health system support

Source for referrals
Professional leadership
Base for outreach activities
Management of primary care

Employment

Inside hospital:
Health professionals
Other health care workers
Outside hospital:
Suppliers
Transport services

Societal

State legitimacy
Political symbol
Provider of social care
Base for medical power
Civic pride

Patient care

Patient care is the defining characteristic of an acute hospital and can be considered in terms of several broad dimensions: emergency or elective care, inpatient or outpatient (ambulatory) care and acute care or rehabilitation. The type of patient a hospital treats, however, differs among hospitals and countries, as the following examples show. Patients in long-term care have been shifted outside the hospital in many high-income countries, as noted in Chapter 2. Patients can refer themselves to hospital in some countries, whereas when the National Health Service was established in the United Kingdom, general practitioners secured an agreement that only they could refer patients to specialists. Hospitals have a major role in providing ambulatory care for patients with complex conditions in most countries, but in Germany, until recently, ambulatory care patients were treated outside hospitals almost entirely by specialists working in their own premises. The following sections explore how patient care is changing within hospitals across Europe.

Inpatient care

Inpatient care remains an essential function of a hospital. Although the total number of hospital beds has fallen in western Europe (as discussed in Chapter 2), admissions have risen steadily, with more people staying for shorter periods of more intensive treatment. The average length of stay in acute care hospitals in European Union countries has declined from 16.5 days in 1970 to 8.6 days in 1996 and has reached 6 days or less in several countries (WHO 2001).

These changes have important implications for hospitals. Shorter lengths of stay and ageing populations mean that those in hospital beds are sicker, and the possibilities arising from new technology enable patients to receive more complex interventions (see Chapter 3). For example, a person admitted to a western European hospital with myocardial infarction in the 1980s could expect little more than monitoring and bed rest, whereas he or she can now expect thrombolytic treatment and possible emergency angioplasty. The changing pattern of care necessitates changes in hospital design, with fewer beds but more facilities for radiology, endoscopy and surgery. It also requires changes in staffing; for example, more people with technical skills such as non-medically qualified endoscopists and more with managerial skills to support complex patient management. At the same time, hospitals must respond to changing patient expectations. Earlier generations of patients may have been content to lie in a row of beds in a ward, whereas now even four-bedded bays are giving way to demands for private rooms in high-income countries.

Ambulatory care

Ambulatory care encompasses a range of activities, including attendance at outpatient clinics and emergency departments, complex treatment such as dialysis or chemotherapy, as well as day surgery. Outpatient care has expanded both because more patients are diverted from inpatient to outpatient care but also because the demand for outpatient care has risen as more complex diagnosis and treatment become available. Comparative statistics on outpatient consultations are fragmentary, but many countries report a steady increase.

There is surprisingly little research on the role of ambulatory care within the health system, such as the proportion of ambulatory care provided in different locations (Berman 2000) or on specific issues such as the optimal management of ambulatory care. The traditional model, in which patients attend a clinic defined by the specialty of its senior physician (surgical, medical, gynaecological and so on), is giving way to integrated management of individuals with common conditions. This is exemplified by the growth of streamlined 'one-stop' clinics in which patients with common conditions, such as breast lumps or rectal bleeding, can have a complete diagnostic work-up involving a team of specialists at a single visit (Waghorn *et al.* 1997).

Ambulatory surgery has increased with developments in short-acting anaesthesia and surgical techniques and, in particular, in minimally invasive surgery. This means that many procedures can now be performed without requiring overnight admission to hospital. Although international comparative data are limited and subject to problems of definition, there appears to be considerable

Figure 4.2 Percentage of cataract extractions performed as day cases in ten industrialized countries (latest available year)

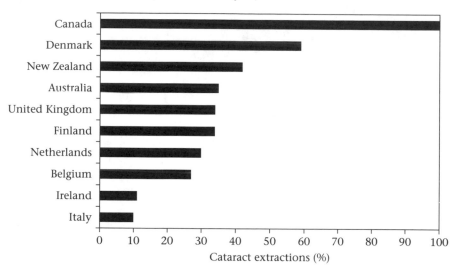

Source: Poullier (2000)

variation in the extent to which these innovations have been taken up, as shown by the example of cataract operations (Figure 4.2).

It is probable that ambulatory surgery will continue to increase in many countries but, as with hospital bed numbers, the potential for change is finite. Some commentators look to the United States as an example of how much care technically can be shifted out of hospitals. This overlooks the fiscal context, as much of this shift was a response to the introduction of prospective payment in the early 1980s, which constrained earnings from inpatient care but allowed costs to rise for ambulatory care. This trend accelerated under pressure from managed-care organizations, but many states in the United States are now legislating to give patients undergoing certain procedures that can be undertaken in an ambulatory setting, such as mastectomies, the right to be treated in hospital if they feel this is appropriate.

The increase in ambulatory care has consequences for hospital design and staffing. Outpatient clinics need to be designed to support new models of integrated care. For example, optimal management of breast lumps requires a team of surgeons, radiologists and cytopathologists. The ratio of operating theatres to beds must increase, and some traditional wards could be converted to day-only use. Most importantly, these new models of care require a high level of organization, with mechanisms for moving patients through the hospital that owe more to airline booking systems than to traditional queues (Waghorn and McKee 2000). These issues are explored in more detail in Chapter 5.

These developments offer the possibility that new forms of ambulatory care, including day surgery, could be provided in purpose-built facilities, separate from traditional hospitals. These ambulatory care centres do not require the same level of facilities that are needed in a hospital receiving emergencies. In addition, they remove the problem of emergency admissions taking up beds intended for non-urgent cases. This is a common cause of cancellation of operations, and thus longer waiting lists, in systems that are already operating at close to full capacity. Such ambulatory care centres can be more dispersed than acute hospitals and thus improve population access to care. They must, however, have adequate back-up mechanisms to cope with the complications that will inevitably occur, no matter how well patients are selected. They must also take account of the environment in which they are established, including levels of training and equipment, and the social support mechanisms available to patients on discharge.

Emergency treatment

A second dimension of an acute care hospital is the differentiation between elective care and emergency care (accident and emergency or casualty departments). Emergency care is a core function of an acute hospital (or the only function if one takes television dramas as a guide). Emergency care in hospital saves lives but only if the patients are stabilized and delivered to the hospital quickly and if the care they then receive is appropriate. As the following discussion shows, many misconceptions surround the organization of emergency care (Gleeson 2000).

The emergency care debate has been shaped by the finding that about 50 per cent of the people dying from trauma in the United States do so at the scene of the injury from unsurvivable injuries, whereas 30 per cent die between 1 and 4 hours later from preventable causes, and 20 per cent die from late complications (Trunkey 1983). Although comparable data are lacking, it is probable that preventable trauma deaths are greater in the parts of Europe where basic emergency services are weak. The observation that so many deaths are preventable has stimulated interest in finding strategies to improve the outcome of care but, as the following examples show, policies that should work in theory may not always do so in practice.

One approach involves paramedics trained in advanced life-support skills. Early intervention should reduce mortality, but research from the United Kingdom found that trauma victims attended by ambulance paramedics actually had a higher death rate than those attended by standard ambulances. Two reasons were suggested. First, the process of resuscitation delays transfer to hospital and, second, improvement in tissue perfusion increases the risk of bleeding on the way to hospital (Nicholl *et al.* 1998). This is not an argument against training ambulance staff in basic life-support skills, but it does emphasize the dilemma of whether to stabilize patients at the scene or to take them rapidly to hospital.

An alternative strategy is to take physicians to the scene of the accident. One question is how to do so quickly? Contrary to most assumptions, except over inaccessible terrain, helicopters are generally slower than ground transport (McKee *et al.* 1993a,b). Helicopter-delivered trauma teams can improve the chances of survival for a small number of seriously injured patients, but medical teams transported by ground transport are similarly effective (Steedman 1990).

The creation of designated trauma centres has increased survival in the United States (Mullins *et al.* 1994). These centres have three features: senior medical staff from a range of specialties are on site at all times; these centres are closely integrated with ambulance services; and they manage 10–20 seriously injured patients each week (American College of Surgeons Committee on Trauma 1990). Largely because of the lower levels of violence and, specifically, the much lower ownership of firearms in Europe, few European hospitals can expect to achieve this volume of cases. Consequently, a trauma facility in the United Kingdom that had been based on the United States concept failed to show the benefits expected (Nicholl and Turner 1997). This suggests that this model may not be appropriate for other European countries.

In each of these examples, interventions that common sense would suggest should be effective are not when transferred to a different setting. This emphasizes the importance of tailoring interventions to the national context. Furthermore, emergency care in one setting may mean something different in another setting. Some countries, especially the countries of the former Soviet Union, created free-standing emergency hospitals; for example, there were 42 in Kazakhstan in 1997 (Kulzhanov and Healy 1999). These cannot, however, be equated with the type of trauma centres in North America and they rarely have advanced diagnostic and therapeutic equipment or recourse to specialist support. Indeed, their continued existence is an obstacle to better-equipped acute care general hospitals and to the development of integrated packages of care.

In most emergency departments, major trauma only comprises a small part of the overall workload, with many patients suffering from what might be considered minor ailments. The extent to which emergency departments become a substitute for inadequate primary care, therefore, is an ongoing concern (Lang *et al.* 1996). Hospital staff regard many of these cases as medically inappropriate or trivial. In contrast, studies that examine attendance from the patient's perspective have found good reasons, albeit in relation to where or when the injury or illness occurred, that make such attendance appropriate (Calnan 1984). One strategy intended to divert less serious cases from casualty is to establish free-standing minor injury units, and patients do choose appropriately where the latter are established (Dale and Dolan 1996). Furthermore, as such units do not need to be located in an acute hospital, they can be made more accessible to patients. Another strategy is to employ primary care physicians within emergency departments, who can provide more cost-effective care than junior hospital physicians, partly because more experienced physicians order fewer unnecessary investigations (Dale *et al.* 1996).

Another strategy is to manage patients who have minor ailments outside the hospital. For example, the United Kingdom has introduced a nationwide telephone service, offering advice from nurses (Pencheon 1998). So far, the service has achieved high levels of patient satisfaction, but, importantly, has not reduced demand for either hospital or primary care (Munro *et al.* 2000), and despite the use of standardized protocols, the telephone advice given varies considerably (Florin and Rosen 1999).

Emergency care exhibits features of a complex system: its effectiveness depends on many external factors; the impact of change is often difficult to predict; it performs multiple functions; and it treats people with conditions ranging from severe to minor. An effective policy response to severe injuries must take account of the many people who die before they reach hospital as well as the system that is in place when they do arrive. Evidence to support the widespread use of expensive interventions such as helicopter evacuation and designated trauma centres is lacking. Instead, greater gains may be achieved simply by identifying the factors contributing to avoidable deaths, for example, by an audit of trauma deaths (Yates *et al.* 1992). This would provide evidence for locally appropriate, targeted interventions; for example, revising hospital treatment protocols, greater use of multidisciplinary trauma teams or improving telephone access in rural areas. Responses to less serious conditions must also reflect local circumstances. In particular, they should take account of the perspective of the patient, remembering that a condition considered trivial by a health professional may be of great importance to a patient, for whom the most appropriate course of action may be far from clear.

Rehabilitation

Rehabilitation is the final element of patient care to consider. The traditional passive model of gradual mobilization, interspersed with lengthy bed rest, is cost-ineffective in terms of patient outcomes. Active rehabilitation programmes, drawing on the skills of multidisciplinary teams, are emerging as much more effective (Dickinson and Sinclair 1998). These are exemplified by multidisciplinary stroke units, which have been shown to improve patient outcomes (Langhorne *et al.* 1993). The question of whether rehabilitation should be undertaken while a patient remains in hospital, however, depends on individual circumstances. Day hospitals allow patients to return to their homes each evening, but for older patients this is not necessarily more cost-effective than inpatient rehabilitation (Forster *et al.* 1999). Rehabilitation in the patient's home is another option but, without empirical research, should not be assumed to be more cost-effective for some groups than rehabilitation in day centres or hospitals (Hensher *et al.* 1996). Rehabilitation should be viewed as an active rather than a passive process, with clear objectives for the patient. Chapter 5 discusses these issues.

Teaching and research

Teaching, research and patient care are highly interdependent. The health care system cannot exist without a supply of trained staff or the knowledge generated by appropriate research. Teaching and research also need health care facilities as settings in which to function and as a source of clinical material.

Teaching hospitals are a key component in any health system. They directly affect the quality of new graduates but also indirectly affect the wider health care system. As training locations, their dominant beliefs and values influence medical and nursing students, many of whom, in their subsequent careers, will work in other parts of the health sector. Despite increased emphasis on primary care in undergraduate medical education in western Europe, the bulk of teaching remains based on hospital patients. As lengths of stay fall, however, and as more health care is provided outside hospitals, the hospital is becoming increasingly less appropriate as the main base for medical education (Hunt *et al.* 1999).

A greater emphasis on ambulatory facilities as settings for training presents challenges for medical educators, not least because many outpatient consultations last only a few minutes (Waghorn and McKee 1999). A few basic changes are needed. Certain clinics should be designated for teaching. These should allow more time for each consultation, be designed with teaching aids and space for students and use teaching methods that enhance the quality of the learning experience (Fields *et al.* 2000).

The changing health care environment has important implications for the co-existence of teaching, research and clinical care. Clinical care traditionally has partly subsidized teaching and research. These subsidies are mostly implicit (Clack *et al.* 1992), but the additional costs to a hospital of teaching and research can be estimated by using methods such as data envelopment analysis (Sherman 1984). Some countries are moving to increase transparency; for example, the United Kingdom National Health Service identifies separate funding streams for teaching and research, for which hospitals and other health care facilities must bid (Bevan 1999). Resources thus follow training and research, which are increasingly undertaken outside designated teaching hospitals. This experience has not been without its problems (Swales 2000), but it does offer valuable lessons to others planning to separate funding streams.

Explicit mechanisms to protect research and training will become more important in the face of growing pressures for 'efficiency' from health care purchasers who may want hospitals to concentrate on their 'core business' of patient care. This is a particular concern in the United States, where managed-care organizations seek ever-higher profits (McKee and Mossialos 1998), and this has led to a crisis in medical education, with several university hospitals facing possible closure. However, it also kindled a debate on the extent to which the increasingly corporate United States health care industry benefits from staff trained and from knowledge generated at the expense of others (Anonymous 2000).

A different issue arises where research, training and health care are rigidly separated. In the countries of the former Soviet Union, medical research was largely separate from undergraduate teaching and patient treatment, which led to fragmentation and two-tier care (Field 1990). Research institutes were established, for example, for cancer and neurology, with only the most complex cases (in theory) referred to these institutions.

A final consideration is the extent to which the hospital itself is a subject of research. Throughout this book, the relative lack of research on hospitals is noted. Consequently, those responsible for national research strategies should place sufficient emphasis on health services research, recognizing the need for a whole-system approach so that the hospital is understood within its wider environment (Peckham 1991).

The message arising from this section is that teaching and research are core roles of the hospital and must be factored into its design and system of rewards. There is a danger that increasing drives for efficiency will squeeze out these roles, which may bring short-term but ultimately unsustainable gains in financial performance.

Figure 4.3 The possible roles of a district general hospital in a health care system

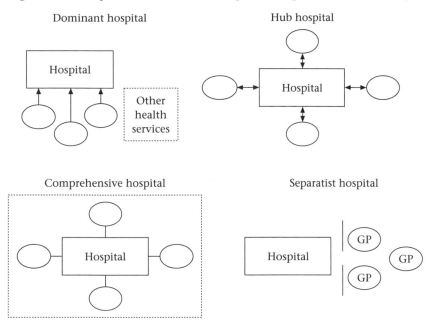

Supporting the health system

Another function of the hospital is to support other health care services; this implies that the hospital should not consume too large a share of resources or dominate the health care system surrounding it. The relationship between the hospital and other health care services varies considerably. At one extreme, typically in rural areas of middle- and low-income countries, the hospital has a central role in the delivery of all types of health care, often with administrative responsibility for outlying facilities. At the other extreme, the United Kingdom has transferred budgets for purchasing hospital care to groups of primary care physicians, thus potentially giving them more power over hospitals (Robinson and Dixon 1999). Within this spectrum, the role of the hospital in the wider health care system can be considered as falling into one of four models: the dominant hospital, the hub hospital, the comprehensive model and the separatist hospital (Figure 4.3).

Dominant hospital

A dominant hospital monopolizes skilled staff and equipment and consumes most of the health care budget, including resources for primary care. Primary care can be defined as 'the first contact with the health system, or the first level of care, or simple treatments that could be delivered by relatively untrained providers, or interventions acting on primary causes of disease' (WHO 2000). Hospitals often take on primary care by default, since many people bypass community providers and go straight to hospitals, as these have the best physicians and most resources. For example, in 1997, one-third of patients attending a tertiary care hospital in Bishkek, the capital of Kyrgyzstan, were self-referred (Sargaldakova *et al.* 2000). Primary care physicians in some health care systems (such as the countries of the former Soviet Union) also refer many of their patients to hospitals and polyclinics rather than diagnose and treat them (Van Lerberghe and Lafort 1990).

The dominant hospital model has been strongly criticized, especially by the community health movement in the 1970s and 1980s, as not satisfactorily addressing the health needs of populations and as undermining rather than supporting primary health care. In the primary health care philosophy embodied in the Declaration of Alma-Ata in 1978 (WHO 1978), the hospital was defined as only one part of a wider health system and the importance of primary care was reaffirmed (Paine and Siem Tjam 1988).

Hub hospital

A general hospital may be the hub of an integrated health system for a defined population catchment area (Van Lerberghe and Lafort 1990). The hospital is involved in planning, administering, supervising and funding (but not providing) community health services. For example, the Soviet health care system placed the hospital at the hub of district health care, and the chief physician of the hospital in the main town administered primary health services in the district. This model can easily transmute into the dominant hospital model unless checks and balances are set in place.

Comprehensive hospital

In the comprehensive model, the hospital undertakes tertiary and secondary as well as primary care and also delivers services outside its walls. District hospitals in the 1970s and 1980s (especially in developing countries) were urged to reach out to the community and to offer primary health care such as immunizations and antenatal care. Hospitals were to become 'a centre of preventive as well as curative medicine' (Van Lerberghe and Lafort 1990). Paradoxically, although some countries have moved to a separatist model of an acute care hospital, many health care providers in the United States are returning to a comprehensive model in which hospitals and other health care facilities (such as rehabilitation services) are owned and managed by the same organization (known as vertical integration). This largely represents a drive for market share, a factor of limited relevance in the mostly publicly owned European hospital sector. Chapter 5 discusses the pressures on hospitals to find substitutes for inpatient care.

Separatist hospital

The separatist hospital is the prevailing model in most high-income countries. The acute hospital divests itself of all but the core functions of short-stay specialist care, providing only services that primary care practitioners and

Table 4.1 Alternative meanings of hospitals

Dimensions	Alternative meanings	
State legitimacy	High-priority policy issue	Low-priority policy issue
Political indicator	Public good	Private commodity
Civic asset	Hospital in every town	Regional facility
Health system indicator	Dominant hospitals	Part of health system
Health care provider	Health and social care	Acute care for critically ill
Medical power	Main power base	One of several power bases

community-based specialists are unable (for various reasons) to undertake. The rationale for concentrating on core business is, first, that hospital staff are trained and hospitals are equipped to provide specialist medical care; second, hospital-based health care is extremely expensive and must be used cost-effectively.

In summary, the importance of these models lies not only in their implications for the hospital but also in their implications for primary and secondary health care. In particular, many countries are seeking to enhance the quality of primary care, but such efforts must take into account the relationship between the hospital and primary care providers. A dominant hospital model makes primary care reform very difficult by attracting the most funds, the best staff and the most patients at the expense of primary care. A weak primary health care system will increase the demands on the hospital and prevent the development of alternative forms of health and social care.

The societal role of the hospital

The previous sections considered the main functions of an acute care hospital, but hospitals are much more than places where patients are diagnosed and treated and health professionals are trained. They also have a societal role and are imbued with many different meanings (Table 4.1). The failure by policy-makers to fully appreciate these diverse roles is a common reason why planned reforms sometimes do not succeed.

A means of creating state legitimacy

One of the functions of the state, and one that enhances its legitimacy, is to ensure the health and welfare of its citizens. As *The World Health Report 2000* (WHO 2000) points out, the ultimate responsibility for the overall performance of a health care system lies with government. Ensuring a good health care system, especially with the hospital as its most visible manifestation, demonstrates that the state has assumed this role. Health care tends to be a low-priority rather than high-priority policy issue, since it does not threaten a state's national interests or those of significant groups (Walt 1994). In some countries, however, health care is a defining national characteristic, as in the United Kingdom, where hospitals are seen as key symbols of the survival of the welfare state.

An indicator of political ideology

Policies towards hospitals are often regarded as an ideological litmus test. The health system choices made by politicians and policy-makers are based on ideological as well as technical factors. One debate is whether health care is a public good or a private commodity. Hospitals fit many of the criteria of a public good. There are benefits for society from a socially cohesive, healthier and more productive population. Public investment in hospitals reaps societal and not just individual gains, such as a healthier and more productive workforce. Universality applies, since few societies exclude people from access: people are generally not turned away to die in the street. Hospital services also can be viewed as a marketable commodity, however, in the sense that there can be buyers (patients or their agents) and sellers (the hospitals). There are many permutations between these two extremes, however, and insights from institutional economics highlight the complexity of these arrangements (Preker *et al.* 2000).

Responsibility for health and social care can be divided between different and overlapping sectors of society (Healy 1998). These sectors include the central and lower levels of government, the voluntary sector (non-governmental and not-for-profit organizations), the community or informal sector (including family care) and the market (commercial or for-profit providers).

Esping-Anderson (1990) identified several models, each of which implies a different approach to hospitals. Under a social democratic model, government is the dominant funder and provider, has universalist policies and funds, and owns and manages many hospitals. Under a liberal and selectivist model, the state funds and regulates lower levels of government, while quasi-government organizations and the voluntary sector run hospitals. Under a conservative-corporatist model, citizens must insure against sickness, so that insurance schemes as third-party payers contract with and fund hospitals (both public and private). Under a market capitalist model, the private for-profit sector funds, owns and manages all hospitals, although the state may regulate. The latter model does not exist in a pure form anywhere, however, even in the United States, where not-for-profit organizations own most hospitals. Under a socialist model, the state funds, owns and manages all hospitals (as formerly in the Soviet Union).

These complex arrangements give rise to many questions as to who is responsible for the many functions involved in running a hospital system, including who can be considered to own the hospitals. Clearly, there is no simple answer to the question of who is mainly responsible for hospitals. Instead, in most health care systems, different sectors and organizations are involved in different aspects of hospital systems and individual hospitals. These issues, involving ideological as well as technical considerations, are taken up in Chapters 7, 8 and 9. The following list illustrates the range of questions about the division of responsibilities within a health system.

- Who formulates hospital policy?
- Who funds capital?
- Who funds recurrent costs?
- Who plans hospitals?
- Who regulates hospitals?
- Who licences staff?
- Who manages hospitals?
- Who delivers the services?
- Who monitors services?
- Who evaluates outcomes?

A civic asset

Hospitals are a symbol of civic pride in many areas, as illustrated by the publicity that typically surrounds their official openings. In the same way that a cathedral once defined a city, the presence of a hospital helps define how a community perceives itself (James 1999). Hospitals are important in attracting residents and industry, and in this way serve an economic development function. The closure of a hospital in an area in economic decline can symbolize a loss of confidence in a region, with implications for other forms of inward investment. The closure of town hospitals, as well as banks and post offices, is seen by many rural communities as yet another factor in their decline.

An indicator of national progress

The number of hospital beds has been used as an indicator of a country's progress in health care, in particular under the Soviet system of central planning, as discussed in Chapter 2. Hospital beds were a key measure of a good health care system (the other being the number of physicians). Normative planning standards (hospital beds per 1000 population) were drawn up in Moscow, and thus the supply of beds was similar across the Soviet Union. This quantitative indicator was highly political, since it was used as proof of a superior health care system (Field 1995). These hospital-centred health care systems became supply-driven; the health system was structured and funded and medicine practised in such a way as to keep these beds full.

A provider of social care

The hospital historically was a source of social care as well as health care. As noted in Chapter 2, this remains the case in many countries. Alternative social care facilities are poorly developed, and problems are therefore medicalized to enable people to receive attention. This situation is sustained by the poor conditions in which much of the population lives. Thus, a conscientious physician may be hesitant to discharge a dependent older patient, admitted after a severe heart attack, home to a third-floor room with no heating or lift, intermittent running water and a pension that is insufficient to buy nutritious food.

A medical power base

Professional power is typically concentrated in the hospital system, with tertiary care hospitals acting as the pinnacle of the modern medical establishment. Hospitals employ a large proportion of health professionals: between one-third and one-half of physicians in Europe and between one-half and three-quarters of nurses (WHO 2001). Furthermore, hospital physicians (who are specialists) have high status, command public respect and also wield political influence. The hospital has been especially important in eastern Europe as a power base for the medical profession in the absence of other alternatives (now emerging), such as associations of physicians and statutory medical bodies.

A source of employment

A hospital is a labour-intensive enterprise and thus also a major employer (Chapter 11). The hospital sector employs, for example, 3.2 per cent of the workforce in Norway and 4.8 per cent in France (OECD 1999). Health care is an important component of public-sector employment. For example, in Kazakhstan, health personnel account for about 40 per cent of government employees (Kulzhanov and Healy 1999). Policy-makers, therefore, focus more explicitly on the role of the hospital as an employer. For example, the Amsterdam Special Action Programme, which was drawn up by the European Investment Bank (1999) in response to the meeting of the Council of the European Union in June 1997, has invested €10 billion in job-creating projects, including health care. Although the core function of a hospital is to treat rather than to employ people, its role as an employer clearly has huge implications for hospital restructuring. A hospital might be a major employer in a small town, so a closure or reduction has serious local socioeconomic consequences. Especially in rural areas, the total impact on employment may be substantially greater than the loss of the jobs provided directly by the hospital because of the effect on local suppliers (Cordes *et al.* 1999). Policy-makers and local politicians must clearly take this issue into account.

Different types of hospitals

The preceding section explored the roles and functions of the hospital. There are considerable differences between types of hospitals, as pointed out in Chapter 1. For example, some hospitals may not engage in teaching or research and, in small communities, the hospital may take on an extended range of social roles. Types of hospitals can be grouped under a hierarchical classification: tertiary care (often a national or regional resource and commonly linked with universities), secondary care (such as district hospitals) and community or rural hospitals. An additional dimension is added by distinguishing between specialist and general hospitals. The limitation of these simple classifications is becoming clearer, especially the division between secondary and tertiary care hospitals, which is increasingly blurred in high-income countries. For example, a 'district' hospital in Germany may have a team of surgeons, each specializing in breast or endocrine surgery, gastrointestinal surgery or vascular surgery, and with specialist support staff. In contrast, in poorer European countries, 'general' surgeons may operate on all of these conditions. Outwardly, these types of hospitals appear similar, but the nature of the care provided is very different.

Second, increasing subspecialization means that it is impossible to specify a single population size to support a single model for a 'tertiary' hospital. Hospital specialties each draw on a different size of catchment area depending on the prevalence of cases in the population; for example, a neurosurgery unit needs to draw from a larger population than a cancer unit. Tertiary hospitals also increasingly specialize among themselves. For example, a country may have ten 'tertiary' hospitals offering cardiac surgery for adults but only one for children; several hospitals may undertake kidney transplants but only one undertakes liver transplants.

Third, as noted earlier, the traditional distinction between teaching hospitals and non-teaching hospitals is breaking down. Training opportunities are being widened for health professionals, a phenomenon that is desirable for a number of reasons. The model of medical education based in a tertiary hospital, which concentrates on very severe or unusual cases, is poor preparation for the majority of medical students, who ultimately work in primary care. Training undertaken in highly specialized settings on atypical patients, using high-technology equipment, has little relevance to routine clinical practice (Britton *et al.* 1999). Finally, such policies can lead to the marginalization of staff working in non-teaching hospitals, with implications for their continuing professional standards.

As old divisions break down, new ones appear, based on different dimensions. These include structural arrangements (such as ownership and funding), functions (such as types of patient care), goals (such as enhancing access or maximizing profit) and how performance might be measured (such as patient satisfaction or low rates of surgical complications). Different issues require different ways of classifying hospitals.

Table 4.2 sets out a list of hospital dimensions and how variables might be measured. These concepts and measures are used throughout this book in discussing hospitals. This (not necessarily exhaustive) list of hospital characteristics and measurements again illustrates the point that a hospital is a complex organization not easily susceptible to being pinned down in a one-dimensional classification. The following paragraphs explore issues that are emerging in relation to these broad categories of hospitals.

Tertiary care hospitals

Tertiary care hospitals are defined, strictly, as those receiving patients referred from secondary care hospitals. Tertiary care hospitals offer the most complex and technologically sophisticated services, are usually linked to a medical school and are generally a regional-level resource. The concept of a tertiary hospital is based on the premise that scarce expertise and expensive equipment need to be concentrated in a few central facilities to which only the patients requiring specialized care are referred. A tertiary care hospital may be

Table 4.2 Describing a hospital: dimensions and measures

Dimensions	Measures
Location	
Geographical level	National, regional, city, district or community
Site structure	Single or multiple site
Governance	
Ownership	Federal, regional or local government; ministry of health or other ministry; autonomous public sector; voluntary sector not for profit; joint stock company; for-profit organization
Management	Managerial, technical, clinical or lay
Finances	
Main source of funds	State, sickness funds, patient charges or other
Cost structure	High cost versus low cost (per patient, patient category, budget year or bed), average salary per staff or staff category
Payment method	Line-item budget, global budget or activity-related budget
Size	
Population coverage	Geographical patient catchment or other (for example, military personnel)
Staff numbers	Total number, per bed, per 100 patients or physician: nurse ratio
Hospital size	Number of beds, inpatients or outpatients
Complexity	
Teaching status	Teaching or non-teaching
Type	Secondary versus tertiary; general versus specialist; acute, convalescent, palliative care or mixed
Specialties	Single or multiple; number and type of specialties
Technology	Type and amount of technology
Performance	
Accreditation	Whether accredited
Outcomes	Ranking on performance indicators
Patient management	Primary nurse, multidisciplinary teamwork
Patient satisfaction	Patient surveys, number of complaints
Responsiveness	Waiting lists and waiting times
Staff satisfaction	Recruitment and retention rates
Activity	High or low
Patient volume	Inpatients, day cases, outpatients, episodes and case mix
Occupancy	Average annual occupied beds
Admissions	Per 100 population
Average length of stay	Number of days
Outcomes	
Clinical performance	30-day mortality, percentage of hospital-caused (nosocomial) infections, percentage of 'medical errors' among patients and emergency readmission within 28 days of discharge

either a general hospital (housing many specialties) or a specialist hospital (concentrating on a population group, illness or technique). A general tertiary hospital typically houses specialties such as cardiac surgery, neurosurgery, transplant surgery and advanced cancer treatment.

The role of the tertiary care hospital has come under increasing scrutiny. First, their monopoly over teaching and research is being challenged, as discussed earlier, since a tertiary hospital is an atypical setting for both teaching and clinical research. Second, tertiary care hospitals often care for many patients who do not require their complex and often expensive services but are people who live nearby who could satisfactorily be diagnosed and treated in a district general hospital (Sanders *et al.* 1998). Third, their monopoly over expensive technology is being challenged, since the rationale for concentrating advanced technology in one place is less compelling with the trend towards diagnostic technology becoming miniaturized and simplified (Chapter 3).

Specialist hospitals

Specialist hospitals proliferated in Europe in the late nineteenth century, reflecting increasing specialization within the medical profession (Porter 1997). These hospitals acquired medical and social status, since they housed the medical elite and were thus regarded as extremely desirable by both staff and patients. Specialist hospitals included maternity, paediatrics, orthopaedic surgery, neurology, ear, nose and throat surgery and ophthalmology. In most western European countries, with a few exceptions, this model gave way to the 'general hospital' from the late 1940s onwards. An example of this process is the merger of many of London's specialist hospitals with nearby general hospitals in the 1990s (Tomlinson 1992). Nevertheless, the argument for rationalizing London hospitals dates back to the 1890s, and rationalization thus took almost a century to implement (Rivett 1986).

Specialist hospitals (that is, single specialties) remain the dominant model for tertiary care (and much secondary care) in the countries of the former Soviet Union, where such hospitals specialize in obstetrics, paediatric care, emergency care, cardiology, psychiatry, cancer, ophthalmology, drug addiction, sexually transmitted diseases and tuberculosis (Chapter 2). This fragmentation exists even in districts with a population of less than 100,000; such districts may have a central district hospital in the main town but also a nearby maternity hospital, paediatrics hospital and possibly a tuberculosis hospital (University of York 1998) (Box 4.1).

District general hospitals

A district general hospital in a high-income country typically serves a population of between 150,000 and 1 million inhabitants. District hospitals treat people for conditions that require more complex treatment than can be provided in a primary care setting or in an ambulatory setting. These hospitals typically have between 200 and 600 beds and usually provide inpatient and outpatient

---

Box 4.1 Specialist hospitals in the central Asian republics

Bishkek, the capital of Kyrgyzstan, has 12 national-level specialist hospitals serving about 500,000 people. Almaty, the former capital of Kazakhstan with a population of 1.2 million, has 17 national specialist hospitals and institutes. The physicians who head these hospitals are well known and influential. Few of the central Asian republics have managed to close specialist hospitals in their capitals during the 1990s.

Sources: Kulzhanov and Healy (1999) and Sargaldakova *et al.* (2000)

---

care, day surgery and an emergency service. They usually include, at the least, departments of medicine, surgery, paediatrics, obstetrics and gynaecology, supported by imaging and pathology services.

Chapter 6 discusses the optimal size of such hospitals, but here we reflect on the implementation of this model in high-income countries. The district general hospital concept was taken up in planning documents in several countries, but the arguments in the 1962 Hospital Plan for England and Wales are typical (Ministry of Health 1962). This sought to redress the previous dominance of the teaching hospitals, which had attracted a disproportionate share of both financial and human resources. It was argued that a district general hospital should be large enough to offer suitable training locations for junior medical staff and to ensure adequate emergency cover at night (McKee and Black 1991), but not so large as to prevent medium-sized towns from having their own hospital.

This model is now being challenged. The Royal College of Surgeons of England (1997) argued that small district hospitals should be replaced by fewer and larger hospitals, each designed to serve a population in excess of 500,000. Such a hospital would typically contain 15 specialist surgeons, 15 specialist orthopaedic surgeons and 30 anaesthetists and would provide capacity for 24-hour operating, an intensive care unit and 24-hour pathology and imaging services (Smith 1999). The Royal College of Physicians of London (1996), in contrast, has argued for smaller district general hospitals serving a population of 150,000 to 300,000. This debate is echoed in many other countries. In general, although there is agreement that a hospital serving fewer than 150,000 people is too small to provide the necessary range of acute care services, there is considerable debate about its most cost-effective upper size.

Community hospitals

Many countries have a lower tier of hospital, sometimes called a community hospital. These typically have 50 beds or less and provide basic diagnostic services, minor surgery and care for patients who need nursing care but not the facilities of a district general hospital.

Small community hospitals exist in some areas because of long distances between scattered communities and the lack of general physicians in remote areas. In Siberia, the small hospitals established during the Soviet period are closing, thus adding to the difficulties facing isolated populations in the far north of the Russian Federation. Elsewhere, such hospitals are a legacy of a bygone era, when the limited scope for medical intervention meant there was no need to concentrate hospital services. In large high-income countries with scattered populations, such as Canada and Australia, small hospitals have closed, but patients needing secondary care are transported long distances by air or, in an emergency, are visited by the flying physician service or air ambulance. As noted in Chapter 2, many high-income countries have closed small hospitals over the last few decades, in some cases converting them into nursing homes. Closures have been difficult, however, since these hospitals are often popular with the local population, perhaps for symbolic as much as practical reasons (White and Williams 1999).

The pendulum may now be swinging back. Community hospitals are being advocated as a means of facilitating discharge from acute care hospitals and as a form of 'step-down' hospital for rehabilitation and convalescence before returning home. For some countries, this would be a return to the old concept of 'a convalescent home'. The main question is whether a community hospital can reduce the need for acute care in general hospitals. A few studies have looked at this issue, mainly in relation to admissions. A study in northern Norway found that districts with community ('general practitioner') hospitals had more than one-quarter fewer admissions to acute care ('general') hospitals than districts without community hospitals (Aaraas *et al.* 1998). Another study from the west of England found that districts with community hospitals had 50 per cent fewer admissions to general and geriatric medicine wards in acute hospitals, but 6 per cent more admissions to hospital overall (Baker *et al.* 1986). A study of total bed use found that the presence of community hospitals increased total admissions by 16 per cent (Round 1997). Chapter 5 points out that there is very limited evidence that community hospitals can substitute for the latter part of an acute hospital stay and thus facilitate earlier discharge. Nevertheless, interest in this option is growing, especially in relation to older patients, who tend to have longer hospital stays.

The changing hospital

Modern acute care hospitals must engage in a continuing process of reconciling several functions: patient care, teaching and research, health system support, employment and wider societal functions. Hospitals in western Europe are busier places, with more and sicker patients being admitted for shorter lengths of time for more intensive treatment. Patient management within the hospital is also changing, with more patients being treated as day cases. In response, the staffing, design of hospitals and organization of work has to be re-engineered. Old ways of classifying hospitals also no longer apply as new technology becomes more widely available to district and not just strictly tertiary care hospitals.

Chapter 5 considers the relationship between the hospital and other health services, especially the issue of substitution: the extent to which services provided in hospitals could be provided in other settings. Chapter 6 examines the optimal size and distribution of hospitals.

References

Aaraas, I., Forde, O.H., Kristiansen, I.S. and Melbye, H. (1998) Do general practitioner hospitals reduce the utilisation of general hospital beds? Evidence from Finnmark County in north Norway, *Journal of Epidemiology and Community Health*, 52(4): 243–6.

American College of Surgeons Committee on Trauma (1990) *Resources for Optimal Care of the Injured Patient.* Chicago, IL: American College of Surgeons.

Anonymous (2000) A case of market failure, *Lancet*, 355: 1657.

Baker, J., Goldacre, M. and Muir Gray, J.A. (1986) Community hospitals in Oxfordshire: their effect on the use of specialist inpatient services, *Journal of Epidemiology and Community Health*, 40: 117–20.

Berman, P. (2000) Organization of ambulatory care provision: a critical determinant of health system performance in developing countries, *Bulletin of the World Health Organization: The International Journal of Public Health*, 78(6): 791–802.

Bevan, G. (1999) The medical service increment for teaching (SIFT): a £400m anachronism for the English NHS?, *British Medical Journal*, 319: 908–11.

Britton, A., McKee, M., Black, N. *et al.* (1999) Threats to applicability of randomised trials: exclusions and selective participation, *Journal of Health Services Research and Policy*, 4: 112–21.

Calnan, M. (1984) The functions of the hospital emergency department: a study of patient demand, *Journal of Emergency Medicine*, 2: 57–63.

Clack, G.B., Bevan, G., Peters, T.J. and Eddleston, A.L. (1992) King's model for allocating service increment for teaching and research (SIFTR), *British Medical Journal*, 305(6845): 95–6.

Cordes, S., van der Sluice, E., Lamphear, C. and Hoffman, J. (1999) Rural hospitals and the local economy: a needed extension and refinement of existing empirical research, *Journal of Rural Health*, 15(2): 189–201.

Dale, J. and Dolan, B. (1996) Do patients use minor injury units appropriately?, *Journal of Public Health Medicine*, 18: 152–6.

Dale, J., Lang, H., Roberts, J.A., Green, J. and Glucksman, E. (1996) Cost effectiveness of treating primary care patients in accident and emergency: a comparison between general practitioners, senior house officers and registrars, *British Medical Journal*, 312(7042): 1340–4.

Dickinson, E. and Sinclair, A. (1998) *Effective Practice in Rehabilitation – Reviewing the Evidence.* London: King's Fund.

Esping-Anderson, G. (1990) *The Three Worlds of Welfare Capitalism.* Oxford: Polity Press.

European Investment Bank (1999) *EIB Initiative on Growth and Employment: Interim Review.* Luxembourg: European Investment Bank.

Field, M.G. (1990) Noble purpose, grand design, flawed execution, mixed results: Soviet socialized medicine after seventy years, *American Journal of Public Health*, 80: 144–5.

Field, M.G. (1995) The health crisis in the former Soviet Union: a report from the 'postwar zone', *Social Science and Medicine*, 41: 1469–78.

Fields, S.A., Ustatine, R. and Steiner, E. (2000) Teaching medical students in the ambulatory setting, *Journal of the American Medical Association*, 283: 2362–4.

Florin, D. and Rosen, R. (1999) Evaluating NHS direct: early findings raise questions about expanding the service, *British Medical Journal*, 319: 5–6.

Forster, A., Young, J. and Langhorne, P. (1999) Systematic review of day hospital care for elderly people: the Day Hospital Group, *British Medical Journal*, 318(7187): 837–41.

Gleeson, A. (2000) Major trauma – major problem, *Journal of Irish Colleges of Physicians and Surgeons*, 29: 69–71.

Healy, J. (1998) *Welfare Options: Delivering Social Services.* Sydney: Allen & Unwin.

Hensher, M., Fulop, N., Hood, S. and Ujah, S. (1996) Does hospital at home make economic sense? Results of an economic evaluation of early discharge hospital at home care for orthopaedic patients in three areas of West London, *Journal of the Royal Society of Medicine*, 89: 595–600.

Hunt, C.E., Kallenberg, G.A. and Whitcomb, M.E. (1999) Trends in clinical education of medical students: implications for paediatrics, *Archives of Paediatric and Adolescent Medicine*, 153: 297–302.

James, A.M. (1999) Closing rural hospitals in Saskatchewan: on the road to wellness?, *Social Science and Medicine*, 49(8): 1021–34.

Kulzhanov, M. and Healy, J. (1999) *Health Care Systems in Transition: Kazakhstan.* Copenhagen: European Observatory on Health Care Systems.

Lang, T., Davido, A., Diakite, B. *et al.* (1996) Non-urgent care in the hospital medical emergency department in France: how much and which health needs does it reflect?, *Journal of Epidemiology and Community Health*, 50: 456–62.

Langhorne, P., Williams, B.O., Gilchrist, W. and Howie, K. (1993) Do stroke units save lives?, *Lancet*, 342: 395–8.

McKee, M. and Black, N. (1991) Hours of work of junior hospital doctors: is there a solution?, *Journal of Management Medicine*, 5: 40–54.

McKee, M. and Mossialos, E. (1998) The impact of managed care on clinical research, *Pharmacoeconomics*, 14: 19–25.

McKee, M., Clarke, A. and Tennison, B. (1993a) Meeting local needs, *British Medical Journal*, 306: 602.

McKee, M., Snooks, H., Nicholl, J.P., Brazier, J.E. and Lees-Mlanga, S. (1993b) Utilisation of the helicopter emergency ambulance services in England and Wales, *Journal of Public Health Medicine*, 18: 67–77.

Ministry of Health (1962) *A Hospital Plan for England and Wales*, Cmnd 1604. London: HMSO.

Mullins, R.J., Veum-Stone, J., Helfand, M. *et al.* (1994) Outcome of hospitalized injured patients after institution of a trauma system in an urban area, *Journal of the American Medical Association*, 271: 1919–24.

Munro, J., Nicholl, J., O'Caithain, A. and Knowles, E. (2000) Impact of NHS Direct on demand for immediate care: observational study, *British Medical Journal*, 321: 150–3.

Nicholl, J. and Turner, J. (1997) Effectiveness of a regional trauma system in reducing mortality from major trauma before and after study, *British Medical Journal*, 315: 1349–54.

Nicholl, J., Hughes, S., Dixon, S., Turner, J. and Yates, D. (1998) The costs and benefits of paramedic skills in pre-hospital trauma care, *Health Technology Assessment*, 2: 1–67.

OECD (1999) *OECD Health Data 99: A Comparative Analysis of 29 Countries*, Paris: Organisation for Economic Co-operation and Development.

Paine, L.H.W. and Siem Tjam, F. (1988) *Hospitals and the Health Care Revolution.* Geneva: World Health Organization.

Peckham, M. (1991) Research and development for the National Health Service, *Lancet*, 338: 367–71.

Pencheon, D. (1998) NHS direct: managing demand, *British Medical Journal*, 316: 215–16.

Porter, R. (1997) *The Greatest Benefit to Mankind: A Medical History of Humanity from Antiquity to the Present.* London: HarperCollins.

Poullier, J.P. (2000) Data and indicators for health care investment, in M. Garcia-Barbero (ed.) *Appraisal of Investments in Health Infrastructure: Proceedings of the European Investment Bank (EIB) and World Health Organization (WHO) Conference on the Appraisal of Investments in Health, Luxembourg, 17–18 June 1999.* Copenhagen: WHO Regional Office for Europe.

Preker, A.S., Harding, A. and Travis, P. (2000) 'Make or buy' decisions in the production of health care goods and services: new insights from institutional economics and organizational theory, *Bulletin of the World Health Organization: The International Journal of Public Health*, 78(6): 779–90.

Rivett, G. (1986) *The Development of the London Hospital System 1823–1982*. London: King's Fund.

Robinson, R. and Dixon, A. (1999) *Health Care Systems in Transition: United Kingdom*. Copenhagen: European Observatory on Health Care Systems.

Round, A. (1997) Emergency medical admissions to hospital – the influence of supply factors, *Public Health*, 111(4): 221–4.

Royal College of Physicians (1996) *Future Pattern of Care by General and Specialist Physicians*. London: Royal College of Physicians.

Royal College of Surgeons of England (1997) *The Provision of Emergency Surgical Services – An Organisational Framework*. London: Royal College of Surgeons.

Sanders, D., Kravitz, J., Lewin, S. and McKee, M. (1998) Zimbabwe's hospital referral system: does it work?, *Health Policy and Planning*, 13: 359–70.

Sargaldakova, A., Healy, J., Kutzin, J. and Gedik, G. (2000) *Health Care Systems in Transition: Kyrgyzstan*. Copenhagen: European Observatory on Health Care Systems.

Sherman, D.H. (1984) Hospital efficiency measurement and evaluation, *Medical Care*, 22: 922–38.

Smith, R. (1999) Editorial. Reconfiguring acute hospital services: no easy answers, but there are principles we should follow, *British Medical Journal*, 319: 797–8.

Steedman, D.J. (1990) Medical teams for accidents and major disasters, *Injury*, 21: 206–8.

Swales, J.D. (2000) Science and health: an uneasy partnership, *Lancet*, 355: 1637–40.

Tomlinson, B. (1992) *Report of the Inquiry into London's Health Service, Medical Education and Research*. London: HMSO.

Trunkey, D.D. (1983) Trauma, *Scientific American*, 249: 28–35.

University of York (1998) *Project Preparation for the Kazakhstan Health Sector Project: Final Report*. Almaty: Ministry of Education, Culture and Health and Fund for Compulsory Health Insurance.

Van Lerberghe, W. and Lafort, Y. (1990) *The Role of the Hospital in the District: Delivering or Supporting Primary Health Care? Current Concerns*, SHS paper No. 2, Division of Strengthening Health Services. Geneva: World Health Organization.

Waghorn, A. and McKee, M. (1999) Surgical outpatients: are we allowing enough time?, *International Journal of Quality Health Care*, 11: 215–19.

Waghorn, A. and McKee, M. (2000) Why is it so difficult to organise an outpatient clinic?, *Journal of Health Services Research and Policy*, 5: 140–7.

Waghorn, A., McKee, M. and Thompson, J. (1997) Surgical outpatients: challenges and responses, *British Journal of Surgery*, 84: 300–7.

Walt, G. (1994) *Health Policy: An Introduction to Process and Power*. London: Zed Books.

White, V. and Williams, S. (1999) Close call, *Health Service Journal*, 4: 26–7.

WHO (1978) *Alma-Ata 1978: Primary Health Care*, Health for All Series, No. 1. Geneva: World Health Organization.

WHO (2000) *The World Health Report 2000. Health Systems: Improving Performance*. Geneva: World Health Organization.

WHO (2001) *WHO European Health for All Database*. Copenhagen: WHO Regional Office for Europe.

Yates, D.W., Woodford, M. and Hollis, S. (1992) Preliminary analysis of the care of injured patients in 33 British hospitals: first report of the United Kingdom major trauma outcome study, *British Medical Journal*, 305: 737–40.

part two

**External pressures
upon hospitals**

chapter five

The hospital and the external environment: experience in the United Kingdom

Martin Hensher and Nigel Edwards

Introduction

Chapter 1 discussed the importance of a whole-system approach to hospitals. Health care analysts and professionals increasingly accept the notion that 'the hospital' is only one, albeit important, link in a complex continuum in which patients move between different levels and types of care. As a result, increasing attention is paid to the concept of the interface: how and where different levels of care intersect and where patients move from one mode of care to another. In the context of the hospital, this attention has focused on the interface between primary and secondary care and between hospital and post-hospital care. Hospitals have multiple functions and therefore a large number of possible interfaces. For example, hospitals concentrate professionals and technology in a single location to deliver specialized patient care; hospitals may serve as organizational hubs, providing a focal point for care providers based outside the hospital; hospitals also educate and train local health care professionals.

The concept of interface has two parts. First, any of the interfaces represent frontiers or boundaries between care providers. As a frontier, the interface may provide an opportunity for the hospital to filter patients and to mediate demand that is considered inappropriate (or that cannot be met). The interface as boundary provides the opportunity to insert physical or process filters (for example, referral systems for non-urgent care and medical assessment units in emergency rooms) that can turn back or re-route patients who do not require acute care. The boundaries may be:

- *Organizational*: responsibility for the care of the patient shifts between organizations, for example, from the general practitioner to hospital.
- *Physical*: the patient has to leave home to be admitted to hospital.
- *Financial*: a different payer or mode of payment may be used for primary and inpatient care.

The second property of the interface is that it comprises a set of interactions, flows and mechanisms by which patients can move from one level of care to another: a bridge across care boundaries. At the core of this notion is the flow of information (in all its forms), on which the smooth and appropriate transition across care boundaries depends. Arguably, changes in both modes of information transfer and attitudes to communication and coordination are at the heart of changing attitudes towards interfaces between hospital and non-hospital care. Clearly, developments in communications technology continue to make information transfers technically easier and cheaper, but more important than the hardware of communication has been a shift in the expectations of health professionals as to what constitutes minimally acceptable levels of communication and coordination. The culture of protocol-driven care makes professionals engage with one another more closely, while simultaneously formalizing information flow requirements at various stages of care.

This chapter uses the experience of the United Kingdom to illustrate some of the issues that face health systems across Europe. During the 1980s, the National Health Service (NHS) in the United Kingdom had been at the forefront of efforts to shift the balance of care between hospitals and primary care and gained extensive experience with a wide range of different policies. We explore some of the key changes that have marked the recent evolution of information flows across care interfaces, with reference to a stylized model of the relationship between general practitioners and hospital-based specialists. We also offer a critique of models in the United Kingdom where this is appropriate.

Approaches to improving the operation of hospital interfaces with the outside world revolve around three fundamental strategies:

- improving the coordination of care;
- shifting organizational and care boundaries; and
- bypassing or substituting for hospital or inpatient care.

The inward interface: preventing admission and bypassing hospital

The inward interface has frontier and boundary points at which patients can be diverted, filtered and channelled. Figure 5.1 presents a stylized representation of the key interfaces between patients being admitted to hospital and types of secondary hospital care.

The hospital as a provider of ambulatory care

Ambulatory care includes outpatients, minor accident cases and day treatment, including surgery, endoscopy and other investigations. This represents the

Figure 5.1 Inward hospital interface links

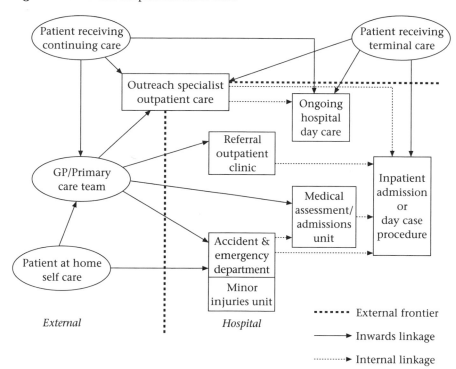

largest single activity of most hospital services in the United Kingdom and most other health systems. As previously noted, despite the very large volume of care provided, there is surprisingly little research into the function, organization or management of ambulatory care.

Overall outpatient activity in the United Kingdom has risen relatively slowly and consistently in recent years. In 1979, there were 28.425 million outpatient attendances across all acute specialties in England; this rose by an average of 1.2 per cent annually to 36.057 million attendances in the fiscal year 1996–97 (Department of Health 1997). This slowly expanding outpatient workload has been spread across a growing number of consultant specialists so that the number of outpatient attendances per consultant has declined steadily (Armstrong and Nicoll 1995).

Systems that allow patients direct access to specialists, as in France, Germany, Sweden and the United States, tend to have higher costs than those that insist on general practitioner referrals, such as Denmark, Finland, the Netherlands and the United Kingdom. The absence of both an agency mechanism and a filter and interpreter of information directly affects hospital activity (Starfield 1994). Furthermore, systems that link in some way to the referring physicians' remuneration are more effective at reducing referrals and encouraging alternative ambulatory care. These include systems that require a referral from primary care to hospital fee-for-service systems, or include fundholding, or where hospital treatment is covered by a capitated allowance. Having said this, the introduction of general practitioner fundholding in the United Kingdom seemed only to slow growth in referrals from capitated fundholders relative to non-fundholders and not to actually reduce referral rates (Surender *et al.* 1995). Yet there are risks to the operation of referral systems, primarily potential underserving and delays in treatment.

> At its best the referral system ensures that most care is contained within general practice, and when specialist care is needed patients are directed to the most appropriate specialist. However, it is also a restrictive practice, initially introduced to protect the interests of doctors, which gives general practitioners a monopoly over primary medical care and restricts patients' freedom of choice.
>
> Coulter (1998: 1974)

In eastern Europe and in systems in which primary care is underdeveloped or has a low status compared with specialist clinics or hospital services, there is less control on the interface with hospital provision. This is a particular problem with chronic conditions that can be managed in primary care with some training and diagnostic support, such as heart failure, hypertension, diabetes, ischaemic heart disease, asthma and chronic obstructive pulmonary disease.

The expectations of the referring physician, specialist and patient often differ substantially in terms of the purpose of the referral to specialist ambulatory care. Coulter (1998) reports widespread misunderstandings. For example, in the United Kingdom, specialists have taken over some patients referred solely for advice on management. Patients may have an entirely different set of expectations about care from both the referrer and the specialist. Financial incentives and protocols are very important in this context for defining the nature of the relationship and making explicit the reasons for referral and may also have the added benefit of reducing the duplication of diagnostic tests.

The practice of the hospital repeatedly calling patients back for further outpatient consultations in the absence of any tangible benefit for the patients is still common, although fundholding did seem to influence this in the United Kingdom. Meanwhile, communication between the ambulatory specialist and the referring physician still commonly causes problems and irritation.

Perhaps the most striking feature of the interface between specialist ambulatory care and primary care in the United Kingdom is the very high variation in referral rates, which may differ by a factor of four for similar populations (Coulter 1998). The following factors account for some of the variation: incentives for general practitioners to shift work to the hospital setting; different levels of competence and diagnostic insight; sociodemographic features of practice populations (Reid *et al.* 1999); and lack of any explicit management or a failure to use protocols. Despite a widespread assumption that general practitioners referring high numbers of patients tend to refer unnecessarily, studies comparing referrals from physicians with high and low referral rates have not confirmed this, and thus greater use of protocols might not significantly affect referral rates (Knotternus *et al.* 1990; Fertig *et al.* 1993). In the

United Kingdom, at least, continuing professional development programmes seldom address known problems of over- or under-referral.

Outpatient care is changing and new models for managing this interface are developing. For example, multidisciplinary outpatient teams can provide a one-stop service for complex diagnosis and treatment (Waghorn *et al.* 1997). Open-access clinics in certain specialties and conditions have also become more common within the NHS (Waghorn *et al.* 1997), although the debate on their appropriateness remains unresolved. Pre-assessment clinics can be used to avoid the need for admission prior to surgery, and the follow-up of post-surgery patients after relatively simple procedures, such as hernia repair, can be dispensed with; but again, rigorous evaluation evidence is limited (Waghorn *et al.* 1997). New technologies also offer the opportunity to undertake many procedures on an outpatient basis that were previously dealt with in hospital. In ambulatory emergency care, a range of models for minor treatment are emerging to treat patients who were previously seen in a primary care setting or in an accident and emergency department. Hospitals appear to be relatively efficient at providing such high-volume low-technology care (Read 1994).

Outside the physical confines of the hospital, specialist outreach clinics increasingly provide mainly consultant-led consultation in primary care locations (Bailey *et al.* 1994). Although consultant outreach clinics are popular among patients, significant questions remain concerning their costs, which are generally higher per patient than traditional outpatient department clinics; they also offer less education and skill benefits to general practitioners (Gillam *et al.* 1995; Anglia and Oxford 1997).

Appropriateness of admission

Most patients admitted to hospital in industrialized countries have no appropriate alternative to hospitalization. At any time, however, studies of acute hospital utilization tend to classify a sizeable minority of admissions (and an even greater proportion of inpatient bed-days) as inappropriate. Depending on the survey instrument and the study population, estimates of the proportion of acute hospital admissions found to be inappropriate in recent studies in the United Kingdom varied considerably. The Oxford Bed Study Instrument found zero inappropriate use (Victor and Khakoo 1994) and the Appropriateness Evaluation Protocol found 6 per cent of emergency medical admissions to be inappropriate (Smith *et al.* 1997). Nevertheless, more than 20 per cent of admissions to a specialty of general medicine and care of elderly people were assessed as being inappropriate using the Intensity-Severity-Discharge review system with Adult Criteria (Coast *et al.* 1995, 1996). A study in Italy using a modified variant of the Appropriateness Evaluation Protocol indicated that as many as 27 per cent of patients in a number of specialties might have been inappropriately admitted (Apolone *et al.* 1997). An earlier review by the authors, however, found that older studies of inappropriate hospital utilization either returned lower (less than 10 per cent) estimates of inappropriate admission or focused exclusively on inappropriate bed use (Edwards *et al.* 1998: 236–60).

A key problem of such appropriateness studies is that, although they identify inappropriate admissions, they cannot by themselves demonstrate that an alternative form of care offering equivalent or better outcome at equivalent or lower cost actually existed for any given patient. Some studies found that only a tiny number of their supposedly inappropriately admitted patients could have gone straight home with no further care; all the others required some form of care beyond that offered routinely in primary care (Coast *et al.* 1995, 1996). The challenge is, therefore, to demonstrate that cost-effective measures can be implemented at the interface between primary and secondary care that ensure that inappropriate hospital admissions are diverted to more appropriate and less costly care locations.

Avoiding inappropriate admission: primary care management

Perhaps the most attractive method of managing the admission interface is to find ways to enable routine primary care management of the patient in the place of admission. Clearly, this can happen without any policy intervention when a new technology (particularly a drug therapy) becomes available to control a condition that would otherwise have required admission. Even within a fixed technology envelope, primary care management of certain acute or sub-acute conditions can still be extended and improved. Critically, the adoption of evidence-based shared-care protocols agreed by local primary care and specialist professionals can promote better disease management, prevent certain acute events from occurring and manage emergencies better when they do occur. Certain chronic conditions such as asthma and diabetes have proved to be particularly fertile ground for such improvements in care coordination.

Managing demand for admission

Growing attention has been paid to inserting filters at the interface between primary and secondary care; the aim is to identify patients who might not (yet) require admission to hospital. One such filter that remains very important is the operation of referral and waiting-list systems. Some conditions may prove to be self-limiting and not require intervention after a period on the waiting list, but others may not subsequently require surgery if the person dies (Marber *et al.* 1991). Waiting lists can clearly be used as a tool to match demand with resource availability over time, but their efficacy, as a long-term demand management tool, remains contentious and unpredictable. Anecdotal evidence suggests that the presence of a waiting list may even increase demand, as patients may be referred early in case their condition deteriorates. The implicit assumption that elective cases are less urgent than emergency cases (and hence can wait) can produce perverse outcomes, whereby patients with urgent surgical needs are forced to wait for care, while people with health emergencies are admitted to hospital when they could have been cared for elsewhere.

An important innovation in recent years has thus been the introduction of medical assessment units and admission units. General practitioners can refer health emergencies directly to medical assessment units, which are geared to providing diagnosis, observation and rapid testing, without the patient having to be admitted immediately. Integration of the medical assessment units with both hospital and community services allows an informed choice to be made as to whether patients require admission or whether they can be managed at home; in this case, the medical assessment units can mobilize and coordinate appropriate resources for home care. Medical assessment units thus sift borderline cases and take appropriate action (Gaspov *et al.* 1994). In parallel, admission units increasingly provide an intensively staffed environment (usually with relatively senior physicians) to allow investigation and active treatment for up to 48 hours and achieve early discharge or transfer to a non-acute setting. In other words, front-loading the acute care content of an episode allows rapid transfer (Audit Commission 1992).

Alternatives to hospital admission

The insertion of filters such as medical assessment units and admission units clearly provides a potential opportunity to divert patients to alternative care locations, thus bypassing hospital. One possible alternative to admission is to provide specialist care outside the hospital. This might involve the provision of specialist physician advice and inputs in a domiciliary setting, such as telephonic monitoring of fetal heart rate in high-risk pregnancies (Dawson *et al.* 1989), home dialysis or home visits by a specialist physician to elderly patients with congestive heart disease (Kornokowski *et al.* 1995). Such approaches focus on delivering technological and specialist care in a non-hospital setting. Alternatively, other groups of patients might be diverted from hospital admission through relatively intensive nursing care in the home setting – this is the hospital-at-home model of care. Unfortunately, problems in study design and programme scale have conspired so far to prevent any robust evaluation of the use of hospital-at-home care in preventing admission (although evidence on early-discharge models is discussed below).

Not all patients who do not need admission to acute hospital can be cared for at home, because of either inappropriate home circumstances (such as poor housing or the lack of an able-bodied care-giver) or the need for continuous surveillance and basic nursing care. Alternatives to acute admission for such patients do exist in the form of admission to an intermediate-care institution. Key examples of intermediate care include community hospitals, respite care in nursing homes, hospice care for the terminally ill and, more controversially, low-intensity wards within hospitals led by general practitioners or nurses. Once again, and with the notable exception of hospice care, very little firm evidence exists to guide policy on whether intermediate care provides a cost-effective alternative to acute hospitalization. As discussed in Chapter 4, community hospitals may provide a cost-effective alternative to acute admission, but they may also effectively add to hospital capacity and increase hospitalization rates (Baker *et al.* 1986). Micro-level evaluation

Table 5.1   NHS inpatient and day case activity in England, 1982–98

	Inpatient cases (thousands)	Day cases (thousands)	Total cases (thousands)	Total per 1000 population	Throughput per bed
All specialties					
1982	5720	707	6427	137.3	16.4
1998	8459	3071	11530	233.9	43.7
Increase	48%	334%	79%	70%	166%
General and acute					
1982	4709	685	5394	115.2	23.7
1998	6514	2439	9549	193.8	47.2
Increase	38%	343%	77%	68%	99%

Sources: Department of Health (1982, 1997); Hensher and Edwards (1999)

Table 5.2   NHS beds in England, 1982 and 1998

Year	All specialties	Acute
1982	348,104	143,535
1998	193,625	107,807
Percentage change	−44%	−25%

Sources: Department of Health (1982), Hensher and Edwards (1999)

evidence on the ability of intermediate care to prevent admission is sorely lacking, and aggregate macro-level data (in the United Kingdom at least) is not adequate to demonstrate whether intermediate care is cost-effective or not.

Day care and day surgery as a substitute for admission

The massive growth in day care and day surgery in many countries is frequently offered as an example of the substitution of inpatient admission by non-inpatient care. However, considerable caution must be exercised in interpreting such claims. Table 5.1 shows the growth in inpatient and day case activity in England between 1982 and 1998. It illustrates vividly that, despite a massive increase in day case activity, inpatient admissions have continued to rise consistently. Thus, a switch towards day case work has not reduced admission rates in England. Over the same period, however, bed numbers have declined substantially (by 25 per cent in the acute hospital sector) and throughput and turnover of acute patients have improved substantially to accommodate a greater number of admissions within a smaller bed stock (Table 5.2). It could be argued, however, that a failure to expand day case activity might have prevented beds from closing and led to even more inpatient admissions than are now occurring. Nevertheless, expanded day care has almost certainly contributed to earlier discharge and hence facilitated the constant increases in patient turnover observed in the NHS.

The rapid growth of day surgery has replaced a wide range of procedures that once required hospitalization, and recent developments in minimally invasive surgery and investigation and in imaging technologies are likely to do the same. Procedures such as cystoscopy, arthroscopy, laparoscopy, varicose vein stripping and inguinal hernia repair are now routinely performed as day procedures. Once again, however, the aggregate picture in the United Kingdom does not square with the limited micro-level evaluation of individual procedures. It appears that the growth in day surgery has contributed to a substantial increase in overall rates of surgery (Raftery and Stevens 1998). Possible explanations for this effect include the introduction of wholly new procedures not previously possible, the possibility of supplier-induced demand and the difficulties of eliminating inpatient surgical capacity; adding facilities for day surgery may simply have increased total surgical capacity within the NHS.

The outward interface: accelerating hospital discharge

Studies of the appropriateness of hospitalization noted a greater proportion of inappropriate bed-days than inappropriate admissions. In other words, even if patients are admitted to hospital appropriately, a high proportion stay in hospital longer than is strictly necessary. The proportion of acute patients said to have ceased to benefit from inpatient care ranged from 14.6 per cent of all specialties excluding psychiatry and obstetrics (Victor *et al.* 1994) to 61.9 per cent of patients treated by a specialty of general medicine or care of elderly people in an urban hospital (Coast *et al.* 1996). The implication of such studies is that there should be rich opportunities for accelerating discharge from hospital. Figure 5.2 presents a stylized diagram of the interfaces between the hospital and post-discharge care services.

Considerable attention has been paid to improving the outward interface between hospital and post-hospital care. Important improvements seem attainable through coordination and planning of individual patient cases and the advance preparation of plans for discharge. Techniques with promise include the use of integrated care pathways or anticipated recovery pathways, which map out an expected course for both hospital and post-hospital care, allowing prior planning of discharge and home-care arrangements. Dedicated discharge coordinators can achieve a similar result by following the progress of each patient in a hospital and consulting relevant external professionals and agencies. Important blockages to patient discharge can often be traced to problems with internal systems and poor discharge planning, although the evidence is not universal. Many problems can also be attributed to the quality of liaison between health and social care agencies regarding expected discharge dates and the services a patient may need to return home, such as home help, home alterations and equipment, or placement in a nursing or residential home. Efforts to improve planning and coordination between agencies have been implemented in several countries other than the United Kingdom.

Figure 5.2 Outward hospital interface links. GP = general practitioner, PHC = primary health care.

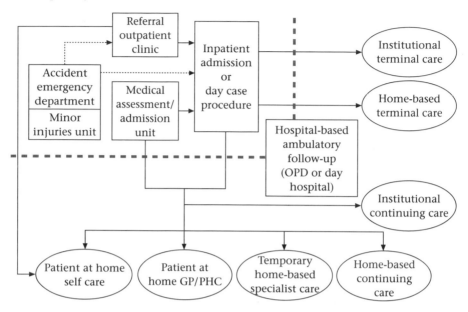

There is some evidence that well-organized rehabilitation services, straddling both hospital and community locations and delivery agencies, can reduce the length of hospital stay while achieving equivalent clinical outcomes (Rudd *et al.* 1997). In a systematic review, Dickinson and Sinclair (1998) found that good rehabilitation services yield positive results in stroke and cardiac care and that comprehensive geriatric assessments can also improve care delivery substantially, but they note that there is little or no costing evidence. Day hospitals have a long-established and pivotal role in providing multidisciplinary assessment and rehabilitation between inpatient and home-based care in the United Kingdom. A systematic review of trials over a 30-year period (Forster *et al.* 1999) found evidence that, while day hospital may lead to some reduction in long-term institutional care, this mode of providing care generally costs as much as or more than both community- and hospital-based alternatives.

As with preventing admission, not every patient's discharge can be accelerated through improved coordination alone. Alternative providers of sub-acute care may be required to allow earlier discharge from acute hospital. Nurse-led inpatient care attempts to provide rehabilitative care in a lower-cost step-down hospital environment (with costs reduced by eliminating physician care), and patient hotels have also been advocated as a halfway house for patients who need observation but not intensive care. A detailed review, however, indicates that rigorous evaluation of these approaches remains largely absent (Steiner 1997). The very limited evidence available on whether community hospitals can replace the last part of an acute inpatient stay suggests that earlier discharge from acute hospital might be achieved through higher overall bed utilization (Baker *et al.* 1986). A vital question, therefore, remains unanswered: Even if institutional intermediate care allows earlier discharge at reduced cost for the individual patient, does it allow an overall reduction in bed use and total costs?

Within the United Kingdom, perhaps the best-evaluated early discharge substitute for hospital care is the hospital-at-home concept. These schemes operate in various specialties and care groups, but all attempt to provide care in the patient's home (usually nursing and rehabilitative therapy) that would otherwise have been provided in hospital. As previously noted, it has proved easier to evaluate hospital-at-home schemes whose objective is to facilitate early discharge than it has to evaluate those seeking to prevent the initial admission. Patient health outcomes from hospital at home are equivalent to those achieved in hospitals (Wilson *et al.* 1997; Richards *et al.* 1998; Shepperd *et al.* 1998a; Shepperd and Illiffe 2000). Hospital-at-home approaches do appear to allow early discharge from hospital, but this may be achieved through a long period of home care (Hensher *et al.* 1996; Shepperd *et al.* 1998b). Cost-minimization analyses of early discharge hospital-at-home care found mixed results. Some studies found hospital-at-home care to be less expensive than standard inpatient care (Wilson *et al.* 1997, Coast *et al.* 1998), whereas others found no difference or even higher costs for hospital-at-home care for certain conditions (Hensher *et al.* 1996; Shepperd *et al.* 1998a).

The continuing care interface

Perhaps oddly, literature on health services research in the United Kingdom has little to say about nursing homes, perhaps the most important means of substituting for hospital care, and certainly one of the key interfaces for the modern hospital. Nursing homes provide individuals with ongoing nursing and personal care in an institutional (but non-hospital) setting.

It is hard to overstate the importance of the relationship between changes in the public hospital sector in the United Kingdom and the mainly privately owned, but publicly funded, nursing home sector. Between 1984 and 1998, the total bed stock of the NHS in England fell from 348,104 to 193,625 across all specialties, a reduction of 154,479 beds. Over the same period, the number of registered nursing home beds in England increased from 32,831 to 185,950, an increase of 153,119 beds. Table 5.3 shows a close statistical association between changes in NHS beds and nursing home beds, both in all specialties and in acute specialties only.

In simple terms, over the last 15 years, for every NHS bed that closed in England, a private nursing home bed opened. Much of this relationship results from a deliberately planned exercise; many patients were transferred from long-term mental illness or learning disability hospitals to smaller units now classified as nursing homes. Nursing homes have also proved vitally important in both allowing the NHS to close continuing-care beds for elderly people and allowing patients who really need continuing care to be discharged from acute beds. The almost equally close correlation between reductions in NHS acute beds and increases in nursing home beds suggests that part of the nursing home sector has provided a very close substitute for acute hospital care.

Table 5.3 Association between positive change in private nursing home bed stock and negative change in NHS hospital bed stock in England, 1984–97

	Total NHS hospital beds	NHS acute hospital beds
Pearson correlation coefficient (r)	−0.998	−0.988
P-value (two-tailed)	< 0.0001	< 0.0001
Linear regression results:		
r^2	0.996	0.976
Slope	−0.848	−0.196
95% confidence intervals of slope	−0.883 to −0.812	−0.216 to −0.175

Source: Adapted from Hensher *et al.* (1999)

The nursing home sector has grown in many countries other than the United Kingdom. Some, such as Belgium, have gone so far as to redesignate acute hospitals as nursing homes, allowing major changes in staffing ratios and skill mixes.

The expansion of the nursing home sector also offers an opportunity to opt for various mixes of public and private provision. The evaluative literature in the United Kingdom is very limited, however, and has focused primarily on long-term mental health and learning disabilities. For example, Beecham *et al.* (1997) found that community-based care for adults with learning disabilities in private nursing and residential homes was, on average, cheaper than long-term hospital care, but total costs varied six-fold among their sample. Knapp *et al.* (1997) emphasized the importance of ensuring that psychiatric care resources released through hospital closure programmes actually reach their intended targets if care quality is to be maintained; this finding is likely to hold across most care areas.

Literature from the United States on the role of nursing homes is much richer than that in the United Kingdom, and a few key themes may well be of importance in the wider European context. Kemper and Murtaugh (1991) estimated that 43 per cent of all people in the United States turning 65 years in the year 1990 would enter a nursing home at some time before they died. Of these, 55 per cent would use a nursing home for more than 1 year, and 21 per cent would have a lifetime use of 5 years or more. Fully 8.5 per cent of all Medicare hospital admissions for persons aged 65 years or over were transfers from nursing homes (Freiman and Murtaugh 1995). Meanwhile, nursing homes transfer a large proportion of their end-of-life residents to die in hospital (Smith *et al.* 1995; Fried *et al.* 1999), and the appropriateness of this practice is questioned. The growing role of nursing homes and the tendency for patients to be discharged to them from hospital sicker and after a shorter stay suggests that the nursing home sector needs more development into comprehensive geriatric centres; this requires a far greater role for physicians than has hitherto been the case (Burton 1994). Arguably, such an option marks a move back towards the traditional geriatric or continuing-care hospital model and may well have implications for the relative cost of nursing home care if adopted.

Changing information flows and relationships

Changing models of service delivery and shifting balances in the location of service delivery will have important effects on the relationships between care providers. Perhaps the key theme is the importance of good care coordination for the individual patient in an increasingly complex system. Table 5.4 illustrates some changes in information flows and interactions, using the example of the interface between general practitioners and hospital specialists in the United Kingdom. An admittedly stereotypical traditional model is presented, but this description is fairly representative of the typical level of interaction in the mid- to late 1980s.

Table 5.4 captures some information flows between only some of the actors at one of the many hospital interfaces with the external world. Closely linked to these information flows are the organizational, logistic and financial mechanisms, which attempt to transfer patients smoothly and appropriately across care boundaries. Technology *per se* has probably not led to notable improvements in information flow and interaction. Improved communication technologies have undoubtedly facilitated communication speed and ease, but quite profound changes in attitudes and assumed roles may be more important. Critically, acceptance of the need for better two-way communication, some reduction in the physical demarcation of roles and growing opportunities for personal and professional interaction between general practitioners and specialists, all mark a sea-change from the traditional model and do not depend on advances in communications and information technology.

Lessons and implications

Any analysis of hospitals must place them within the wider system of community care, social care, primary care, specialist ambulatory care and tertiary services. This whole-system approach to planning is not to be confused with a normative model, in which planners seek to ascribe a set role to each part of the system and to define parameters for their operation. The whole-system approach requires a sophisticated and subtle recognition of the complex interactions and information exchanges that take place within the hospital and between the hospital and its wider community.

Failing to appreciate the incentives, information flows and expectations that govern the behaviour of the different interfaces and behaviour within hospitals themselves will produce policy with often undesirable and unanticipated consequences. Predicting the responses of hospitals and clinicians to changes in the interfaces is difficult. The example of the creation of a new area of work by the introduction of day surgery is a salutary example of how systems can respond in ways that can contradict the intentions of policy-makers.

Failing to understand the expectations of, and influences on, the behaviour of different actors is a major obstacle to effective hospital management, whether one is arranging a specialist outpatient appointment or discussing major change in a hospital system. Filters, protocols and other methods of making the information exchange and expectations of actors explicit are probably as

Table 5.4 Changes in information flows and interaction between general practitioners and hospital consultants across the interface between primary care and hospital

Type of flow or interaction	Traditional model	Evolving model
Personal contact	Mainly informal, via education and professional associations Some general practitioner sessional specialists in hospital	Joint preparation of care protocols Commissioning and planning of services General practitioner beds More general practitioner sessional work (such as in accident and emergency departments) Consultant outreach clinics in general practice
Telephone contact	Possible, but probably quite dependent on mutual familiarity	Still true for general practitioner or consultant But patients increasingly able to contact specialist direct for advice post-discharge Urgent admission or consultation can be booked by telephone Nursing staff likely to consult by telephone with primary care team in advance of discharge
Written communication	General practitioner referral letter required to obtain outpatient appointment Consultant's discharge letter to general practitioner (sometimes sporadic)	Fax and electronic transfer speeds all written communication Referral letter may not be necessary: for example, when urgent outpatient slots are available for general practitioner's telephone referral Content of discharge letter formalized to provide agreed minimum data
Clinical data transfer	Clinical records unlikely to be transferred to general practitioner	Copy of clinical records may accompany or follow discharge letter Moving towards automatic, electronic access?
Imaging transfer	X-rays might accompany discharge letter	Copies of imaging more likely to accompany records General practitioner can have direct access to X-ray Moving towards electronic access with patient records?

important a set of policy instruments for managing interfaces as the more traditional financial incentives. Both sets of instruments are required to achieve changes in behaviour.

Once the role of primary care in managing chronic disease and some acute conditions is agreed and in operation, the hospital-discharge interface is likely to yield more opportunities to change the use of hospital facilities than are further attempts to prevent inappropriate admissions. Changing the discharge interface will have important side-effects by creating hospital capacity that could allow increased admissions. The implications for primary and social care providers need to be considered but are often ignored when the hospital is the unit of planning rather than the whole health economy. This may mean that the search for the lowest cost bed-day and the multiplication of alternative providers, each with fixed costs and assets, could increase the total cost of the health system.

Treating technocratic leadership of hospitals as though they are closed systems was never appropriate and is even less relevant today, since hospital care is increasingly a short episode in a longer patient career rather than an isolated event. An unanticipated consequence of reforms of the 1990s that broke up provider systems into stand-alone business units was the failure to achieve change in hospitals as isolated units. Hospitals have lost, or are losing, some of the prestige and power that allowed them to operate in isolation from the rest of the health care system and indeed from each other. The future leaders of hospitals need to work across all the interfaces, to communicate and to collaborate with other providers as well as to compete. They need the personal skills to influence their clinical colleagues and to persuade primary and social care providers to do the same. This may require a different type of person and approach from traditional types of hospital management.

References

Anglia and Oxford Intermediate Care Project (1997) *Opportunities in Intermediate Care: Summary Report from the Anglia and Oxford Intermediate Care Project.* Milton Keynes: NHS Executive Anglia and Oxford.

Apolone, G., Fellin, G., Tampieri, A. *et al.* (1997) Appropriateness of hospital use: report from an Italian study, *European Journal of Public Health*, 7: 34–9.

Armstrong, D. and Nicoll, M. (1995) Consultants' workload in outpatient clinics, *British Medical Journal*, 310: 581–2.

Audit Commission (1992) *Lying in Wait: The Use of Medical Beds in Acute Hospitals.* London: HMSO.

Bailey, J., Wilkin, D. and Black, E. (1994) Specialist outreach clinics in general practice, *British Medical Journal*, 308: 1083–6.

Baker, J., Goldacre, M. and Muir Gray, J.A. (1986) Community hospitals in Oxfordshire, their effect on the use of specialist in-patient services, *Journal of Epidemiology and Community Health*, 40: 117–20.

Beecham, J., Knapp, M., McGilloway, S. *et al.* (1997) The cost effectiveness of community care for adults with learning disabilities leaving long-stay hospital in Northern Ireland, *Journal of Intellectual Disabilities Research*, 41: 30–41.

Burton, J. (1994) The evolution of nursing homes into comprehensive geriatrics centres: a perspective, *Journal of the American Geriatric Society*, 42: 794–6.

Coast, J., Inglis, A., Morgan, K. *et al.* (1995) The hospital admissions study in England: are there alternatives to emergency hospital admission?, *Journal of Epidemiology and Community Health*, 49: 194–9.

Coast, J., Inglis, A. and Frankel, S. (1996) Alternatives to hospital care: what are they and who should decide?, *British Medical Journal*, 312: 162–6.

Coast, J., Richards, S., Peters, T. *et al.* (1998) Hospital at home or acute hospital care? A cost minimisation analysis, *British Medical Journal*, 316: 1802–6.

Coulter, A. (1998) Managing demand at the interface between primary and secondary care, *British Medical Journal*, 316: 1974–6.

Dawson, A., Middlemiss, C., Coles, E., Gough, N. and Jones, M. (1989) A randomised study of a domiciliary antenatal care scheme: the effect on hospital admissions, *British Journal of Obstetrics and Gynaecology*, 96: 1319–22.

Department of Health (1982) *Health and Personal Social Services Statistics for England*. London: The Stationery Office.

Department of Health (1997) *Statistical Bulletin 1996*. London: Government Statistical Service.

Dickinson, E. and Sinclair, A. (1998) *Effective Practice in Rehabilitation – Reviewing the Evidence*. London: King's Fund.

Edwards, N., Hensher, M. and Werneke, U. (1998) Changing hospital systems, in R. Saltman, J. Figueras and C. Sakellarides (eds) *Critical Challenges for Health Care Reform in Europe*. Buckingham: Open University Press.

Fertig, A., Roland, M., King, H. and Moore, T. (1993) Understanding variation in rates of referral among general practitioners: are referrals inappropriate and would guidelines help to reduce rates?, *British Medical Journal*, 318: 1467–70.

Forster, A., Young, J. and Langhorne, P. (1999) Systematic review of day hospital care for elderly people: the Day Hospital Group, *British Medical Journal*, 318(7187): 837–41.

Freiman, M. and Murtaugh, C. (1995) Interactions between hospital and nursing home use, *Public Health Reports*, 110: 546–54.

Fried, T., Pollack, D., Drickamer, M. and Tinetti, M. (1999) Who dies at home? Determinants of site of death for community-based long-term patients, *Journal of the American Geriatric Society*, 47: 25–9.

Gaspov, J., Lee, T., Weinsteing, M. *et al.* (1994) Cost-effectiveness of a new short-stay unit to 'rule-out' acute myocardial infarction in low risk patients, *Journal of the American College of Cardiology*, 24: 1249–59.

Gillam, S., Dunne, H., Ball, M. *et al.* (1995) Investigation of benefits and costs of an ophthalmic outreach clinic in general practice, *British Journal of General Practice*, 45: 649–52.

Hensher, M. and Edwards, N. (1999) Hospital provision, activity, and productivity in England since the 1980s, *British Medical Journal*, 319: 911–14.

Hensher, M., Fulop, N., Hood, S. and Ujah, S. (1996) Does hospital at home make economic sense? Results of an economic evaluation of early discharge hospital at home care for orthopaedic patients in three areas of West London, *Journal of the Royal Society of Medicine*, 89: 595–600.

Hensher, M., Fulop, N., Coast, J. and Jefferys, E. (1999) The hospital of the future: better out than in? Alternatives to acute hospital care, *British Medical Journal*, 319: 1127–30.

Kemper, P. and Murtaugh, C. (1991) Lifetime use of nursing home care, *New England Journal of Medicine*, 324: 595–600.

Knapp, M., Chisholm, D., Astin, J., Lelliott, P. and Audini, B. (1997) The cost consequences of changing the hospital–community balance: the mental health residential care study, *Psychological Medicine*, 27: 681–92.

Knotternus, J., Joosten, J. and Daams, J. (1990) Comparing the quality of referrals of general practitioners with high and average referral rates: an independent panel review, *British Journal of General Practice*, 40: 178–81.

Kornokowski, R., Zeeli, D. and Averbuch, M. (1995) Intensive home care surveillance prevents hospitalization and improves morbidity rates among elderly patients with severe congestive heart failure, *American Heart Journal*, 129: 762–6.

Marber, M., MacRae, C. and Joy, M. (1991) Delay to invasive investigation and revascularisation for coronary heart disease in South West Thames region: a two-tier system?, *British Medical Journal*, 302: 1189–91.

Raftery, J. and Stevens, A. (1998) Day case surgery trends in England: the influences of target setting and of general practitioner fundholding, *Journal of Health Services Research and Policy*, 3: 149–52.

Read, S. (1994) *Patients with Minor Injuries: A Literature Review of Options for their Treatment Outside Major A&E Departments or Occupational Health Settings*. Sheffield: Sheffield Centre for Health and Related Research.

Reid, F., Cook, D. and Majeed, A. (1999) Explaining variation in hospital admission rates: cross sectional study, *British Medical Journal*, 319: 98–103.

Richards, S., Coast, J., Gunnell, D. *et al.* (1998) Randomised controlled trial comparing effectiveness and acceptability of an early discharge hospital at home scheme with acute hospital care, *British Medical Journal*, 316: 1796–801.

Rudd, A., Wolfe, C., Tilling, K. and Beech, R. (1997) Randomised controlled trial to evaluate early discharge scheme for patients with stroke, *British Medical Journal*, 315: 1039–44.

Shepperd, S. and Iliffe, S. (2000) Hospital-at-home versus in-patient hospital care, *Cochrane Database of Systematic Reviews*, 2: CD000356.

Shepperd, S., Harwood, D., Jenkinson, C. *et al.* (1998a) Randomised controlled trial comparing hospital at home care with inpatient hospital care I: three month follow up of health outcomes, *British Medical Journal*, 316: 1786–91.

Shepperd, S., Harwood, D., Gray, A., Vessey, M. and Morgan, P. (1998b) Randomised controlled trial comparing hospital at home care with inpatient hospital care II: cost minimisation analysis, *British Medical Journal*, 316: 1791–6.

Smith, H., Pryce, A., Carlisle, L. *et al.* (1997) Appropriateness of acute medical admissions and length of stay, *Journal of the Royal College of Physicians of London*, 31: 527–32.

Smith, W., Kellerman, A. and Brown, J. (1995) The impact of nursing home transfer policies at the end of life on a public acute care hospital, *Journal of the American Geriatric Society*, 43: 1052–7.

Starfield, B. (1994) Is primary care essential?, *Lancet*, 344: 1129–33.

Steiner, A. (1997) *Intermediate Care: A Conceptual Framework and Review of the Literature*. London: King's Fund.

Surender, R., Bradlow, J., Coulter, A., Doll, H. and Stewart Brown, S. (1995) Prospective study of trends in referral patterns in fundholding and non-fundholding practices in the Oxford region, *British Medical Journal*, 311: 1205–8.

Victor, C. and Khakoo, A.A. (1994) Is hospital the right place? A survey of 'inappropriate' admissions to an inner London NHS trust, *Journal of Public Health Medicine*, 16(3): 286–90.

Victor, C., Nazareth, B., Hudson, M. and Fulop, N. (1994) The inappropriate use of acute hospital beds in an inner London District Health Authority, *Health Trends*, 25(3): 94–7.

Waghorn, A., McKee, M. and Thompson, J. (1997) Surgical outpatients: challenges and responses, *British Journal of Surgery*, 84: 300–7.

Wilson, A., Parker, H., Wynn, A. *et al.* (1997) Hospital at home is as safe as hospital, cheaper and patients like it more: early results from a randomised controlled trial, *Journal of Epidemiology and Community Health*, 51(5): 593.

chapter six

Are bigger hospitals better?

John Posnett

Introduction

Hospital services can be provided in many different ways within the overall health care system. In particular, they can be highly concentrated, with care being provided from a few very large facilities, or they can be diffuse, with care located in many small ones. The precise choice must reflect the geographical context but should also take into account evidence on whether bigger hospitals are better in their own right and whether concentrating or distributing hospital care affects patient access.

Optimum hospital scale is a function of the interaction between patient access, economies of scale and volume as a determinant of patient outcome. The current trend in many countries has been towards larger hospitals because average costs are believed to decline with size and because patient outcomes are believed to be better in hospitals in which clinicians see a larger volume of cases. The trade-off is that greater concentration leads, inevitably, to reduced patient access. This chapter reviews the research evidence on each of these factors.

Economies of scale

It is tempting to believe that larger hospitals must have lower unit costs than smaller hospitals because of the operation of economies of scale. The evidence suggests that this is unfounded. Economies of scale refer to a situation in which long-term average costs fall as the scale or volume of activity rises. Economies are expected to characterize a situation in which fixed costs are high relative to variable costs. As the volume of activity increases, average costs fall as fixed costs are spread over a larger base. Figure 6.1 shows a typical long-term average cost curve. Note that, at some point, average costs begin to

Figure 6.1   Theoretical long-term average cost curve

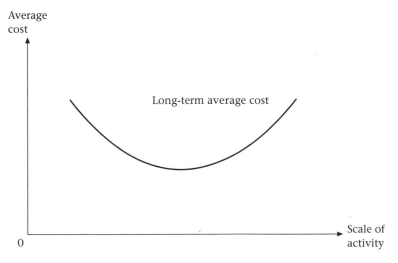

Source: Adapted from Aletras *et al.* (1997)

rise with size as economies are exhausted and additional costs generate diseconomies of scale.

Applying this concept to the acute hospital sector requires distinguishing between the effect on the average cost of increasing the rate of activity in a facility
that is currently operating at less than full capacity and comparing average
costs in two facilities of different sizes. If a hospital is staffed to a certain level, all
costs are effectively fixed up to that level; increasing activity generates economies
of scale until the capacity ceiling is reached. However, this is not the point at
issue. The belief that larger hospitals are more efficient than smaller hospitals is
based on the assumption that average costs are higher in the smaller hospital
even if both hospitals are operating at full capacity. If this belief were justified,
evidence would be expected of significant economies of scale in studies comparing unit costs between otherwise similar hospitals of different size.

In a recent systematic review of the economic literature on economies of
scale, Aletras *et al.* (1997) identified more than 100 studies. Methods varied
from studies of hospital cost functions, through econometric production function studies, to data envelopment analysis and survival analysis.

Studies of hospital cost functions are designed to identify the main determinants of the differences in observed costs between hospitals, including hospital size. Rejection of the null hypothesis (that cost does not depend on size)
is consistent with the existence of economies or diseconomies of scale. Such
studies are based on the assumption that hospitals operate in an environment
that is consistent with minimizing costs, so that observed differences in cost
are a reflection of underlying differences in efficiency.

Published studies vary in the quality of their underlying methods, and the
results of these studies must be interpreted in this light. Three important
considerations are an appropriate unit of measurement, adjustment for case
mix and adjustment for input prices.

- *An appropriate unit of measurement.* As a measure of relative efficiency, cost per case is superior to cost per day, and studies that use cost per case as the dependent variable are more robust. Because hospital costs are typically higher in the first few days after admission, a hospital that improved efficiency by reducing average lengths of inpatient stay may have higher average costs per day than a neighbouring hospital that was relatively less efficient.
- *Adjustment for case mix.* One of the most obvious determinants of differences in cost per case between hospitals is difference in case mix. Studies that do not adequately adjust for differences in resource intensity between hospitals are difficult to interpret, especially in relation to economies of scale. If larger hospitals attract a more resource-intensive workload, unit costs may be higher even in the presence of economies of scale.
- *Adjustment for input prices.* Costs are a function of the input mix and the price of individual inputs. Without adequate adjustment, differences in the cost of inputs may confound any true underlying relationship between size and efficiency.

Studies of the hospital production function have also been used to test hypotheses about economies of scale by estimating the relationship between input and output. If output increases more than an equal proportional increase in all inputs, this is obvious evidence of economies of scale. The same criteria apply in judging the quality of a production function study as in the case of cost studies.

Data envelopment analysis uses observed production relations in a sample of hospitals to construct an efficiency frontier. The relative efficiency of a particular hospital is judged by its position in relation to the frontier. Models have been developed that indicate the existence of increasing, decreasing or constant returns to scale, and these models can be used to estimate a minimum efficient scale (Banker 1984).

Survival analysis focuses attention on the process of competition and its effect in shaping the observed size distribution of hospitals in a local or national market. Underlying this type of analysis is the assumption that hospitals that prosper over time (increase market share) are in the optimum size category. Hospitals that are either too small or too large relative to the market will tend to lose market share.

Early hospital cost studies tended to be poorly controlled for differences in case mix, and most focused on cost per day as the dependent variable. Almost without exception, studies that use cost per case as the unit of analysis, and in which adjustment for case mix is adequate, show evidence of constant cost or diseconomies of scale. Pauly (1978) corrected for differences in case mix and differences in non-physician input prices and reported constant returns to scale for a sample of hospitals with a mean size of 180 beds. Evans and Walker (1972) found modest diseconomies in a sample of hospitals of various sizes from less than 25 beds to more than 1000 beds, whereas economies were reported only for hospitals with fewer than 100 beds.

Most more recent cost studies, which are better defined and adjusted for differences in case mix, also show constant cost or diseconomies of scale (Eakin and Kniesner 1988; Vita 1990; Pangilinan 1991; Kemere 1992; Scuffham *et al.* 1996). Evidence from these studies is consistent with the view that, if there are economies of scale in hospital production, such economies are exhausted at a relatively small size: in the range of 100–200 beds. Kemere (1992) reported constant returns to scale for hospitals of around 300 beds; Scuffham *et al.* (1996) found that economies of scale were fully exploited in hospitals of no more than 125 beds and Vita (1990) found evidence of diseconomies at 180 beds.

If the assumption that hospitals minimize costs is warranted, information on economies of scale can be derived from either the cost function or the production function. Econometric studies of hospital production are relatively rare, but most have shown constant or decreasing returns to scale (Feldstein 1967; Lavers and Whynes 1978; Jensen and Morrisey 1986). Little evidence is available from studies of this kind on the size of hospital at which economies are fully exploited.

Studies reporting results from data envelopment analysis generally agree that hospitals with fewer than 200 and more than 620 beds are scale-inefficient. Smaller hospitals exhibit economies of scale and larger hospitals exhibit diseconomies. There is less agreement about optimum size. Banker *et al.* (1986) and Byrnes and Valdemis (1994) estimated the optimum size to be between 220 and 260 beds. A study of French hospitals by Derveaux *et al.* (1994) suggested a higher optimum at between 500 and 520 beds. Evidence from one study (Maindiratta 1990) showed that diseconomies of scale occur slowly in relation to optimal size: a hospital needs to be very much bigger than the optimum before it is efficient to apportion activity to smaller hospitals (up to 1.8 times optimal scale).

The results from survival studies are difficult to interpret, since the observed success of a hospital in relation to other hospitals in the same market may result from factors other than the effect of size and relative efficiency. For this reason, the results of these studies should be given less weight than the results of cost or production function studies that are well controlled for case mix and other confounding factors. Most survival studies suggest that hospitals with fewer than 200 beds are scale-inefficient (Mobley 1990; Lille-Blanton *et al.* 1992; Frech and Mobley 1995). The studies by Mobley and Frech (1994) and Frech and Mobley (1995) suggest an optimum scale of 325 and 200–370 beds respectively.

The literature is extensive and covers a wide range of statistical techniques, and the results are remarkably consistent. Most studies report constant or increasing unit costs for these acute hospitals. If economies of scale are evident, these economies appear to be fully exploited at a relatively low level (in the range of 100–200 beds). Diseconomies of scale are a significant feature of hospital production, although it is difficult to generalize the level at which unit costs may be expected to rise. Somewhere in the range of 300–600 beds is consistent with the evidence. These results are not consistent with the hypothesis that larger hospitals are more efficient.

Figure 6.2 shows the general shape of the long-term average cost curve suggested by the literature. What is it about the technology of hospital production that gives rise to a long-term cost curve of this kind? Suppose a general acute hospital is defined as a grouping of complementary medical, diagnostic

Figure 6.2 Observed long-term average cost curve

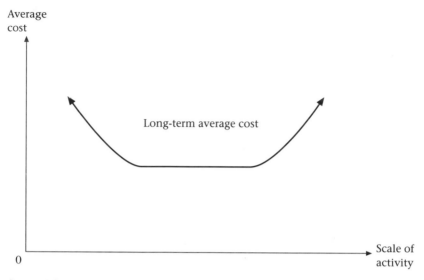

Average
cost

Long-term average cost

0

Scale of
activity

Source: Adapted from Aletras *et al.* (1997)

and support services. Once the configuration and size of the hospital is determined, appropriate staffing and equipment levels follow. Suppose further that there is a minimum scale of staffing and equipment necessary to provide all of the necessary specialties and support services characteristic of a general hospital, and that the maximum capacity of such a hospital is *x* (cases) per year. There will be unexploited economies of scale in any hospital with capacity less than *x*. The literature suggests that the minimum size of a general acute hospital is about 200 beds. However, most of the literature relates to the United Kingdom or the United States. It is important to recognize, however, that this minimum size is not the result of any inexorable technical relationship, but rather is the result of a judgement about what constitutes the minimum scale of staffing and equipment required to provide the core of complementary services that define a general hospital. This judgement may vary substantially in different countries.

As the size of the hospital increases beyond this level, staffing and equipment costs become variable. The existence of economies of scale now depends on the way in which costs rise as capacity is increased. Some costs (such as the costs of management and administration) may be fixed well beyond the minimum capacity, but most costs (such as the costs of medical, nursing and technical staff) will probably rise approximately in proportion to the increase in capacity. If this is the case, few, if any, economies of scale will be evident in larger hospitals: unit costs will be constant over this range (200 or more beds).

Diseconomies of scale become evident if some of the resources necessary to operate the hospital are not increased sufficiently to accommodate the increase in capacity. Average costs then begin to rise as excess utilization leads to inefficiency in management, higher rates of staff absence or more frequent equipment breakdown (somewhere in the range of 300–600 or more beds).

Table 6.1 Distribution of acute hospitals in England by size (including acute sites in combined National Health Service trusts)

Number of beds	Acute hospitals		Beds in acute hospitals	
	n	%	n	%
< 100	90	22.0	5 002	3.5
100–200	59	14.4	8 491	6.0
200–300	51	12.5	12 513	8.9
300–400	55	13.4	19 260	13.7
400–500	48	11.7	21 147	15.0
500–600	39	9.5	21 224	15.1
> 600	67	16.4	53 320	37.8

Source: NHS Centre for Reviews and Dissemination and Nuffield Institute for Health (1996)

To place this discussion in context, Table 6.1 shows the distribution of hospitals by size in the National Health Service in England in 1997. About 50 per cent of acute hospitals had 300 or fewer beds, but 50 per cent of capacity was in hospitals larger than 400 beds.

Volume and outcome

It has also been argued that better clinical outcomes are achieved in units with higher volumes of activity. This view is apparently supported by a large body of literature and by a number of literature reviews (Luft *et al.* 1979; Black and Johnston 1990; Banta and Bos 1991; Stiller 1994).

The process by which outcomes are improved in larger units is imperfectly understood. Possible hypotheses are that outcomes are related to the experience of individual physicians, to the skills and experience of the clinical team, or to the availability of appropriate complementary medical and support services on site. Most of the literature has focused on the first of these factors. Nevertheless, the possible existence of a relationship between volume and outcome does not necessarily suggest that outcomes are better in larger hospitals. It suggests that, for services in which a positive relationship between volume and outcome has been demonstrated, outcomes will be better if activity is concentrated in departments (or specialties) that can meet minimum volume criteria.

Most studies in this area are cross-sectional studies that compare outcomes for patients treated in one group of hospitals with low volume with those for patients treated in another group of hospitals with higher volume. A positive relationship between volume and outcome is said to exist if outcomes are better in higher-volume hospitals.

In most cases, patient outcomes are proxied by in-hospital or short-term (30-day) mortality. Procedure volumes are measured either at the level of the hospital or, less commonly, at the level of the individual clinician, and definitions of what constitutes high and low volume differ between studies. Some studies impose a volume threshold to distinguish between high and low volume; others treat volume as a continuous variable and employ regression techniques to test for the statistical significance of volume as a determinant of outcomes.

All these variants in study design are relevant in interpreting the results of published studies, but most important is the adequacy of adjustment for differences in case mix. Any observed relationship between volume and outcome will be confounded by unadjusted differences in patient prognosis. High-quality studies adjust for all of the factors likely to affect patient outcomes such as age, severity, co-morbidity and other relevant socioeconomic characteristics. Studies that adjust for risk on the basis of detailed analysis of clinical data will be the most reliable.

A systematic review (Sowden et al. 1997) has demonstrated conclusively that most of the studies in this area are either uncontrolled or poorly controlled for differences in patient prognosis. When case mix is adequately controlled, the size of the apparent relationship between volume and outcome is therefore diminished or disappears completely.

One study examined the relationship between mortality and the volume of patients admitted to adult intensive care units in the United Kingdom (Jones and Rowan 1995). Average volumes ranged from 8.3 to 37.7 cases per month. Using unadjusted mortality data, a relationship was evident between higher volume and lower mortality. However, using scores on the APACHE II Severity of Disease Classification System (Knaus et al. 1985) with further adjustments for age and chronic ill-health as a predictor of mortality for each patient, the relationship disappeared. Differences in mortality between units were no longer statistically significant. In another study, hospitals performing less than 100 coronary artery bypass procedures per year were found to have significantly greater mortality rates than hospitals performing more than 100, but the difference disappeared with adequate adjustment for differential risk (Shroyer et al. 1996). In a study of outcomes for patients treated before and after the introduction of a stroke unit, analysis of crude (unadjusted) rates of mortality suggested that the introduction of the unit had reduced mortality. However, after adjustment for age, sex and other prognostic indicators, differences in mortality were no longer significant (Davenport et al. 1996). These examples illustrate the importance of critical judgement in interpreting the results of published studies.

The systematic review by Sowden et al. (1997) summarizes evidence on the relationship between volume and quality from studies with adequate adjustment for differences in case mix (Table 6.2). The main results from this review are as follows. The sheer volume of articles showing a positive relationship between volume and outcome is misleading. Once adequate account is taken of potential confounders, the relationship either disappears or is greatly reduced. If a positive relationship remains after adjustment, the implicit volume threshold is relatively low. For example, the evidence is consistent with the hypothesis that outcomes of surgery for coronary artery bypass grafting are better in hospitals undertaking more than 200 procedures a year. However, in England, no more than 0.04 per cent of these procedures are carried out in hospitals below this threshold (NHS Centre for Reviews and Dissemination

Table 6.2 Evidence of relationship between volume and quality for various health care procedures or services or conditions from the best-quality studies

Procedure, service or condition	Evidence
Coronary artery bypass graft surgery	Slightly reduced risk of in-hospital mortality in hospitals carrying out more than 200 procedures per year (odds ratio = 0.90; 95% confidence interval = 0.82–0.98)
Paediatric heart surgery	Reduced death rate in hospitals with more than 300 cases per year compared with hospitals with less than 10 cases (odds ratio = 0.125) and more than 300 cases (odds ratio = 0.33)
Acute myocardial infarction	No significant difference for in-hospital mortality but higher 6-month mortality and lower rate of re-infarction in hospitals with more than 300 beds (mortality 17% versus 12%) Significant negative relationship between in-hospital mortality and physician volume but not hospital volume
Cardiac catheterization	No relationship with physician volume found. Mortality declines by 0.1% for every 100 increase in the annual number of hospital procedures (average number of treatments = 400)
Percutaneous transluminal coronary angioplasty	No significant association between physician volume and angiographic or clinical success Reduction in major complications when volume exceeds 400 per year (odds ratio = 0.66) No relationship with physician volume found for mortality, but more complications, emergency coronary artery bypass graft surgery and longer length of stay in physicians carrying out more than 50 procedures per year
Abdominal aortic aneurysm	Standardized mortality rate 30% higher in hospitals with more than 14 patients per year, but no relationship with surgeon volume found 12% mortality for hospitals with less than 6 procedures versus 5% for those with more than 38 per year. Low-volume surgeons had twice the mortality (< 6) of high-volume surgeons (> 26) Mortality declines by 1% for an increase of 4 operations per year per hospital (average number of treatments = 23 per year). No evidence of an effect of surgeon volume 2% increased odds of dying if surgery is in hospital with less than 21 cases compared with more than 21. This risk difference greater for ruptured aneurysms
Amputation of lower limb (no trauma)	Standardized mortality rate 16% higher in hospitals with below-average annual volume (average number of treatments = 10.5)
Gastric surgery	No significant difference between hospitals with annual volume below and above average (average number of treatments = 24 per year)

Table 6.2 (cont'd)

Procedure, service or condition	Evidence
	Mortality declines by 1% for each increase by 17 in the annual number of hospital operations (average number of treatments = 38 per year). No relationship between physician volume and mortality (average number of treatments = 8 per year)
	Surgeons carrying out one procedure annually associated with higher mortality rate than those doing more than one
	No relationship between physician volume and mortality (average number of treatments = 8)
Cholecystectomy	Standardized mortality rate 26% higher in hospitals with below-average annual volume (average number of treatments = 109 per year)
	Hospitals performing more than 168 procedures per year had a mortality rate of 1.52% compared with 1.21% in those with higher volume. No significant association with surgeon volume found
Intestinal operations (excluding cancer)	Hospital mortality higher (8.3%) when more than 40 operations performed per year compared with less than 40 operations (5.9%). Surgeons with annual volume exceeding 8 also associated with lower mortality
Gall bladder (non-surgical)	Standardized mortality rate 14% lower in hospitals with below-average annual volume (average number of treatments = 73)
Ulcer (non-surgical)	No statistically significant effect of volume
Knee replacement	Higher hospital volume associated with lower risk of complications (average number of treatments = 35)
Hip fracture	No significant effect of hospital volume on mortality (average number of treatments = 45)
Neonatal care	Infants < 28 weeks gestation had better survival in intensive care units (> 500 days of ventilation per year) than in special care units (< 500 days of ventilation per year). No difference for more mature infants
Paediatric intensive care	No statistically significant association found between mortality and monthly volume
Adult intensive care	No association between the percentage dying and monthly unit volume
Prostatectomy	No statistically significant differences found
Trauma care	No statistically significant association between mortality from major trauma and volume across accident and emergency departments with volumes ranging from less than 10 to more than 90 per year in three regions with and without an experimental trauma system
	No difference in mortality in a tertiary trauma unit for patients with mainly blunt injuries as it doubled in volume over a 4-year period

Table 6.2 (cont'd)

Procedure, service or condition	Evidence
Cataract surgery	Surgeons carrying out more than 200 operations per year had a greater rate of adverse events (especially posterior capsular opacification, odds ratio = 2.5)
AIDS	Risk of 30-day mortality was 2.5 times as high when treated in hospitals with less experience (less than 43 patients) than in a hospital having treated more than 43 patients (relative risk for 30-day mortality = 2.5)
Breast cancer	Mortality reduced by 15% among surgeons treating more than 29 new cases per year, but no advantage of more than 50 compared with more than 29
Colon and rectal cancer	Mortality rate 20% higher in hospitals with below-average annual volume (average number of treatments = 17)
Laparotomy with colorectal resection (for cancer and non-cancer diagnoses)	No significant association between volume and in-hospital mortality (average number of treatments = 50) or surgeon volume (average number of treatments = 8)
Laparotomy with colorectal resection (for cancer and non-cancer diagnoses)	No statistically significant differences in mortality or morbidity between surgeons with volumes ranging from 44 to 110 cases per year
Stomach cancer	No statistically significant association between mortality and either hospital or surgeon volume
Malignant teratoma	Mortality after 5 years 60% lower in patients treated at a cancer unit that treated more than 50% of patients with this type of cancer in the area
Oesophageal cancer	Operative mortality rate 17% lower in surgeons performing less than three operations annually Mortality after 5 years reduced by 4% among surgeons treating more than 5 new cases per year, mostly explained by reduced operative deaths
Pancreatic cancer	Patients treated by surgeons with the highest volume (76 cases in 20 months) had the lowest risk of complications (fistula) compared with lower-volume surgeons in the same hospital

Note: Outcomes in this table are adjusted for case mix. The results of studies with less adequate adjustment for case mix are not summarized here. Odds ratio is the ratio of the odds of an adverse event occurring in a higher-volume unit compared to a low-volume unit; if the odds ratio is less than 1, then there is less risk of a poor outcome in the higher-volume unit.

Source: NHS Centre for Reviews and Dissemination and Nuffield Institute for Health (1996)

and Nuffield Institute for Health 1996). An experience effect should be evident in a positive relationship between outcomes and physician volume. Of the 16 studies identified by Sowden *et al.* (1997) that included a measure of physician volume (Table 6.2), nine found no significant differences in mortality or rates of complications associated with annual physician volumes. Another six reported a positive association between volume and outcomes and one suggested that surgeons carrying out more than 200 cataract operations annually had a higher rate of adverse events.

Other studies have found a positive relationship between outcomes and hospital volumes. Most of these studies did not include a measure of physician volume, but four studies reported a significant relationship between outcomes and hospital volume but no relationship with the volumes of individual clinicians. Kelly and Hellinger (1986) found a hospital volume effect but no physician volume relationship for cardiac catheterization. Two studies (Flood *et al.* 1984; Kelly and Hellinger 1986) have found a significant relationship for abdominal aortic aneurysm with hospital volumes but not with the volumes of individual clinicians. Hannan *et al.* (1989) reported a similar result for cholecystectomy.

One of the most important conclusions to emerge from the existing evidence is that a good deal more needs to be understood about the processes associated with better clinical outcomes. On its own, volume of activity is too crude an indicator to be useful in planning clinical services.

After controlling for patient characteristics affecting prognosis, outcomes are likely to be determined by a range of factors. These include the skill and experience of individual clinicians, the composition and experience of the medical and nursing team, appropriate training, availability of complementary medical and support services, and the range of diagnostic and surgical procedures in use. Most of the research literature has focused on the importance of clinical experience, proxied by volume, to the exclusion of all other factors, and this focus has been very influential in the trend towards greater concentration of services into larger hospitals. Nevertheless, outcomes could be improved without the need to concentrate services through better training, effective teamwork and the development of evidence-based protocols for diagnosis and treatment.

Patient access

The trend towards greater centralization of services into larger hospitals implies a reduction in patient access, as small local hospitals are closed. The potential negative effect of reduced geographical access on health status should not be overlooked. From an individual viewpoint, a decision to seek health care will be a function of cost, the perceived severity of the condition (relative to 'normal health') and the expected effectiveness of treatment. Other things being equal, the greater the costs of access, the less severe the condition and the less effective treatment is perceived to be, the lower will be the rate of utilization.

In a health care context, access is primarily about the social and economic costs of utilization. Social costs include those costs associated with inconvenient opening hours (such as for those in work), or particular costs imposed on users from different ethnic backgrounds (such as language barriers). Economic costs include user charges, travel costs and the opportunity cost of time. The greater the costs of use, the less accessible the service.

The relative accessibility of health care facilities is expected to have effects at three levels: the initial decision by the patient to consult (to seek a primary diagnosis); the decision of the primary care clinician to refer for specialist assessment; and the patient's decision to comply with treatment.

Higher access cost is likely to have its greatest impact on the initial decision to consult or on the use of diagnostic services (including primary care consultation, screening and some outpatient services). This is because a patient is more likely to perceive the benefits of care after diagnosis than in the symptomatic or pre-symptomatic stages of disease. In this context, access to primary care is one of the most important dimensions of the accessibility of health care services.

High costs of access to secondary or tertiary care are expected to have a lower impact in deterring referral and compliance because, assuming that treatment is perceived to be of value, the expected benefits are more likely to offset the costs. However, it is important to recognize that, when accessibility is reduced, the effect is to shift some of the costs of health care to patients and their care-givers. The response to this increase in cost is not expected to be uniform across the population, and studies that show no significant deterrent effect overall may mask significant effects for particular groups, such as those with low income or restricted personal mobility.

The published research in this area focuses almost exclusively on the relationship between observed rates of utilization and distance, or travel time as a proxy for access. This is a partial approach because, as noted above, distance is only one of a number of factors affecting access.

Most studies of patient access are cross-sectional, comparing rates of utilization between populations living at different distances from a health care facility. Most are poorly controlled for the potential effect of confounders such as differences in health care needs. For example, if populations living in inner-city areas have higher rates of utilization than populations living in outlying suburbs, this is not conclusive evidence of a deterrent effect of distance. It may simply reflect the fact that inner-city populations need more health care. Few studies have examined the effect of access on health outcomes. Carr-Hill *et al.* (1997) have reviewed studies of patient access, and this summary draws heavily on that review.

There is evidence of a deterrent effect of increasing distance on primary care consultations for both urban and rural populations (Parkin 1979; Whitehouse 1985; Bentham and Haynes 1992; Veitch 1995). Evidence from France (Launoy *et al.* 1992) of more severe symptoms on diagnosis in the rural population, especially women, may reflect delayed presentation caused by the higher costs of access in rural areas. Jones (1996) found increased mortality from neoplasm of the female breast in areas with less access to primary care services.

There is also evidence of a negative association between distance and rates of self-referral to accident and emergency departments (Magnusson 1980; Bentham and Haynes 1985; McKee *et al.* 1990). In a study of attendances at an accident department in Scotland, Campbell (1994) found a clear deterrent effect on self-referral but no distance effect when a patient was referred by their primary care physician.

Evidence relating to the take-up of screening services indicates a negative effect of distance in the case of opportunistic cytology screening (Bentham *et al.* 1995) and mammography (Haiart *et al.* 1990; Hurley *et al.* 1994). A study by Majeed *et al.* (1994) illustrates that distance is not the only important dimension of access, the uptake of cervical smear tests being higher in practices with a female physician.

A number of studies have suggested that rates of hospital utilization are lower in communities living further from hospitals. The hypothesis about the determinants of utilization suggests that the effect of distance will be greatest for diagnostic procedures and for conditions in which there is disagreement about the benefits of treatment.

Goodman *et al.* (1994) found that utilization of inpatient medical services for children under 15 years declines with travel time to the hospital. Gittelsohn and Powe (1995) found that a distance of more than 130 km was significant in determining the rates of coronary artery bypass graft surgery and other discretionary surgical procedures. In France, Launoy *et al.* (1992) found that patients living further from the referral centre were less likely to receive specialist treatment for colorectal cancer. Wood (1985) found that hospital utilization declined when the patients lived more than 5 km from their primary care physician and when the practice was more than 56 km from the hospital. Black *et al.* (1995) found that rates of coronary revascularization increase with the presence of a local cardiologist and decrease with increasing distance from the specialist centre. Slack *et al.* (1997) found a significant inverse relationship between rates of hospitalization and travel times to the nearest hospital.

However, not all the research evidence suggests that distance reduces access. Grumbach *et al.* (1995) compared coronary artery bypass graft surgery rates in New York, California, Ontario and British Columbia. They found that greater distance was not associated with lower rates of coronary artery bypass graft surgery in Canada, whereas in the United States, where overall rates of surgery were higher, there was evidence of a distance effect. Anderson and Lomas (1989) also found no evidence that rates of coronary artery bypass graft surgery in Ontario were affected by distances ranging from 24 to 190 km. Other studies have found no relationship between distance and utilization for admissions for heart disease (Gittelsohn and Powe 1995) and hip replacement (Roos and Lyttle 1985).

It is difficult from this evidence alone to identify the separate effects of patient access on the referral behaviour of physicians and on the willingness of patients to comply with medical advice. If physicians act as agents for their patients, it is perfectly rational for a physician's referral decision to be influenced by the access costs faced by patients. A few studies have focused on the referral behaviour of physicians. Greenberg *et al.* (1988) found that referral of lung cancer patients for specialist treatment was strongly related to the distance between the referral centre and the patient's home (from 25 to more than 120 km). Roos and Sharp (1989) found physicians in Western Manitoba reluctant to refer patients to Winnipeg for coronary artery bypass graft surgery. In contrast, Clarke *et al.* (1995) found that referrals of patients with testicular cancer to specialist cancer centres were similar throughout Scotland and were not affected by distance.

Part of the reason for apparent lower rates of hospitalization in communities living further from health services may be that patients themselves decide not to comply with recommended referral or follow-up. If this is the case, it should be evident in attendance at outpatient appointments, clinics or pre-booked elective admissions. The evidence is mixed.

Drop-out rates at clinics for alcoholism and diabetes have been shown to increase with distance (Prue *et al.* 1979; Graber *et al.* 1992; Fortney *et al.* 1995). Haynes and Bentham (1979) found that attendance at outpatient clinics declined with distance (> 16 km); Bentham and Haynes (1985) reported a similar result. Kaliszer and Kidd (1981) found that women living more than 7 km from an antenatal clinic presented on average 3 weeks later for a first appointment. Other studies have reported no apparent effect of distance on attendance for paediatric allografts (Meyers *et al.* 1995), investigation after breast screening (Kohli *et al.* 1995), radiotherapy (Junor *et al.* 1992) and day case cataract surgery (Strong *et al.* 1991).

Studies of the relationship between access and patient outcomes are rare. Some studies have found that reduced access increases the rates of mortality for road traffic accidents, diabetes mellitus and asthma (Jones and Bentham 1995; Jones 1996) and acute medical post-neonatal syndromes in children under 5 (Kelly and Munan 1974). There appears to be no such association for breast cancer, cervical cancer, hypertension and stroke or peptic ulcer (Jones 1996).

Reduced access to health care facilities increases the costs of utilization. The research evidence suggests that increased cost will have the greatest effect on the use of diagnostic, outpatient and screening services, especially primary care. Health outcomes are reduced to the extent that delayed presentation is associated with greater severity and a poorer prognosis, or where the condition is immediately life-threatening. Local access to primary diagnostic services and emergency treatment should be a priority.

Evidence of the impact of distance on the use of secondary and tertiary services is mixed. Some studies have suggested that rates of referral and intervention are lower in populations living further from a hospital. Other studies have shown no significant effect of distance on rates of hospital utilization.

Most of the literature relates to the United Kingdom or North America. It is important when interpreting these results to consider their relevance to the local context. In particular, the magnitude of the distances involved should be considered relative to the availability of transport and levels of income. A study carried out in a small, affluent and relatively densely populated country such as the United Kingdom may be of little relevance elsewhere.

Even if no overall disincentive effect of distance is apparent, effects may be significant for specific groups in the population, notably those with low incomes or restricted personal mobility. Reducing access by centralizing hospital services will have the greatest effect on the health outcomes of those in the most vulnerable groups and is likely to increase existing inequity in health status.

Optimum hospital scale

The first conclusion that follows from the research literature is that costs cannot generally be presumed to be lower or outcomes better in larger hospitals. The literature on economies of scale suggests that scale economies are fully exploited in the range of 100–200 beds. The vast literature on the relationship between volume and outcome has identified volume gains for some specific procedures, but these gains are achieved at a relatively low threshold.

The determinants of patient outcome are poorly understood, and the emphasis on volume as a proxy for the skill and experience of individual clinicians is probably misplaced. A good deal more needs to be understood about the processes that drive good outcomes. The importance of on-going training, teamwork, adherence to evidence-based protocols and appropriate support services should not be overlooked.

The research evidence suggests that the optimal scale of an acute hospital depends on the interaction between the health care needs of a local population and the extent of interrelationships between specialties within the hospital. The evidence on economies of scale suggests that the optimal hospital size is determined by the minimum core of complementary medical, surgical and support services necessary to provide the range of health services required. This is important: optimal hospital size is a direct function of the health care needs of the local population that it is designed to serve.

Once the range of services required by the local population is determined, the size of the hospital then depends on the extent of necessary complementary and support services (links between specialties). Support services include pathology, imaging, catering, pharmacy, building maintenance and personnel. Complementary services are the medical or surgical services required to support other specialties; for example, general surgery, paediatrics, general medicine and elderly medicine support an accident and emergency department. Appropriate space, equipment and staffing follow from the defined range of services.

Although guidelines have been produced in a number of countries, the precise relationship between inter-specialty links and patient outcomes is poorly understood. In most countries, guidelines are based on the opinions of the medical profession rather than on research evidence, and the same is true of staffing norms. Better research evidence is needed in this area.

In the absence of compelling evidence of the benefits of scale in hospital provision, the potential trade-off between access, efficiency and outcomes becomes less stark. Current research offers no convincing argument against the proposition that small hospitals can be efficient and can produce good outcomes for patients. However, despite the research evidence, increasing concentration in hospital services (often through mergers) continues to be a major aim of health policy in a number of countries. This is not entirely irrational. In a private health care market, hospital mergers may be justified primarily as a means of reducing competition and enhancing profitability.

In a public system, mergers may be justified for two reasons. The first is where hospitals are currently operating at less than full capacity. The evidence is consistent with the expectation that costs can be reduced by the elimination of duplication and excess capacity through merger and rationalization. However, elimination of excess capacity has little to do with economies of scale. The second reason is if rationalizing clinical services is justified by evidence of the relationship between service organization and patient outcomes. Furthermore, medical and surgical associations often press for minimum levels of consultant staffing that are difficult to achieve in small hospitals, and rationalization may be easier to achieve if clinician teams are part of a single organization. Thus, mergers may be justified as a least-cost means of achieving changes in clinical practice.

The burden of proof must be with those who propose concentration to quantify the expected benefits and costs and to explain the process by which benefits will be realized in practice.

References

Aletras, V., Jones, A. and Sheldon, T. (1997) Economies of scale and scope, in B. Ferguson, T. Sheldon and J. Posnett (eds) *Concentration and Choice in Healthcare*. London: Royal Society of Medicine.

Anderson, G.M. and Lomas, J. (1989) Regionalization of coronary artery bypass surgery: effects on access, *Medical Care*, 27: 288–96.

Banker, R.D. (1984) Measuring most productive scale size using data envelopment analysis, *European Journal of Operational Research*, 17: 35–44.

Banker, R.D., Conrad, R.F. and Strauss, R.P. (1986) A comparative application of data envelopment analysis and translog methods: an illustrative study of hospital production, *Management Science*, 32: 30–44.

Banta, D. and Bos, M. (1991) The relation between quantity and quality with coronary artery bypass graft (CABG) surgery, *Health Policy*, 18: 1–10.

Bentham, G. and Haynes, R. (1985) Health, personal mobility and the use of health services in rural Norfolk, *Journal of Rural Studies*, 1: 231–9.

Bentham, G. and Haynes, R. (1992) Evaluation of a mobile branch surgery in a rural area, *Social Science and Medicine*, 34: 97–102.

Bentham, G., Hinton, J., Haynes, R. *et al.* (1995) Factors affecting non-response to cervical cytology screening in Norfolk, England, *Social Science and Medicine*, 40: 131–5.

Black, N. and Johnston, A. (1990) Volume and outcome in hospital care: evidence, explanations and implications, *Health Services Management Research*, 3: 108–14.

Black, N., Langham, S. and Petticrew, M. (1995) Coronary revascularisation: why do rates vary geographically in the UK?, *Journal of Epidemiology and Community Health*, 49: 408–12.

Byrnes, P. and Valdemis, V. (1994) Analysing technical and allocative efficiency in hospitals, in A. Charnes, W.W. Cooper, A.Y. Lewin and L.M. Seiford (eds) *Data Envelopment Analysis: Theory, Methodology and Applications*. Dordrecht: Kluwer.

Campbell, J.L. (1994) General practitioner appointment systems, patient satisfaction and use of accident and emergency services: a study in one geographical area, *Family Practice*, 11: 438–45.

Carr-Hill, R.A., Place, M. and Posnett, J. (1997) Access and the utilisation of healthcare services, in B. Ferguson, T. Sheldon and J. Posnett (eds) *Concentration and Choice in Healthcare*. London: Royal Society of Medicine.

Clarke, K., Howard, G.C.W., Elia, M.H. *et al.* (1995) Referral patterns within Scotland to specialist oncology centres for patients with testicular germ cell tumours, *British Journal of Cancer*, 72: 1300–2.

Davenport, R.J., Dennis, M.S. and Warlow, C.P. (1996) Effect of correcting outcome data for case-mix: an example from stroke medicine, *British Medical Journal*, 312: 1503–5.

Derveaux, B., Leleu, H., Lebrun, T. and Boussemart, J.P. (1994) Construction d'un indice de production pour le secteur hospitalier public: Version provisoire [Construction of an index of production for the public hospital sector: Provisional version], *Xvemes Journees des Economistes de la Santé*, 20–21 Janvier.

Eakin, K.B. and Kniesner, T.J. (1988) Estimating a non-minimum cost function for hospitals, *Southern Economic Journal*, 54: 583–97.

Evans, R.G. and Walker, H.D. (1972) Information theory and the analysis of hospital cost structure, *Canadian Journal of Economics*, 5: 398–418.

Feldstein, M.S. (1967) *Economic Analysis for Health Services Efficiency: Econometric Studies of the British National Health Service*. Amsterdam: North-Holland.

Flood, A.B., Scott, W.R. and Ewy, W. (1984) Does practice make perfect? 1: The relation between hospital volume and outcomes for selected diagnostic categories, *Medical Care*, 22: 98–114.

Fortney, J.C., Booth, B.M., Blow, F.C. and Bunn, J.Y. (1995) The effects of travel barriers and age on the utilization of alcoholism treatment aftercare, *American Journal of Drug and Alcohol Abuse*, 21: 391–406.

Frech, H.E. and Mobley, L.R. (1995) Resolving the impasse on hospital scale economies: a new approach, *Applied Economics*, 27: 286–96.

Gittelsohn, A. and Powe, N.R. (1995) Small area variations in health care delivery in Maryland, *Health Service Research*, 30: 295–317.

Goodman, D.C., Fisher, E.S., Gittelsohn, A. *et al.* (1994) Why are children hospitalized? The role of non-clinical factors in pediatric hospitalizations, *Pediatrics*, 93: 896–902.

Graber, A.L., Davidson, P., Brown, A.W. *et al.* (1992) Dropout and relapse during diabetes care, *Diabetes Care*, 15: 1477–83.

Greenberg, E.R., Dain, B., Freeman, D. *et al.* (1988) Referral of lung cancer patients to university hospital centres: a population based study in two rural states, *Cancer*, 62: 1647–52.

Grumbach, K., Anderson, G.M., Luft, H.S. *et al.* (1995) Regionalization of cardiac surgery in the United States and Canada: geographic access, choice and outcomes, *Journal of the American Medical Association*, 274: 1282–9.

Haiart, D.C., McKenzie, L., Henderson, J. *et al.* (1990) Mobile breast screening: factors affecting uptake, efforts to increase response and accessibility, *Public Health*, 104: 239–47.

Hannan, E.L., O'Donnell, J.F., Kilburn, H. *et al.* (1989) Investigation of the relationship between volume and mortality for surgical procedures performed in New York State hospitals, *Journal of the American Medical Association*, 262: 503–10.

Haynes, R.M. and Bentham, C.G. (1979) *Community Hospitals and Rural Accessibility*. Farnborough: Saxon House.

Hurley, S.F., Huggins, R.M., Jolley, D.J. *et al.* (1994) Recruitment activities and socio-demographic factors that predict attendances at a mammographic screening program, *American Journal of Public Health*, 84: 1655–8.

Jensen, G.A. and Morrisey, M.A. (1986) The role of the physician in hospital production, *Review of Economics and Statistics*, 63: 432–42.

Jones, A.P. (1996) *Health Service Accessibility and Health Outcomes*. Norwich: University of East Anglia.

Jones, A.P. and Bentham, G. (1995) Emergency medical service accessibility and outcome from road traffic accidents, *Public Health*, 109: 169–77.

Jones, J. and Rowan, K. (1995) Is there a relationship between the volume of work carried out in intensive care and its outcome?, *International Journal of Technology Assessment in Health Care*, 11: 762–9.

Junor, E.J., Macbeth, F.R. and Barrett, A. (1992) An audit of travel and waiting times for outpatient radiotherapy, *Clinical Oncology*, 4: 174–6.

Kaliszer, M. and Kidd, M. (1981) Some factors affecting attendance at ante-natal clinics, *Social Science and Medicine*, 15: 421–4.

Kelly, A. and Munan, L. (1974) Epidemiological patterns of childhood mortality and their relation to distance from medical care, *Social Science and Medicine*, 8: 363–7.

Kelly, J.V. and Hellinger, F.J. (1986) Physician and hospital factors associated with mortality of surgical patients, *Medical Care*, 24(9): 785–800.

Kemere, P. (1992) *The Structure of Hospital Costs: An Econometric Analysis of Short Term General Hospitals in Maryland*. Washington, DC: Howard University.

Kohli, H.S., Teo, P.Y., Howie, F.M. and Dobson, H.M. (1995) How accessible is the breast screening assessment centre for Lanarkshire women?, *Health Bulletin*, 53: 153–8.

Knaus, W.A., Draper, E.A., Wagner, D.P. and Zimmerman, J.E. (1985) APACHE II: a severity of disease classification system, *Critical Care Medicine*, 13: 818–29.

Launoy, G., Le Coutour, X., Gignoux, M., Pottier, D. and Dugleux, G. (1992) Influence of rural environment on diagnosis, treatment and prognosis of colorectal cancer, *Journal of Epidemiology and Community Health*, 46: 365–7.

Lavers, R.J. and Whynes, D.K. (1978) A production function of English maternity hospitals, *Socio-economic Planning Sciences*, 12: 85–93.

Lille-Blanton, M., Felt, S., Redmon, P. *et al.* (1992) Rural and urban hospital closures 1985–88: operating and environmental characteristics that affect risk, *Inquiry*, 29: 332–4.

Luft, H.S., Bunker, J.P. and Enthoven, A.C. (1979) Should operations be regionalized? The empirical relationship between surgical volume and mortality, *New England Journal of Medicine*, 301: 1364–9.

Magnusson, G. (1980) The role of proximity in the use of hospital emergency departments, *Sociology of Health and Illness*, 2: 202–14.

Maindiratta, A. (1990) Largest size-efficient scale and size efficiencies of decision-making units in data envelopment analysis, *Journal of Econometrics*, 46: 57–72.

Majeed, F.A., Cook, D.G., Anderson, H.R. *et al.* (1994) Using patient and general practice characteristics to explain variations in cervical smear uptake rates, *British Medical Journal*, 308: 1272–6.

McKee, C.M., Gleadhill, D.N. and Watson, J.D. (1990) Accident and emergency attendance rates: variation among patients from different general practices, *British Journal of General Practice*, 40: 150–3.

Meyers, K.E., Weiland, H. and Thompson, P.D. (1995) Paediatric renal transplantation non-compliance, *Pediatric Nephrology*, 9: 189–92.

Mobley, L.R. (1990) *Multihospital Systems in California: Behaviour and Efficiency*. Santa Barbara, CA: University of California at Santa Barbara.

Mobley, L.R. and Frech, H.E. (1994) Firm growth and failure in increasingly competitive markets: theory and application to hospital markets, *Journal of the Economics of Business*, 1: 77–93.

NHS Centre for Reviews and Dissemination and Nuffield Institute for Health (1996) Hospital volume and health care outcomes, costs and patient access, *Effective Health Care*, 2(8): 1–16.

Pangilinan, M.B. (1991) Production/cost inefficiency and flexible cost functions: the case of New York State hospitals, 1981–1987. PhD dissertation, State University of New York at Albany, Albany, NY.

Parkin, D. (1979) Distance as an influence on demand in general practice, *Epidemiology and Community Health*, 33: 96–9.

Pauly, M.V. (1978) Medical staff characteristics and hospital costs, *Journal of Human Resources*, 13(suppl.): 77–111.

Prue, D.M., Keane, T.M., Cornell, J.E. and Foy, D.W. (1979) An analysis of distance variables that affect aftercare attendance, *Community Mental Health Journal*, 15: 149–54.

Roos, N.P. and Lyttle, D. (1985) The centralization of operations and access to treatment: total hip replacement in Manitoba, *American Journal of Public Health*, 75: 130–3.

Roos, N.P. and Sharp, S.M. (1989) Innovation, centralization and growth: coronary artery bypass surgery in Manitoba, *Medical Care*, 27: 441–52.

Scuffham, P.A., Devlin, N.J. and Jaforullah, M. (1996) The structure of costs and production in New Zealand public hospitals: an application of the transcendental logarithmic variable cost function, *Applied Economics*, 28: 78–85.

Shroyer, A.L., Marshall, G., Warner, B.A. *et al.* (1996) No continuous relationship between Veterans Affairs hospital coronary artery bypass grafting surgical volume and operative mortality, *Annals of Thoracic Surgery*, 61: 17–20.

Slack, R., Ferguson, B. and Ryder, S. (1997) Analysis of hospitalisation rates by electoral ward: relationship to accessibility and deprivation data, *Health Services Management Research*, 10: 24–31.

Sowden, A.J., Watt, I. and Sheldon, T.A. (1997) Volume of activity and healthcare quality: is there a link?, in B. Ferguson, T.A. Sheldon and J. Posnett (eds) *Concentration and Choice in Healthcare*. London: Royal Society of Medicine.

Stiller, C.A. (1994) Centralised treatment, entry to trials and survival, *British Journal of Cancer*, 70: 252–62.

Strong, N.P., Wigmore, W., Smithson, S. *et al.* (1991) Day case cataract surgery, *British Journal of Ophthalmology*, 75: 731–3.

Veitch, P.C. (1995) Anticipated response to three common injuries by rural and remote area residents, *Social Science and Medicine*, 41: 739–45.

Vita, M.G. (1990) Exploring hospital production relationships with flexible functional forms, *Journal of Health Economics*, 9: 1–21.

Whitehouse, C.R. (1985) Effects of distance from surgery on consultation rates in an urban practice, *British Medical Journal*, 290: 359–62.

Wood, P.W. (1985) *Geographical Equity and Inpatient Hospital Care: An Empirical Analysis.* Aberdeen: Health Economics Research Unit, University of Aberdeen.

chapter seven

Investing in hospitals

Martin McKee and Judith Healy

Introduction

The World Health Report 2000 (WHO 2000) identified three overall goals of a health care system: achieving good health for the population, ensuring that health services are responsive to the public and ensuring fair payment systems. The hospital has a central role in achieving these goals. The hospital does not, however, act alone. Government, and those acting on its behalf, have a responsibility to create the conditions in which hospitals can function and that ensure the long-term sustainability of a hospital system. In other words, governments and other societal institutions must invest wisely in improving the performance of hospitals. Specifically, *The World Health Report 2000* maintained that governments have a 'stewardship' function in that they retain ultimate responsibility for a country's health care system and that they, or those acting on their behalf, should set and monitor the overall goals of a health care system.

Hospitals are, therefore, increasingly subject to pressure to improve performance from central, regional or local governments and their agents, such as social insurance funds, and from other external bodies, such as professional associations and consumer groups. Hospitals must also comply with legislative requirements across a range of areas. Paradoxically, as hospital managers gain greater autonomy in how they run their hospitals, they are required to pursue externally defined goals and to account for their progress in achieving them.

Hospitals require an array of inputs to function effectively. Earlier work on the relationship between inputs and outputs of hospitals (the production function) (Montford 1981) focused on narrow outputs such as the numbers of patients treated, adjusted for case mix (Jensen and Morrisey 1986). Consequently, these models concentrated on the classical economic inputs of physical and human capital. In the new context, where the focus of policy-makers has shifted to the health gain that the hospital achieves and to the other goals of the hospital such as training and research, the inputs need to expand to

Figure 7.1   External levers to improve hospital performance

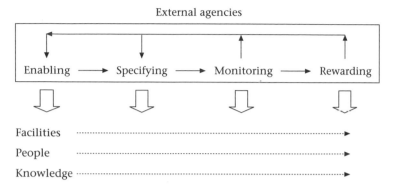

encompass intellectual capital (knowledge) (Buxton and Hanney 1996). In addition, recognition is growing of the need to include social capital in any consideration of institutional performance (Putnam 1992). Chapter 14 discusses the role of social capital in the health sector in relation to organizational culture.

Many of these inputs are the products of systems that are external to the hospital. Thus, there are many points at which external authorities can influence both the establishment and the ongoing functioning of a hospital. This chapter examines the means by which external bodies seek to influence hospital performance. We offer a framework for considering how these external bodies might act on the inputs that hospitals require using selected strategies as examples (Figure 7.1).

External authorities can pursue a range of strategies that address one or more sets of inputs. Here, we identify and discuss some of the main strategies for improving hospital performance. These are intended as illustrations rather than as an exhaustive list. Other strategies might include pharmaceutical regulation, health and safety regulations, building regulations and many others that, although they are important, are less specific to the work of the hospital. Our selected strategies are classified (in Table 7.1) according to the type of resource

Table 7.1   Inputs and policy levers: examples of strategies

Inputs	Enabling	Specifying	Monitoring	Rewarding
Facilities	Access to capital	Directing investment		Incentives to invest
People	Training and education	Workforce size and mix Revalidation Patients' rights	Performance monitoring	
Knowledge	Research and development	Population needs assessment Guidance on effectiveness		

and type of policy action and provide a framework for the format of this chapter. Many strategies involve a combination of inputs and a combination of actions, and we argue that success is more likely if action is coordinated. This chapter first discusses these strategies according to the input involved. Here, physical capital is encapsulated by the term 'facilities', human capital by 'people' and intellectual capital by 'knowledge'. Social capital, or culture, influences relationships between the hospital and external agencies (Saltman *et al.* 2001). Based on the evidence from other sectors, benefits are likely from long-term collaborative arrangements between external agencies and hospitals, based on trust (Fukuyama 1992) rather than confrontational, short-term interactions. However, the health-sector research on this topic primarily considers the role of trust within the hospital. Consequently, social capital is not discussed in this chapter but is examined in Chapter 10, which deals with the hospital's internal environment. We then examine three activities that bear on multiple inputs: accreditation, strategic purchasing and integrated quality programmes.

Facilities

Ownership

Improving health care facilities requires discussing hospital ownership, an issue subject to much misunderstanding. In the past, a simple taxonomy was sufficient, encompassing government, voluntary-sector and for-profit hospitals (Roemer 1993). More recently, a variety of models has emerged with the distinctions between them becoming increasingly blurred (Box 7.1). In Europe, most models can be considered to lie within the broadly defined public sector, although this also encompasses non-governmental bodies that essentially act on behalf of governments, from whom they often obtain a considerable proportion of their capital funding.

This taxonomy illustrates the wide variety of models that exists. However, it also raises fundamental questions about what is meant by a hospital and by ownership. Although hospitals that are fully privately owned are rare in Europe, fully publicly owned hospitals are also becoming less frequent. Is a hospital defined in terms of physical buildings and equipment or in terms of clinical service delivery? In some countries, one may be public but the other private. What is the difference between for-profit and not-for-profit owners in the non-governmental sector? What is the difference between private ownership in a relatively unregulated system and in a highly regulated one?

In response to these questions, Chapter 9 proposes a classification of hospitals according to five dimensions: autonomy, market exposure, degree of financial responsibility, accountability and social functions. A hospital might be located at a different point along the continuum for each of these dimensions, and might be classified as a budgetary, autonomized, corporatized or privatized hospital (Harding and Preker 2001). For the present purposes, the key point is that most hospitals in Europe remain dependent primarily on government, in some form or other, for funds for investment.

Box 7.1 Models of hospital ownership

Government-owned and -managed hospitals
Government (central, regional or local) ownership exists in all parts of Europe. Such hospitals are accounting units within the relevant tier of government. Managers and other staff may be employed as civil servants. This model is common in countries in which health care is funded from taxation, as in Scandinavia, where hospitals are owned by county councils, but it also exists in countries with social insurance systems. In France, for example, the government owns 65 per cent of hospital beds. In many countries in central and eastern Europe, ownership has been transferred from central to local government during the 1990s.

Public-sector autonomous hospitals
Public-sector autonomous hospitals offer a mechanism by which governments retain ultimate ownership of assets but give some autonomy to hospital management. The hospital may have an independent legal status to enable it to enter into a contract with a health insurance fund, although, in the United Kingdom, the extent to which these contracts can be enforced in law may be restricted. A commonly cited example is the creation in the United Kingdom from 1990 onwards of National Health Service trusts (Robinson and Dixon 1999). Similar models have been adopted in some parts of central and eastern Europe.

Geographically defined health boards
Geographically defined health boards exist in several countries that organize their health care systems along regional lines, such as Ireland. Governments act through boards that manage groups of hospitals. The boards may be elected, appointed or a combination of both. Regional boards offer greater opportunities to coordinate services in neighbouring hospitals but may constrain the scope of local decision-making.

State-owned enterprises
A state-owned enterprise is registered under law as an autonomous legal entity entitled to raise and keep some of its own revenue. In Kazakhstan, from 1997 onwards, former government hospitals could seek independent legal and financial status. The expectation was that about one-quarter of health facilities would become state-owned enterprises, but the distinction between for-profit and not-for-profit status remains confused (Kulzhanov and Healy 1999).

Public not-for-profit hospitals
Public not-for-profit hospitals are owned by voluntary groups, such as religious organizations and trade unions. In many cases, funds for investment are still provided by government and they often act within a highly constrained regulatory environment.

Joint stock hospitals
Joint stock hospitals have been developed in Georgia, in part in response to that country's problems in financing health care. Hospitals are owned jointly by government and private for-profit companies.

Private management of publicly owned hospitals
Publicly owned and privately managed hospitals exist in Portugal and some other countries. The state retains ownership of hospital assets, but the management of the facility is contracted to the private sector.

Public management of privately owned hospitals
The private sector can be responsible for financing, constructing and maintaining hospital buildings and equipment but the public sector provides clinical services from these facilities. This is becoming an important means of securing acute hospital services in the United Kingdom under a mechanism known as the Private Finance Initiative (see Box 7.2).

Private for-profit hospitals
Private for-profit hospitals are widespread in the United States, where many formerly not-for-profit hospitals have changed their status, but are less common in Europe. Such hospitals do, however, account for up to one-fifth of hospital capacity in countries such as France, Portugal and Spain (Busse *et al.* 2002).

Investing in facilities

The first step in achieving the desired outcome of high-quality, cost-effective care is ensuring that the right physical structures are in place. Given the continually changing nature of the health sector, this requires ongoing investment in new and updated facilities and equipment. Such investment offers the policy-maker scope to shape hospital performance through investment decisions, although, as already noted, the precise opportunities depend on the ownership, funding and regulatory systems within which the hospital exists.

Over the coming decades, Europe is likely to see greatly increased investment in health care facilities. In western Europe, failure to invest in new facilities while allowing existing facilities to depreciate was a major contributor to the containment of health care costs during the 1990s. In some countries, this has created an enormous backlog of maintenance and refurbishment. In eastern Europe, the situation is much worse; even the facilities built in the 1980s are already obsolete. Much needed reconfigurations of hospital systems across Europe will require many new or renovated buildings if they are to respond to changing health needs and offer new treatment methods, as described in Chapters 3 and 4.

Those responsible for health care systems thus face several challenges. The first is to ensure that hospital managers have access to funds that permit them to invest in facilities. The second is to ensure that they invest adequately and wisely. Many existing budgeting systems create perverse incentives that make it more attractive to cover revenue deficits by allowing facilities to run down or by failing to invest in new facilities.

The third challenge is to ensure that any investment in facilities is appropriate to the health needs of the population, is based, where possible, on evidence of effectiveness, and is considered in the context of surrounding health care services. New hospitals are expensive to build but, much more importantly, once built they generate even greater revenue needs. As resources for health care are finite, new hospital facilities should not be considered in isolation. They must be looked at in relation to neighbouring facilities, drawing on the evidence reviewed in Chapter 6, and in the context of what services can be provided in different settings, as discussed in Chapter 5. Careful investment choices will enable hospitals to position themselves to take advantage of advances in diagnosis and treatment, such as ensuring sufficient operating theatres to expand day surgery. Conversely, new equipment may bring prestige to an individual hospital but may do little to improve care for the population and, by deflecting resources from more worthy initiatives, may even harm it.

The fourth challenge is to give hospital managers the freedom to respond rapidly and appropriately to changing needs that they will be in the best position to identify. This is, however, not the only reason to give hospitals greater scope to manage their capital stock. If purchasers remove discretion over assets from providers, they allow an excuse for failure. Also, a hospital may be in a better position than a health care payer to balance the competing, and equally legitimate, demands on its infrastructure of patient care, teaching and research (Ferguson *et al.* 1997).

Together, these challenges pose a dilemma. Those working in hospitals are in the best position to know what they need to do their jobs properly. Conversely, they are less well placed to take a whole-system perspective. What is needed is a more devolved system of capital management than is present in many countries but within a well-developed regulatory framework that is informed by evidence of health need and effectiveness and that takes account of the local context.

One further issue requires attention. The building of hospitals and the purchase of complex equipment offer lucrative opportunities to unscrupulous individuals. These activities can only work well where corruption in public procurement has been eradicated, as discussed in a companion volume (Saltman *et al.* 2002).

Public–private partnership

Change requires money. The method of financing investment in hospitals is critically linked to the issues of ownership and governance (Box 7.1). Privately owned hospitals, by definition, raise capital for investment from private sources. This is not the predominant model in Europe, where most hospitals remain dependent primarily on government, in some form or other, for funds for investment. This has traditionally come from government revenues, either in the form of grants or repayable loans. However, given the many pressures on budgets, this has been a perennial problem in many countries. An emerging alternative to government directly financing the capital needs of public-sector health services is a public–private partnership. In this model, the public sector contracts with a private partner to build, manage and maintain a facility for a period of time. When the contract expires, the hospital will either be transferred to the public sector or retained by the private owners depending on the contractual agreement. In practice, most hospitals are likely to be transferred back to the public authorities; few private enterprises would wish to retain a hospital building for which there are few alternative uses. The transfer of hospitals back to the public sector is a key feature of the Private Finance Initiative hospital contracts concluded in the United Kingdom, which have been at the forefront of this means of procurement.

Such partnerships are superficially attractive to the state sector in that they provide money up front, eliminating the need for one-off capital allocations, by converting these into a commitment to make future streams of annual payments to the private operator. Their main attraction is, however, their scope to transfer the risks of the non-clinical operation of hospitals to the private sector. Thus, hospital managers should seek to transfer the risk associated with tasks such as building and maintaining the hospital to an organization that has made these its core business. The private-sector partner will expect to be compensated for taking on this risk. From the public-sector perspective, the key to success is, therefore, to transfer maximum risk at least cost. This is easier said than done.

In Europe, public–private partnerships have been used most often to finance major infrastructure projects; examples include the Tagus Bridge in Portugal and bridges in Greece. The United Kingdom's Private Finance Initiative has, however, extended their scope considerably, especially in the health and education sectors, and this is now the principal means of paying for new, large hospitals in the United Kingdom. The only other example in the health sector so far is the building of a 250-bed public hospital in the Valencia Region of Spain. This was financed by a private consortium, which will manage it for 10 years before transferring ownership to the Regional Ministry of Health.

The United Kingdom Private Finance Initiative stands out both in terms of its magnitude and in the amount of critical scrutiny it has attracted (Gaffney *et al.* 1999a,b). For these reasons, it is useful to examine it in more detail (Box 7.2). Public–private partnerships may become an important new way of funding the development of hospitals. Thus, it is essential that lessons be learned from the experience so far.

Incentives for investment

Securing access to funds is only a first step. How can policy-makers create incentives for hospitals to invest at all? This requires an appropriate accounting system, as well as sufficiently flexible planning controls. In many health care systems, both the cost and value of capital are ignored, thus removing any incentive to manage assets efficiently. This is especially likely where revenue and capital funding streams are separated, as is the case in much of Europe. Ignoring the opportunity cost of capital stock can allow potentially valuable space to be under-utilized.

Giving autonomy to hospitals will only achieve results if it is accompanied by a more permissive planning system. This should allow alternative use of otherwise unproductive facilities, such as the capacity to sell assets or to rent space for alternative uses, although this should be within a clearly defined overall framework for land use. Achieving such a regimen offers scope for constructive engagement by health policy-makers with local government planning departments. This can ensure wider recognition of the contribution that health care facilities make to local economic development. It can also ensure that health gets onto the wider agenda, for example, by ensuring that new facilities are served by good public transport and cycle lanes.

Box 7.2 United Kingdom Private Finance Initiative

The Private Finance Initiative (PFI) is a partnership programme intended to encourage private investment in the public sector. The United Kingdom National Health Service can now fund hospital capital costs with private capital instead of drawing on public-sector borrowing or taxation revenue. The PFI was introduced under the Conservative government, but the Labour government is also committed to the initiative.

The PFI arose from a situation in which one-third of health authorities and trusts were in serious financial difficulties by the mid-1990s (Pollock *et al.* 1999) but had a substantial need for new investment in facilities. Under the PFI scheme, a publicly owned hospital enters into a contract with a private consortium, in which the consortium builds and maintains the hospital building. The hospital management pays a performance-adjusted annual fee, which is fixed for the life of the contract (typically about 30 years) at the outset. The potential financial advantages to the hospital are two-fold. First, it does not need to raise the entire cost of the building at the outset. Second, and more importantly, it transfers the financial risks associated with the future maintenance and operation of the facility to the private company. It has also been argued, more contentiously, that private-sector management will ensure lower construction and operating costs. Advocates of the PFI argue that the incentives to the private sector of having to consider the whole-life costs of the building and, in some cases, the non-clinical services that will be delivered in it, will achieve greater efficiency. Experience of contracting with external providers for domestic services suggests that this may be difficult.

The operation of the PFI in the health sector has attracted considerable criticism. One issue is the cost of financing. The private-sector partner will have to borrow money to fund the project but at a rate that will almost certainly be higher, because of the greater risk involved, than the rate at which governments could borrow. The private sector charges the National Health Service fees equivalent to between 11 and 19 per cent of construction costs, whereas the Treasury could borrow at a 3.5 per cent real rate of annual interest (Gaffney *et al.* 1999a, b). This comparison does not, however, take account of the cost of maintenance over the life of the contract or that the Treasury borrowing rate reflects only the interest component, and not the repayment, of loans. As the private consortium will be handing the hospital over to the public sector – in good condition and without further charge – at the end of the contract, it clearly needs to ensure that the fees it charges cover the repayment of capital loans and not simply the interest on them. Second, it has been argued that the private-sector partner is rewarded disproportionately for the often low risk it has to bear. This argument has some justification. Third, and most importantly, business cases prepared by health authorities initially were shrouded in commercial confidentiality, so that many overly optimistic assumptions remained unchallenged and contrary views were not considered (Pollock *et al.* 1999).

The expertise required to make PFI projects a success should not be underestimated. Those negotiating on behalf of the public sector must define in considerable detail exactly what they want the project to deliver, specifying the nature and quality of the facilities, the standards to which they will be maintained and the nature and quality of the services provided in them. Finally, one of the main concerns about public–private partnerships in the health sector is the high transaction cost, often involving considerable legal and other advisers' fees, as each side seeks to minimize its risk. In the future, this is likely to be reduced by developing standardized project documentation.

The editor of the *British Medical Journal* may be going too far in labelling the PFI as Perfidious Financial Idiocy, but it clearly has some important weaknesses as presently designed (Smith 1999). These result from specific features of the various schemes, often including the lack of open discussion about the assumptions involved. Despite the secrecy that surrounds individual projects, the intense scrutiny to which the overall programme has been subjected means that the PFI offers many lessons, both good and bad, for other countries.

Capital charging

One type of incentive, known as capital charging, was introduced in the United Kingdom in 1990, whereby self-governing hospitals, while remaining in public ownership, were required to value their assets and pay to the Treasury a 6 per cent charge. Although hospital funding allocations were adjusted to cover these costs, the process focused managerial attention on how assets were used and whether additional investment or disposal of existing stock was required. In many cases, obsolete facilities that had been lying vacant were sold and public space within hospitals was rented to shops. This is of mutual benefit: hospital entrances have high flows of people, making them attractive sites for shops, and the shops also provide enhanced facilities for staff and patients. Nevertheless, just as some airports seem confused about whether they are a shopping mall or a transport facility, careful balancing is needed. Similar models apply in other countries; in Stockholm County, Sweden, private companies operate hospitals owned by the county council. Hospital rents are designed to encourage managers to make the best use of capital assets, disposing of those that are unnecessary.

Specifying, monitoring and rewarding investment

Because of the considerable consequences for the economy, many governments have retained some control over the specification of major capital investment in hospitals, even where they are not the formal owners. For example, Germany has dual financing of hospitals, with revenue costs paid by the sickness funds but investment funded by the *Länder* (states), with major decisions made within the framework of regional hospital plans (Busse 2000). The Netherlands has freed up investment to a greater extent than most countries, as the voluntary-sector hospitals can borrow on the financial markets, although, until recently, government underwrote their loans. Nevertheless, hospitals are constrained by the Hospital Facilities Act, which requires government approval for most new facilities to ensure that the resulting distribution is equitable and reflects need (Maarse 1996). In Canada, where hospitals are largely autonomous not-for-profit entities run by community boards, partnerships with private-sector companies have increased, but provincial governments retain tight control over capital spending.

The outcome of good investment – that is, high-quality care – should be monitored and rewarded within a general framework of performance management, and this should incorporate assessment of structures and processes as well as outcomes (Donabedian 1966). The creation of public–private partnerships does offer an additional instrument to encourage adequate investment. In the United Kingdom Private Finance Initiative, ownership of the hospital is transferred to the National Health Service at the end of the contract, typically after 30 years, but payment of the full fee is conditional on the hospital being maintained in good condition throughout this period.

Investing in people

Effective health care also depends on a supply of trained staff armed with up-to-date knowledge of clinical effectiveness and with appropriate managerial skills. Those responsible for health care systems have a clear responsibility to ensure that appropriate education and training systems are in place to ensure the existence of a knowledgeable and skilled health care workforce. As with capital, the short-term pressure faced by hospitals can provide a disincentive to invest in staff. This is also a complex process that requires negotiation with a wide range of external bodies such as universities, ministries of education and professional associations.

Developing the health care workforce

Unfortunately, the planning of human resources in the health care sector remains weak in many countries (World Bank 1993), even though health workers are a significant group as a large and growing proportion of the total workforce. For example, the health sector employs 4–10 per cent of the workforce in the Group of Seven (G7) leading industrialized countries (OECD 1999). The health care workforce in these countries expanded rapidly during the 1970s and 1980s, a time of expansion for the service sector of the economy, although growth began to slow in most countries during the 1990s. In contrast, the number of health-sector personnel has fallen in some central and eastern European countries (Healy and McKee 1997; International Labour Organization and Sectoral Activities Programme 1998).

Workforce planning aims to ensure that the right number of people with the appropriate knowledge and skills are available at the right time and place to deliver the appropriate services to people who need them (Armstrong 1991). The main planning issues relate to the balance of different groups within the overall workforce (Egger *et al.* 2000; WHO 2000):

- numerical imbalances, with an excess supply of physicians in some European countries and insufficient supply in others;
- skill-mix imbalances with, for example, a shortage of qualified nurses, technical occupational groups and trained managers, plus increasing inter-

est in the possibilities for substitution between health care professionals; and

- distribution imbalances, with urban versus rural inequity in the distribution of health care professionals a common problem.

Getting the balance right is extremely difficult, for reasons that are discussed in Chapter 11. Normative staffing guidelines that set staff : population ratios have little place in modern health systems. Although many policy documents cite such figures, guidelines date quickly and depend on the context. For example, legislation in Germany set out nursing time standards, whereby the amount of nursing time for which each unit was reimbursed was adjusted according to how dependent the patients are, with allocations of between 52 and 215 minutes of nursing per patient per day. The regulation succeeded in increasing the numbers of nurses but was abolished after 3 years because it was costly and restrictive for hospitals (Busse and Schwartz 1997; Busse 2000). As Carr-Hill and Jenkins-Clarke (1995) commented, 'there is no evidence that [nursing workload measures] are anything more than an expensive numbers game'.

Arriving at the right number by means of workforce comparisons between countries (such as physicians per 1000 population) must also be regarded with caution, since occupational definitions, training levels and expectations vary. This is especially true for nursing; in some countries nursing is a graduate-level profession, but others only require high school training (Salvage and Heijnen 1997).

Production of physicians has received most attention, in part because they are the most expensive group of health care professionals. Furthermore, the mobility of physicians across the European Union has brought increasing convergence in medical education, although important differences still remain. The greying of the physician workforce across Europe combined with controls on university entry suggest that the number of active physicians may begin to decline after 2005 (Eysenbach 1998), although there is great variation among countries. Most countries seek to control the production of physicians (Mossialos and Le Grand 1999). In those that have not managed to do so, such as Italy, there has been over-production, with many gaining only limited clinical experience. This is not only wasteful of resources but is also unfair to the individuals concerned. In a few countries, low levels of investment in training, combined with dependence on migrants from developing countries, have led to shortages.

The numbers of nurses required is also poorly planned, especially in countries in which nurse training has progressed little in recent decades, in part because of the dominance of the medical profession (Salvage and Heijnen 1997). Such nurses often have limited skills and thus weak capacity to deliver modern health care.

Professional development and revalidation

In the past, a medical or nursing qualification, achieved in one's early twenties, was considered sufficient to allow one to practise. Even 50 years ago this was not justifiable, but it is even less appropriate now given the rapidity with which new knowledge is generated.

Continuing education in most countries remains a voluntary activity, although it may be linked to acquisition or retention of specialist status. It is left to the individual health professional to ensure that he or she keeps up to date with changes in clinical practice. In some countries, systems are being developed that will require certain health professionals to demonstrate that they are keeping their knowledge and skills up to date. Individuals will have to develop learning plans, with clear objectives and demonstration of activities to achieve those objectives. This often involves a combination of attendance at training courses or conferences, participation in quality assurance activities and self-directed learning. Schemes in which participation is initially voluntary tend to become obligatory. Several initiatives are also underway within Europe to exchange experience on different schemes and, in some cases, to establish systems by which credits can be accrued based on attending an event in a different country.

Mandatory continuing education is less common, in part because of the lack of effective sanctions for transgressors. It can, however, be enforced through a system of revalidation. Revalidation involves health professionals applying to retain their professional status, having demonstrated that they remain competent to practise. Although long established in some state and national specialty boards in the United States, revalidation is only beginning to be discussed in Europe. One example is the United Kingdom, where the General Medical Council, in association with the Royal Colleges, is developing a system under which all practising physicians must undergo an assessment every 5 years. This will be based on evidence such as participation in continuing professional development, quality assurance programmes, assessment of clinical outcomes, relationships with patients and other professionals and their response to untoward events (Buckley 1999).

Pressure for revalidation has emerged from concerns about the existing system of professional self-regulation. In most countries, however, the regulation of hospitals and staff is invoked only as a last resort for the most glaring failures, and this depends on professional regulatory bodies and the courts to exert the ultimate sanction against malpractice. First, recourse to the courts as a means of action to redress errors arising from malpractice is a very unsatisfactory approach, since there is little evidence that fear of being sued for malpractice is especially effective at changing clinical practice (Black 1990). Second, legal systems handle cases of medical negligence in very different ways. For example, in Catalonia in Spain, the Barcelona College of Physicians has instituted a system that seeks to reduce claims by preventing the circumstances that give rise to them as well as by mediating if this fails (Trilla and Bruguera 2000). This has been associated with a sustained reduction in malpractice claims. In contrast, allegations of medical negligence in Italy often are dealt with by the criminal courts. The system is highly confrontational and unsatisfactory for all involved (Jourdan et al. 2000). It has been associated with a dramatic increase in claims. Best practice must provide lessons in this area, with systems based on mediation and risk management to be preferred to those based on suspicion and blame. Continuing education and revalidation

Box 7.3 The Bristol hospital enquiry

A 1998 hearing by the General Medical Council into paediatric heart surgery at the Bristol Royal Infirmary found three physicians guilty of professional misconduct. Two had continued to operate despite high mortality rates among their patients. A third, although not involved in the operations, was judged to have erred because he was managerially responsible for physicians in the hospital and had failed to act when he became aware of problems, thus raising the issue of responsibility for addressing problems among one's colleagues. A subsequent independent public inquiry in 1999 into the standards of paediatric heart surgery in Bristol highlighted the lack of effective monitoring of medical standards in the United Kingdom. It exposed weaknesses in regulation by physicians, by their employer (a National Health Service Trust), by statutory professional bodies such as the General Medical Council and by the Department of Health.

The Bristol case has had several outcomes. The General Medical Council introduced an enhanced system to detect poorly performing physicians. After investigation and assessment, the General Medical Council may suspend the physicians' registration or recommend remedial training. The Department of Health announced an integrated quality programme in 1999 intended to ensure higher standards in the National Health Service (see Chapter 10).

Sources: Dunn (1998), Egan (1998), Smith (1998), Treasure (1998) and Cummings (1999)

issues are important in the European Union, given the freedom of movement of health professionals under the European Union Treaties.

The intensity of the debate on professional self-regulation and clinical competence in the United Kingdom reflects a series of high-profile events in which these systems were found to be lacking (Box 7.3).

Monitoring performance

Some countries have assembled an impressive body of experience in monitoring the performance of public-sector organizations against specified criteria and goals. However, few would suggest that this is easy, not least because of the need to pursue sometimes competing goals (Wildavsky 1979; Pollit *et al.* 1999; Pollit and Bouckaert 2000).

Monitoring the performance of a hospital and its staff requires skilled people, information and resources. Those undertaking monitoring should: understand how health care is delivered; have evaluation skills that encompass both quantitative and qualitative approaches; understand the methodological limitations; be familiar with how health care organizations respond to different incentives; and have access to relevant and accurate information. Many of the usual statistics, such as the numbers of patients treated, with no differentiation between specialties or conditions, are almost useless. The following section examines one approach to performance indicators, the publication of clinical performance indicators.

Box 7.4 Clinical performance indicators: England

The Department of Health reports on the performance of each NHS trust in terms of six main clinical indicators. These include measures such as deaths in hospital within 30 days of surgery, deaths in hospital within 30 days of emergency admission with hip fracture for patients aged 65 years and over, and rates of emergency readmission to hospital within 28 days of discharge. A set of 41 high-level performance indicators focus on issues such as reported deaths, length of waiting lists and emergency psychiatric readmission, as well as progress towards targets set out in the national health strategy *Our Healthier Nation* (Department of Health 1998a) in four areas (cancer, heart disease, accidents and suicides). The indicators used to assess health authorities include length of waiting lists and 5-year survival rates for breast and cervical cancer.

Source: Department of Health (1999)

Clinical performance indicators

Publication of indicators of clinical performance has attracted the attention of policy-makers in some countries for two reasons. One is that it enables patients and those referring them to hospital to make choices about which hospital to use, although this presupposes that a choice exists, which is rarely the case. The second is that the process of 'naming and shaming' may encourage failing hospitals to improve their performance.

Performance indicators can take several forms. The broad approach looks at various measures of hospital performance encompassing responsiveness to patients, clinical outcomes and efficiency. The second approach focuses on clinical outcomes. The following sections examine the development of performance indicators and some of the criticisms levelled against them.

Among European countries, England has introduced the most developed system of performance indicators, as central to the government's commitment to delivering high-quality care. Furthermore, a statutory duty was placed on all health organizations to seek quality improvement (Department of Health 1997), as part of a spectrum of activities directed at improving standards of care (Scally and Donaldson 1998; Dixon and Preker 1999).

Performance indicators in England measure each hospital trust against a set of criteria, and the published results allow hospitals and the public to compare hospital performance. The national performance assessment framework sets out measures of quality and efficiency of services in six main areas: improvements in people's health, fair access to services, the delivery of effective care, efficiency, the experiences of patients and their care-givers, and health outcomes. These indicators include measures of inputs, process, outputs, efficiency and outcomes, all over different time frames (Box 7.4).

The experience in England demonstrates the many challenges involved in the use of performance indicators (New 1998). Their publication may have improved clinical and organizational practices, but their achievements have been under-researched. Second, the interpretation of indicators is widely contested; for example, hospitals in poorer areas generally perform less well, suggesting insufficient allowance for increased population illness and fewer resources. Third, some hospitals modified their data collection when it became apparent that their reported performance was very different from their perceptions. The process also has highlighted the problems of combining relevance, simplicity and data availability. This is especially problematic with composite measures that combine data on related but different types of activity (McKee and Sheldon 1998).

The public disclosure of rankings of clinical outcomes achieved by hospitals or physicians ('league tables') raises some specific issues. It is seen as a strategy both for improving standards and for empowering customers or patients. Although superficially attractive, 'naming and shaming' has many critics, on both technical and managerial grounds. For example, a recent review concluded that 'the current official support for output league tables, even adjusted, is misplaced' (Goldstein and Spiegelhalter 1996).

The first concern is that substantially fewer resources are devoted to collecting clinical data in Europe than in the United States, where league tables are used extensively and where the culture puts a high value on informing consumers. Even the countries that have undertaken major investments in data quality still have considerable problems (McKee and Hunter 1995). In many European countries, routinely collected data are insufficient to construct such tables.

The second concern is whether the data are adequate to control for patient characteristics. Both primary and secondary diagnoses must be recorded because the latter are required to adjust for differences in patient severity (McKee *et al.* 1999). The denominator must be recorded, since adverse outcomes must be linked to patients not admissions (Clarke and McKee 1992). Adverse outcomes arising after discharge must also be identified. A measure such as 30-day mortality should ideally be used, since otherwise a hospital that discharges patients very early may have a spuriously positive outcome. True differences in case severity are hard to measure, and several studies have shown how increasingly detailed adjustment for severity leads to substantial changes in rankings (Green *et al.* 1991; Rockall *et al.* 1995; Davenport *et al.* 1996).

The third technical concern is that such studies are possible only with high-volume hospitals and physicians, since the number of cases must be sufficient for one to be statistically confident that the outcomes are a true reflection of practice and not have simply arisen by chance (Marshall *et al.* 1998).

League tables are intended to lead eventually to higher average standards. The response by the various stakeholders is therefore important. Ideally, a lagging hospital would search for the causes of failings followed by remedial action. In practice, it is as likely to massage the data to ensure that the ranking improves the next time (Smith 1993; Edhouse and Wardrope 1996; Savill 1996). This phenomenon has received most attention in the United States. For example, New York State developed report cards on death rates among those operated on by cardiac surgeons (Green and Owen 1995). Their introduction was accompanied by a substantial increase in the reported severity of patients having chronic obstructive pulmonary or congestive heart failure, although this was not matched by more objective markers of chronic disease. After adjustment for the apparently increasingly poor health of the patients concerned, outcomes seemed to improve. It was impossible to ascertain whether this was real or the combined effect of more rigorous selection of patients and the exaggeration of patient severity (Hannan *et al.* 1994).

Another concern is that the information may not improve clinical performance. In Pennsylvania, where death rates for individual surgeons are published, a survey found that 87 per cent of cardiologists reported that the information had no or minimal influence on their referral decision to surgeons (Schneider and Epstein 1996). The study also found that less than 10 per cent reported discussing the information with more than one in ten of their patients who were contemplating surgery. Although these findings suggest that publication is neither beneficial nor harmful, the survey also found that cardiologists were experiencing greater difficulty in finding surgeons willing to operate on high-risk patients, which was consistent with reports from the cardiac surgeons.

This is not to argue that hospital clinical outcomes should not be monitored; we certainly endorse the principle of monitoring the performance of health systems. We want to sound a cautionary note, however, that publication of hospital rankings is problematic and can create perverse incentives. It is important that those responsible for health care establish monitoring systems that recognize the uncertainty intrinsic to health care, that improve current measurement techniques, that highlight broad differences rather than precise rankings and that seek continuing improvement and act on serious failings.

Patients

Patients are the second group of people who interact with the hospital and have long been the neglected element in hospital planning. The benefits to be gained from a situation in which patients are partners in the process of care are increasingly recognized. They include not only more satisfied patients but also better outcomes (McPherson and Britton 1999). Thus, informed patients can be considered to make an important impact on health care outcomes, and external agencies are becoming much more explicit about the rights that patients have in relation to hospitals.

Patients' rights

Explicit recognition of the rights of patients provides a framework within which the hospital system can operate and can enable the public to have a voice in how that care is provided. In ideal circumstances, hospitals would be highly responsive to the needs of their patients. In reality, this is rarely so (Weatherall 1994). Patients are in a weak position. They are in an unfamiliar setting, vulnerable because of their illness and their lack of information and dependent on others. Consequently, some governments and other organizations responsible for hospital systems have sought to redress this balance, at least in part, by safeguarding patients' rights and by requiring that patients be involved in making decisions about their own care.

The potential influence of the patient on the hospital can be considered in terms of 'exit' and 'voice' (Hirschman 1970). Voice is a political concept that refers to a person's ability to influence an organization while continuing to use its services. The citizen participation model that emerged in the 1970s in many high-income countries aimed to empower people to have some say over public-sector organizations and to ensure that their rights as users were recognized. Exit is an economic concept that refers to a person's ability to leave an organization and seek services or products elsewhere. However, the patient's power of exit is usually extremely limited, whether because of the urgency of the situation, the absence of competition or administrative rules that limit choice. For these reasons, strategies to enhance the role of patients have focused on strengthening their voice.

Most European countries are subject to international treaties that have consequences for patients' rights; the most important is the European Convention on Human Rights and Fundamental Freedoms (Hewson 2000). In addition, a number of documents, while not legally binding, carry some moral authority. These include the Amsterdam Declaration on the Promotion of Patients' Rights from 1994. The World Health Organization included the principle of patients' rights in its 21 targets within the health for all policy framework for the twenty-first century for the European Region. Target 16 on managing for quality of care calls for the measurement of patient satisfaction (WHO 1999). Especially in northern and western Europe, a range of national legislation has emerged to protect and enforce patients' rights (Leenen *et al.* 1993).

The Nordic countries have been particularly active in passing legislation that formalizes relationships between physicians and patients. An Act on Patients' Rights, passed in Norway in 1999, includes the right to choose a hospital, to access to specialist evaluation within 30 days of referral, to a second opinion, to be fully informed, to give informed consent and to complain (Myklebust 2000).

The growing complexity of health care and the need for a neutral authority to mediate between hospitals and patients has led to the establishment of a hospital ombudsman in several European countries (Swingedau 2000). The ombudsman, an office developed in the Nordic countries, deals with complaints by individuals and aims to improve services on behalf of the public. An ombudsman first mediates between the patient and the hospital. If this fails, the ombudsman might be empowered to take the case to court (as in Finland) or to a mediation centre or tribunal (as in France and the Netherlands).

Patient's rights can also be defined formally in patients' charters, which might set out formal grievance procedures. Patients' charters have been produced in several countries from the early 1970s onwards, notably in France, the Netherlands and the United Kingdom (Massion 2000). For example, the Patient's Charter for England, launched in 1991, set out ten rights and codified the standards that a patient could expect from the National Health Service (Department of Health 1995). These rights and standards, however, are not enforceable under law. In contrast, in some states of the United States, patients' bills of rights have legislative force, although fines are rare, for example, occurring only 12 times in 5 years in New Jersey (Silver 1997).

National or regional patient surveys are another mechanism intended to encourage the hospital system to take patients' views into account. For example, the Department of Health in England undertakes an annual national survey of patient and user experience, the results of which feed into national performance indicators (Department of Health 1998b). Although it is entirely legitimate to seek the views of those using hospitals, these surveys must be interpreted with great caution (Carr-Hill 1992; Williams 1994). Surveys of patient satisfaction with health services generally obtain over 80 per cent satisfaction ratings, but these levels of approval are often strikingly discordant with more focused evaluations.

Various other mechanisms enable a patient's voice to be heard. These include citizen representation on hospital boards, a patient advocate within a hospital and formal grievance procedures. Such grievance procedures provide a formal avenue for complaint and can also be a method for monitoring hospital performance. For example, in Spain, patients' complaints have fed into audit programmes since 1984 (Sunol *et al.* 1991). Patients' complaints will also be taken into account in the system of medical revalidation in the United Kingdom.

Investing in knowledge

A modern hospital system must be able to take advantage of advances in knowledge. Those with responsibility for stewardship of the health care system should, therefore, ensure that a national or regional research and development strategy is in place that can, at least, undertake research on issues of greatest local importance.

For this reason, six of the 15 European Union countries had established formal national programmes on health technology assessment by late 1999. There are also some international programmes. The EUR-ASSESS project was set up as a coordinating network for the European Union countries plus Switzerland (Banta 1997). The activities promoted by technology assessment centres and professional associations have created a large body of 'systematically developed statements to assist practitioner and patient decisions about appropriate health care for specific clinical circumstances' (NHS Centre for Reviews and Dissemination and Nuffield Institute for Health 1994).

Some countries have set up national committees for high-technology planning that attempt to implement a system with certificates of need. For example, in Germany, legislative and corporatist bodies have attempted to control the introduction of expensive technology. Between 1987 and 1997, the German states (*Länder*) used planning committees consisting of representatives of the hospitals, physician associations, sickness funds and state government. These committees were abolished in 1997, since they had failed to halt the substantial increase in technological devices over the previous decade, despite the argument that the increase may have been even greater without regulation by these external bodies (Perleth *et al.* 1999).

External bodies must also ensure that hospital staff are aware of research; that is, that they have access to the research that they need (increasingly available via the Internet) as well as the skills to interpret it. This process has been facilitated enormously by the Cochrane Collaboration (1991). This international collaboration has established a procedure for undertaking and disseminating systematic literature reviews of the effectiveness of a range of interventions, spanning health care, prevention and health promotion, with the database available on the Internet (http://www.cochrane.org). An understanding of the principles and methods of evidence-based health care should be part of the basic training of all health professionals and managers.

Assessing the needs of the population

If a hospital is to provide an appropriate spectrum of care, it must know something about the health needs of the population it serves. Recent years have seen a marked increase in understanding the methods available to assess the health needs of the population and their strengths and limitations. Three broad approaches can be used: epidemiological, comparative and corporate (Stevens and Raftery 1994).

Epidemiological needs assessment involves several steps. The first is defining the clinical indications for a particular form of treatment. One example is the level of urinary symptoms above which a prostatectomy would be considered appropriate (Sanderson *et al.* 1997). The second step is to measure, by means of a survey, how many men in the population fall into this category. Knowledge of how the condition varies by age, ethnicity or other parameters makes it possible to extrapolate the results to other populations.

The second approach is comparative, looking at variation in the provision of health care in different populations and making a judgement about the appropriate level. Where possible, this approach should be adjusted for known measures of disease frequency. For example, Figures 7.2 and 7.3 show that the

Figure 7.2 Cardiac surgery procedures (bypasses, stents and angioplasties) per million population

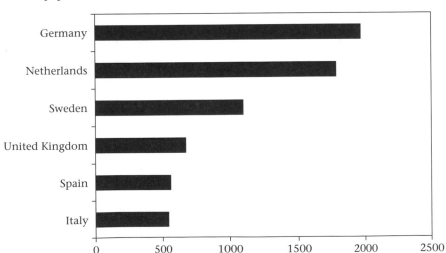

Source: http://www.escardio.org (accessed 21 January 2001)

Figure 7.3 Cardiac surgery procedures (bypasses, stents and angioplasties) per million population as a proportion of deaths from ischaemic heart disease

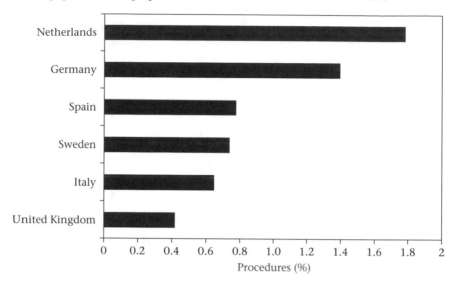

Source: http://www.escardio.org (accessed 21 January 2001)

Box 7.5 Steps in assessing needs for a health care intervention

- Defining what is included (describing the condition and the services involved in its management
- Identifying relevant subcategories requiring different packages of care (such as mild or severe stroke)
- Measuring the prevalence or incidence (as appropriate) of those in need
- Identifying the services available and the gaps
- Assessing the effectiveness and cost-effectiveness of alternative strategies
- Developing evidence-based models of care
- Identifying outcomes and setting targets

Source: Stevens and Raftery (1994)

United Kingdom performs cardiac surgery procedures at about the average rate for western Europe, but that adjustment for the burden of disease places it below other countries. The third approach, referred to as corporate, essentially involves a judgement by key stakeholders (patients, professionals and purchasers) on the services that a hospital will provide. All these methods require considerable capacity in both epidemiology and the appraisal of evidence of effectiveness.

These approaches have been combined in a standardized format in the United Kingdom, where the evidence related to a wide variety of interventions and services has already been assembled (Stevens and Raftery 1994) (Box 7.5).

Assessing the needs of a population is a method by which those who are ultimately responsible for organizing and delivering health care can establish the basic goals of effective and equitable treatment. The complexity of health care and the asymmetry of information means that the health care professional and the patient together must decide on the optimal management of the particular case. Conversely, this must be balanced by a strategic vision that looks to the needs of those who have not been able to access care as well as to the sustainability and overall cost-effectiveness of the system.

Guidance on clinical effectiveness

Need for health care has been defined as 'ability to benefit' from an intervention (Acheson 1978). Thus assessment of health needs depends on knowledge of which interventions work. Consequently, another role for government or its agents is the development and dissemination of locally relevant guidance on new technology, specific interventions and models of care based on available research.

In many cases, the evidence base may be limited. Formal consensus methods can often be used, however, to agree on guidance based on the best available evidence (Black *et al.* 1999). This method has been used most in Germany, the Netherlands, the Nordic countries and the United Kingdom.

One of the weakest links in the chain is dissemination of research to those who make the decisions (Granados *et al.* 1997). Even where this information is made available, physicians incorporate new evidence-based information in their routine clinical practice only to a limited extent (Chapter 13). Clinical behaviour is quite resistant to change where only a single strategy is used, whether this is the dissemination of clinical protocols or short training courses. These findings suggest that improving clinical performance requires a package of approaches involving both external and internal interventions.

Coordinated strategies

So far, this chapter has considered how a policy lever acts mainly on one of the inputs required for high-quality care. To revert to the systems model set out in Chapter 1, the various inputs that enable a hospital to function are interdependent, so that optimum health care requires that each of these subsystems is effectively linked. Consequently, a variety of policy mechanisms has been developed that combine these inputs. Three are considered here: accreditation, strategic purchasing and integrated quality programmes.

Hospital accreditation

Accreditation is an external activity that evaluates the overall ability of the hospital to provide quality care and looks at facilities, staff, equipment, processes and sometimes outcomes. It involves an independent body evaluating the degree of compliance by a hospital with previously determined standards and, if the hospital is adequate, awarding a certificate (Robinson 1995; Bohigas *et al.* 1996; Scrivens 1998).

Accreditation systems are most developed in countries that separate financing and delivery (Scrivens 1995). In terms of policy leverage, the key distinction is whether hospital accreditation is compulsory or voluntary. If compulsory (as in France and Spain), it is mainly an enabling and regulatory policy that carries entitlement to receive funding and is a means of ensuring that all hospitals provide care of an acceptable standard. If voluntary (as in Australia, Canada and the United States), it provides a means of specifying and rewarding, through public and professional recognition, the hospitals that have met appropriate criteria. Accreditation thus is a mark of achievement that may make it easier to attract and retain staff and may give a competitive advantage in negotiations with purchasers.

Some features are common to both models. The accrediting body should be independent, although hospitals usually pay a fee to be accredited. The process is undertaken by health care professionals, either employees elsewhere in the health system or independent consultants, trained in evaluating compliance with a set of standards (Bohigas *et al.* 1998). Accreditation is awarded for a period of typically about 3 years.

The ethos underlying accreditation is changing. Existing systems have focused primarily on structures and processes and have been criticized for neglecting clinical effectiveness (Purdy and Rich 1995; Robinson 1995). Well-designed hospital structures and processes have been assumed to produce good clinical outcomes (despite the absence of hard evidence). In future, accreditation systems will face pressure to place more emphasis on measurable clinical effectiveness (Scrivens 1997, 1998).

Successful voluntary schemes can attract high levels of participation. The United States system, which is the oldest, has a single independent body, the Joint Commission on Accreditation of Healthcare Organizations, which accredits most hospitals (80 per cent), having survived competitive challenges (Scrivens 1995). In Canada, accreditation is voluntary under the Canadian Council on Health Facilities Accreditation, but 95 per cent of hospitals are accredited (Caillet and Baillet 2000). The Australian Council on Healthcare Standards is an independent body that stresses that its role is 'evaluative and educative rather than inspectorial or judgmental'. It awards accreditation for 1, 3 or 5 years, after an on-site survey, which reflects a hospital's demonstrated ability to maintain quality of care, with 40 per cent of public hospitals in Australia, mostly large hospitals, accredited (Australian Institute of Health and Welfare 1998).

A compulsory system arguably changes the role of accreditation from recognition to regulation, from a professional model of education to one of control, while the surveyors change from professional educators to inspectors. In Spain, where regional health authorities finance and provide most hospital care, Catalonia developed the country's first accreditation system in 1981, prompted by its high proportion of private beds, before legislation in 1984 made assessment systems mandatory in all hospitals in Spain (Sunol *et al.* 1991). France introduced compulsory accreditation in 1999 and expects all 4000 hospitals to be audited by 2004 (Caillet and Baillet 2000). An independent public agency funded by the government conducts accreditation (Agence Nationale d'Accreditation et d'Evaluation en Santé 1998).

Accreditation has two different but related goals. The first is to provide a guarantee that a hospital meets a defined minimum standard; the second is a developmental process in which best practice can be exchanged and promoted (Scrivens 1995). It appears axiomatic that accreditation can contribute to the former, but there is little empirical evidence about the cost-effectiveness of accreditation as a means for raising standards.

The success or failure of an accreditation system depends on its effective implementation. A successful scheme is likely to be one that sets realistic but challenging goals, recognizes the constraints that the hospital faces and seeks to be helpful rather than negative and punitive. An important issue is that resources are required, since someone must pay for the process, often the hospital involved. The identifiable costs may be only a small proportion of the total if the process requires a substantial volume of preparatory work by each hospital. In each case, the costs must be weighed against the benefits. It may be that many elements of an accreditation programme could be obtained within a system of strategic purchasing, possibly with pooling of resources among purchasers. There is also a case for any system being firmly embedded within a broader quality strategy (as discussed later in this chapter).

Strategic purchasing

Throughout this book, we have argued that the state, or those acting on its behalf, such as sickness funds, have a responsibility to specify the nature of the hospital care that should be provided to the population. Some health care professionals would challenge this view, however, since professional autonomy is jealously guarded in many parts of western Europe. From that perspective, the health care professional is accountable only to his or her patient, and the role of the social insurance fund or regional health authority is limited to paying for treatment provided. A similar view is held in many parts of eastern Europe, although this reflects a different history: a reaction to the previous system, whereby the state as employer set out in minute detail exactly how each type of patient should be managed. This allowed little flexibility to adapt or update treatment to the needs of the individual patient.

Europe, therefore, had two quite different systems in the 1980s. One was *laissez-faire*, providing only a minimalist legal framework within which hospitals and health professionals were expected to operate. The second, exemplified by the Soviet model, was highly regulated, based on command and control and allowing almost no discretion. Neither encouraged the provision of health care that combined cost-effectiveness, responsiveness and equity. By the early 1990s, many countries were moving towards a middle course. This involved assessing the health needs of the population, identifying whether these needs were being met and seeking to bridge any gaps using mechanisms such as contracting for services. These activities have been termed 'strategic purchasing'.

Strategic purchasing has been identified as an effective means of aligning the external incentives acting on providers to enhance the quality of care (WHO 2000). It implies the reorientation of the many incentives within payment systems to achieve goals such as enhancement of health and improved responsiveness, all within an overall health strategy. It is a complex task, as attested by the growing literature on the topic (Øvretveit 1995). Strategic purchasing involves a continuous search for the best interventions to purchase, the best providers and the best payment and contracting mechanisms. The process of assessing need and defining packages of care requires highly skilled staff with access to appropriate data. A health service product is difficult to specify, there is enormous scope for opportunistic behaviour by providers and there is continuing tension between the level of detail desired and the transaction costs involved.

For many countries, this model remains an aspiration. Some previously *laissez-faire* systems have made considerable progress in replacing simple reimbursement, albeit within broadly agreed rules, with a more active purchasing process based on evidence of effectiveness. Greater specification can, however, provoke considerable opposition from a medical profession that guards its autonomy. In the formerly highly regulated systems of eastern Europe, health professionals have gained more autonomy, which, while in some cases allows innovative models of care to emerge, has yet to be matched by the creation of sophisticated evidence-based regulatory schemes.

Specifying hospital services

The precise nature of strategic purchasing depends on the features of the health care system. Where purchasing and provision have been separated, this is likely to involve some system of contracting. However, where the two functions remain combined, some principles of contracting can still be embedded in service agreements.

Even within superficially similar systems, contracting may mean very different things. Some contracts may be formal and detailed, with payment withheld if the provisions are not met (purchase-of-service contracting). Others may be a looser agreement on the broad pattern of care. Since the topic of contracting is dealt with in another book in this series (Mossialos *et al.* 2002), only some basic concepts are discussed here.

Public contract models have become more common in western Europe in the late 1990s, as countries with previously integrated systems have introduced splits between purchasers (typically geographically based health authorities) and hospitals and other providers (Mossialos and Le Grand 1999). Although the public contract model has long been used in countries with social insurance systems, the new version involves a more proactive process of specifying what type of care should be provided, with a focus on effectiveness and equity. At the risk of simplification, earlier systems had been largely payment systems within rules that concentrated on cost containment.

Contracting for health care offers several potential advantages. Contracts can specify what types of services will be provided, to whom and in what manner. If contracting is combined with sophisticated assessment of population needs,

Figure 7.4 An integrated quality programme: the quality framework in England

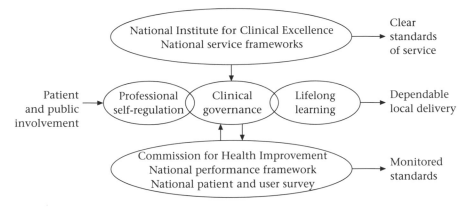

Source: Department of Health (1998b)

this can support the provision of effective and equitable care. It is argued that efficiency is enhanced, as the purchaser can choose between competing providers. In reality, however, choice is often highly constrained because of the barriers to market entry – a new hospital cannot be created overnight. The threat of loss of contracts, or contestability, however, may stimulate better care at lower cost (Ham 1996). Regular contracting rounds offer the scope to reassess what is being purchased in the light of new developments.

There are also disadvantages. These include high transaction costs that typically are underestimated, although these may be reduced in contracts that span several years; on the other hand, long contracts also reduce the scope to adapt to emerging circumstances. High transaction costs mean that monopoly situations may be consolidated, since the cost of market entry is often high.

The type of purchasing that can enhance health outcomes and responsiveness requires high levels of managerial skills, investment in information technology and access to nationally relevant research on both clinical and organizational innovations. Few European countries have managed to achieve this.

Integrated quality programmes

Although ensuring that the inputs needed for high-quality health care are in place is clearly important, policies directed at only one element of the overall system often achieve somewhat disappointing results. For example, as described in Chapter 13, publication of evidence-based guidelines is an important step but is not sufficient to change clinical practice. Similarly, encouraging invest-ment in facilities does not mean that those working within them are competent. Monitoring outcomes in the absence of real commitment to quality by pro-fessionals is as likely to lead to the distortion of data as it is to real improve-ments in the quality of care. For these reasons, some countries are seeking integrated approaches to high-quality care.

The recently established system of performance management in the National Health Service in England illustrates the essential elements of such a system (Department of Health 1998b) (Figure 7.4). The first element is the development of standards by the National Institute for Clinical Excellence (Rawlins 1999). As well as making decisions on specific treatments, such as advising health authorities on the cost-effectiveness of certain anti-cancer drugs, it has prepared a series of national service frameworks, which are compilations of evidence on the overall management of certain conditions, spanning prevention, treatment and rehabilitation. An early example was a guideline on the management of cardiovascular disease (Department of Health 1998b). These national service frameworks specify the optimal package of care and therefore the required facilities, equipment and skills.

These frameworks, and other evidence of good practice, are to be implemented locally, building on new systems of professional regulation, continuing professional development and clinical governance. Clinical governance is a means of integrating traditional managerial and quality assurance activities, to ensure that managers place quality of care high on their agendas and that those seeking to ensure quality care have command over the resources they need. Clinical governance is described in more detail in Chapter 10.

The success of these activities will be monitored by means of a national survey of the views of patients, by a series of clinical performance indicators derived from administrative data and by inspections. The inspections will involve site visits as well as the collection of quantitative data and will be undertaken by a new body, the Commission for Health Improvement. This Commission will undertake many of the functions normally seen in accreditation agencies but, in addition, will also be responsible for supporting development of clinical governance capacity in hospitals.

As such models are still at an early stage, it is too early to assess their success. They do, however, recognize the importance of interconnections between different parts of the health system. They also recognize that it is not enough simply to specify what must happen without establishing mechanisms by which standards can be implemented and monitored.

Lessons and implications

This chapter has identified various prerequisites for high-quality care. Although an individual hospital has a major role to play in securing such resources, it cannot do so alone. Thus, governments and those acting on their behalf have a responsibility to create the conditions necessary for hospitals to improve their performance.

In most cases, governments are already actively involved in these activities through their promulgation of rules on ownership and investment, their support for universities and their funding of health care, both capital and revenue. We simply argue that these activities should be aligned to achieve certain objectives: enhancing health outcomes and making services more responsive to patients. These external bodies should create the conditions that enable hospitals to perform well and should also play a greater role in specifying how hospitals should deliver health care.

There is experience with a wide range of tools across Europe. Some focus on specific resources, such as ensuring the existence of an appropriately trained workforce, or offering the capital that hospitals need to invest in facilities and equipment. As a first step, governments should evaluate the extent to which they have mechanisms in place that secure these resources. On their own, however, these individual activities are not enough. Well-designed buildings will not provide excellent care without well-trained staff, supported by the appropriate equipment. Even if all resources are in place, external agencies should be involved in guiding the hospital's activities so that it meets the health needs of the population it serves, in monitoring its achievements and in rewarding them accordingly. The challenge for the future is how to bring these activities together, with integrated programmes to promote high-quality care and sophisticated purchasing systems that can specify health needs and ensure that these are met in the most appropriate way.

References

Acheson, R.M. (1978) The definition and identification of need for health care, *Journal of Epidemiology and Community Health*, 32: 10–15.

Agence Nationale d'Accreditation et d'Evaluation en Santé (1998) *A Propos de l'Accreditation* [*On accreditation*]. Paris: Agence Nationale d'Accreditation et d'Evaluation en Santé.

Armstrong, M. (1991) *A Handbook of Personnel Management*. London: Kogan Page.

Australian Institute of Health and Welfare (1998) *Australian Hospital Statistics 1996–97*. Canberra: Australian Institute of Health and Welfare.

Banta, D. (1997) Report from the EUR-ASSESS project, *International Journal of Technology Assessment in Health Care*, 13: 133–340.

Black, N. (1990) Medical litigation and the quality of care, *Lancet*, 335: 35–7.

Black, N., Murphy, M., Lamping, D. *et al.* (1999) Consensus development methods: a review of best practice in creating clinical guidelines, *Journal of Health Service Research and Policy*, 4: 236–48.

Bohigas, L., Smith, D., Brooks, T. *ct al.* (1996) Accreditation programs for hospitals: funding and operation, *International Journal for Quality in Health Care*, 8: 583–9.

Bohigas, L., Brooks, T., Donahue, T. *et al.* (1998) A comparative analysis of surveyors from six hospital accreditation programmes and a consideration of the related management issues, *International Journal for Quality in Health Care*, 10: 7–13.

Buckley, G. (1999) Revalidation is the answer, *British Medical Journal*, 319: 1145–6.

Busse, R. (2000) *Health Care Systems in Transition: Germany*. Copenhagen: European Observatory on Health Care Systems.

Busse, R. and Schwartz, F. (1997) Financing reforms in the German hospital sector: from full cost cover principle to prospective case fees, *Medical Care*, 35(19): 40–9.

Busse, R., van der Grinten, T. and Svensson, P-G. (2002) Regulating entrepreneurial behaviour in hospitals: theory and practice, in R.B. Saltman, R. Busse and E. Mossialos (eds) *Regulating Entrepreneurial Behaviour in European Health Care Systems*. Buckingham: Open University Press.

Buxton, M. and Hanney, S. (1996) How can the payback from health services research be assessed?, *Journal of Health Services Research and Policy*, 1: 35–43.

Caillet, R. and Baillet, S. (2000) Accreditation: the French experience, *Hospital: Official Journal of the European Association of Hospital Managers*, (1): 23–4.

Carr-Hill, R.A. (1992) The measurement of patient satisfaction, *Journal of Public Health Medicine*, 14: 236.

Carr-Hill, R.A. and Jenkins-Clarke, S. (1995) Measurement systems in principle and in practice: the example of nursing workload, *Journal of Advanced Nursing*, 22(2): 221–5.

Clarke, A. and McKee, M. (1992) The consultant episode: an unhelpful measure, *British Medical Journal*, 305: 1307–8.

Cochrane Collaboration (1991) *Commission on Health Research for Development. Health Research: Essential Link to Equity in Development.* Oxford: Oxford University Press.

Cummings, M. (1999) Look at this case again, *British Medical Journal*, 318: 1009.

Davenport, R.J., Dennis, M.S. and Warlow, C.P. (1996) Effect of correcting outcome data for case-mix: an example from stroke medicine, *British Medical Journal*, 312: 1503–5.

Department of Health (1995) *NHS: The Patient's Charter: A Charter for England.* London: HMSO.

Department of Health (1997) *The New NHS: Modern, Dependable.* London: The Stationery Office.

Department of Health (1998a) *Our Healthier Nation: A Contract for Health.* London: The Stationery Office.

Department of Health (1998b) *A First Class Service: Quality in the New NHS.* London: The Stationery Office.

Department of Health (1999) *The NHS Performance Assessment Framework.* London: Department of Health.

Dickinson, E. (1998) Clinical effectiveness for health care quality improvement, *Journal of Quality in Clinical Practice*, 18(1): 37–46.

Dixon, J. and Preker, A. (1999) Learning from the NHS, *British Medical Journal*, 319: 1449–50.

Donabedian, A. (1966) Evaluating the quality of medical care, *Millbank Memorial Fund Quarterly*, 44: 169.

Dunn, P. (1998) The Wisheart affair: paediatric cardiological services in Bristol, 1990–5, *British Medical Journal*, 317: 1144–5.

Edhouse, J.A. and Wardrope, J. (1996) Do the national performance tables really indicate the performance of accident and emergency departments?, *Journal of Accident and Emergency Medicine*, 13: 123–6.

Egan, J. (1998) Concept of collective responsibility is important, *British Medical Journal*, 317: 811.

Egger, D., Lipson, D. and Adams, O. (2000) *Achieving the Right Balance: The Role of Policy-Making Processes in Managing Human Resources for Health Problems*, document WHO/EIP/OSD/00.2. Geneva: World Health Organization.

Eysenbach, G. (ed.) (1998) *Medicine and Medical Education in Europe.* Stuttgart: Thieme.

Ferguson, B., Sheldon, T. and Posnett, J. (1997) *Concentration and Choice in Health Care.* Glasgow: Royal Society of Medicine Press.

Fukuyama, F. (1992) *Trust: The Social Virtues and the Creation of Prosperity.* New York: Free Press.

Gaffney, D., Pollock, A.M., Price, D. and Shaoul, J. (1999a) PFI in the NHS: is there an economic case?, *British Medical Journal*, 319: 116–19.

Gaffney, D., Pollock, A.M., Price, D. and Shaoul, J. (1999b) The politics of the new private finance initiative and the new NHS, *British Medical Journal*, 319: 249–53.

Glanville, J., Haines, H. and Auston, I. (1998) Finding information on clinical effectiveness, *British Medical Journal*, 317(7152): 200–3.

Goldstein, H. and Spiegelhalter, D.J. (1996) League tables and their limitations: statistical issues in comparisons of institutional performance, *Journal of the Royal Statistical Society*, 159: 385–443.

Granados, A., Jonsson, E., Banta, D. *et al.* (1997) EUR-ASSESS project subgroup report on dissemination and impact, *International Journal of Technology Assessment in Health Care*, 13: 220–86.

Green, A. and Owen, D. (1995) The labour market aspects of population change in the 1990s, in R. Hall and P. White (eds) *Europe's Population: Towards the Next Century*. London: UCL Press.

Green, J., Passman, L.J. and Wintfeld, N. (1991) Analyzing hospital mortality: the consequences of diversity in patient mix, *Journal of the American Medical Association*, 265: 1849–53.

Ham, C. (1996) Contestability: a middle path for health care, *British Medical Journal*, (312): 70–1.

Hannan, E.L., Kilburn, H., Racz, M., Shields, E. and Chassin, M.R. (1994) Improving the outcomes of coronary artery bypass surgery in New York State, *Journal of the American Medical Association*, 271: 761–6.

Harding, A. and Preker, A.S. (2001) A conceptual framework for organizational reforms of hospitals, in A.S. Preker and A. Harding (eds) *Innovations in Health Services. Vol. 1: The Corporatization of Public Hospitals*. Baltimore, MD: Johns Hopkins University Press.

Healy, J. and McKee, M. (1997) Health sector reform in central and eastern Europe: the professional dimension, *Health Policy and Planning*, 12(4): 286–95.

Hewson, B. (2000) Why the Human Rights Act matters to doctors, *British Medical Journal*, 321: 780–1.

Hirschman, A. (1970) *Exit, Voice and Loyalty: Responses to Decline in Firms, Organizations and States*. Cambridge, MA: Harvard University Press.

International Labour Organization and Sectoral Activities Programme (1998) *Terms of Employment and Working Conditions in Health Sector Reforms*. Geneva: International Labour Office.

Jensen, G.A. and Morrisey, M.A. (1986) Medical staff specialty mix and hospital production, *Journal of Health Economics*, 5: 253–76.

Jourdan, S., Rossie, M.L. and Goulding, J. (2000) Italy: medical negligence as a crime, *Lancet*, 356: 1268–9.

Kulzhanov, M. and Healy, J. (1999) *Health Care Systems in Transition: Kazakhstan*. Copenhagen: European Observatory on Health Care Systems.

Leenen, H., Gevers, S. and Pinet, G. (eds) (1993) *The Rights of Patients in Europe: A Comparative Study*. Dordrecht: Kluwer.

Maarse, H.A.M. (1996) Fixed budgets in the inpatient sector: the case of the Netherlands, in F.W. Schwartz, H. Glennester, R.B. Saltman and R. Busse (eds) *Fixing Health Budgets: Experience from Europe and North America*. Chichester: John Wiley.

Marshall, E.C., Spiegelhalter, D.J., Sanderson, C. and McKee, M. (1998) Reliability of league tables of *in vitro* fertilisation clinics: retrospective analysis of live birth rates. Commentary: how robust are rankings? The implications of confidence intervals, *British Medical Journal*, 316: 1701–5.

Massion, J. (2000) The ethical characteristics of patients' rights in Europe, *Hospital: Official Journal of the European Association of Hospital Managers*, 2(1): 11–13.

McKee, M. and Hunter, D. (1995) Mortality league tables: do they inform or mislead?, *Quality Health Care*, 4: 5–12.

McKee, M. and Sheldon, T. (1998) Measuring performance in the NHS: good that it's moved beyond money and activity but many problems remain, *British Medical Journal*, 316: 322.

McKee, M., Coles, J. and James, P. (1999) 'Failure to rescue' as a measure of quality of hospital care: the limitations of secondary diagnosis coding in English hospital data, *Journal of Public Health Medicine*, 21: 453–8.

McPherson, K. and Britton, A. (1999) The impact of patient treatment preferences on the interpretation of randomised controlled trials, *European Journal of Cancer*, 35: 1598–602.

Montford, A.P. (1981) Production functions of general hospitals, *Social Science and Medicine*, 15: 87–98.

Mossialos, E. and Le Grand, J. (1999) Cost containment in the EU: an overview, in E. Mossialos and J. Le Grand (eds) *Health Care and Cost Containment in the European Union*. Aldershot: Ashgate.

Mossialos, E., Dixon, A., Figueras, J.E. and Kutzin, J. (2002) *Funding Health Care: Options for Europe*. Buckingham: Open University Press.

Myklebust, A. (2000) Patients' rights in the 1999 reforms in Norway, *Hospital: Official Journal of the European Association of Hospital Managers*, 1: 16.

New, B. (1998) Accountability and performance, in R. Klein (ed.) *Implementing the White Paper*. London: King's Fund.

OECD (1999) *OECD Health Data 99: A Comparative Analysis of 29 Countries*. Paris: Organisation for Economic Co-operation and Development.

Øvretveit, J. (1995) *Purchasing for Health*. Buckingham: Open University Press.

Perleth, M., Busse, R. and Schwartz, F. (1999) Regulation of health-related technologies in Germany, *Health Policy*, 46: 105–26.

Pollit, C. and Bouckaert, G. (2000) *Public Management Reform: A Comparative Analysis*. Oxford: Oxford University Press.

Pollit, C., Girre, X., Lonsdale, J. *et al.* (1999) *Performance or Compliance: Performance Audit and Public Management in Five Countries*. Oxford: Oxford University Press.

Pollock, A.M., Dunnigan, M.G., Gaffney, D., Price, D. and Shaoul, J. (1999) The private finance initiative: planning the 'new' NHS: downsizing for the 21st century, *British Medical Journal*, 319(7203): 179–84.

Purdy, S. and Rich, G. (1995) Accrediting hospitals, *British Medical Journal*, 311: 456.

Putnam, R.D. (1992) *Making Democracy Work: Civic Traditions in Modern Italy*. Princeton, NJ: Princeton University Press.

Rawlins, M. (1999) In pursuit of quality: the National Institute for Clinical Excellence, *Lancet*, 353: 1079–82.

Robinson, R. (1995) Accrediting hospitals, *British Medical Journal*, 310: 755–6.

Robinson, R. and Dixon, A. (1999) *Health Care Systems in Transition: United Kingdom*. Copenhagen: European Observatory on Health Care Systems.

Rockall, T.A., Logan, R.F., Devlin, H.B. and Northfield, T.C. (1995) Variation in outcome after acute upper gastrointestinal haemorrhage: the national audit of acute upper gastrointestinal haemorrhage, *Lancet*, 346: 346–50.

Roemer, M.I. (1993) Health facilities, in *National Health Care Systems of the World*, Vol. 2. New York: Oxford University Press.

Saltman, R.B., Busse, R. and Mossialos, E. (eds) (2002) *Regulating Entrepreneurial Behaviour in European Health Care Systems*. Buckingham: Open University Press.

Salvage, J. and Heijnen, S. (eds) (1997) *Nursing in Europe: A Resource for Better Health*, WHO Regional Publications, European Series, No. 74. Copenhagen: WHO Regional Office for Europe.

Sanderson, C., Hunter, D.J., McKee, M. and Black, N. (1997) Limitations of epidemiologically based needs assessment: the case of prostatectomy, *Medical Care*, 35: 669–85.

Savill, R. (1996) Targets being put ahead of patients says resigning health manager, *Daily Telegraph*, 25 April, p. 6.

Scally, G. and Donaldson, L.J. (1998) Clinical governance and the drive for quality improvement in the new NHS in England, *British Medical Journal*, 317: 61–5.

Schneider, E.C. and Epstein, A.M. (1996) Influence of cardiac-surgery performance reports on referral practices and access to care: a survey of cardiovascular specialists, *New England Journal of Medicine*, 335: 251–6.

Scrivens, E. (1995) *Accreditation: Protecting the Professional or the Consumer?* Buckingham: Open University Press.

Scrivens, E. (1997) Putting continuous quality improvement into accreditation: improving approaches to quality assessment, *Quality in Health Care*, 6: 212–18.

Scrivens, E. (1998) Policy issues in accreditation, *International Journal for Quality in Health Care*, 10(1): 1–5.

Silver, M.H.W. (1997) Patients' rights in England and the United States of America: the Patient's Charter and the New Jersey Patient Bill of Rights: a comparison, *Journal of Medical Ethics*, 23: 213–20.

Smith, P. (1993) Outcome related performance indicators and organisational control in the public sector, *British Journal of Management*, 4: 135–51.

Smith, R. (1998) All changed, changed utterly, *British Medical Journal*, 316: 1917–18.

Smith, R. (1999) PFI: perfidious financial idiocy: a 'free lunch' that could destroy the NHS, *British Medical Journal*, 319: 2–3.

Stevens, A. and Raftery, J. (1994) *Health Care Needs Assessment*, Vol. 1. Oxford: Radcliffe.

Sunol, R., Delgado, R. and Esteban, A. (1991) Medical audit: the Spanish experience, *British Medical Journal*, 303: 1249–51.

Swingedau, O. (2000) The Ombudsman: mediating on behalf of patients, *Hospital: Official Journal of the European Association of Hospital Managers*, 2(1): 14–15.

Treasure, T. (1998) Lessons from the Bristol case. More openness – on risks and on individual surgeons' performance, *British Medical Journal*, 316: 1685–6.

Trilla, A. and Bruguera, M. (2000) Spain: avoiding law suits, *Lancet*, 356: 1266–7.

Weatherall, D. (1994) The inhumanity of medicine, *British Medical Journal*, 309: 1671–2.

WHO (1999). *HEALTH21: The Health for All Policy Framework for the WHO European Region*, European Health for All Series, No. 6. Copenhagen: WHO Regional Office for Europe.

WHO (2000) *The World Health Report 2000. Health Systems: Improving Performance*. Geneva: World Health Organization.

Wildavsky, A. (1979) *Speaking Truth to Power: The Art and Craft of Policy Analysis*. Boston, MA: Little, Brown & Company.

Williams, B. (1994) Patient satisfaction: a valid concept?, *Social Science and Medicine*, 38: 509.

World Bank (1993) *World Development Report 1993: Investing in Health*. New York: Oxford University Press.

chapter eight

Hospital payment mechanisms: theory and practice in transition countries

John C. Langenbrunner
and Miriam M. Wiley

Introduction and overview

The rationale for provider payment policies for hospitals is to change behaviour. If this is managed carefully, performance can improve, leading to both lower costs and higher quality. This, in short, is the premise behind policy changes in hospital payment methods around the world, especially in more mature health care delivery systems.

Payment system changes create new incentives for motivating providers of care and for driving overall organizational changes related to the role of the hospital in the delivery of services. The financing of the hospital sector and the search for more efficient and effective tools and techniques is now a feature of the health systems of most members of the Organisation for Economic Co-operation and Development (OECD). The recent trends in these countries are just the beginning of a longer-term transition for hospitals and their role in health care delivery.

This chapter examines the evolving changes in hospital payment policies, with particular attention to countries in eastern Europe, defined in this chapter as the countries of central and eastern Europe, the countries of the former Soviet Union plus Turkey. The Czech Republic (1995), Hungary (1996), Poland (1996) and Turkey (1961) are also members of the OECD.

These countries face a new and challenging environment. Severe health-sector problems exist related to both total funding for health care and the efficiency of their health care services. In the late 1980s, it became clear that poor performance and declining health outcomes were caused not only by underfunding, but also by inadequate management of health care resources (Sheiman 1993; Ensor 1997). The lack of efficiency incentives were compounded by low levels of spending. The share of gross domestic product devoted to health was traditionally small, ranging from 3 to 6 per cent (Preker and Feachem 1996) versus 6–9 per cent in OECD countries (Poullier *et al.* 1994). The chronic underfunding was exacerbated in the transition to a more market-based economy when health funding fell precipitously (Klugman and Schieber 1996; University of York 1998).

Another area of concern was the bias of hospital care over primary care, compounded by the inefficiency of outpatient physicians. The lack of competition and choice as well as the lack of efficiency incentives encouraged physicians to act as indifferent dispatchers in referring patients to hospitals. Referral rates to hospitals ran as high as 25–30 per cent of first visits to clinics in countries of the former Soviet Union in the early 1990s (Sheiman 1993) relative to 8.6 per cent in the United Kingdom and 5.2 per cent in the United States (Sandier 1989). Hospital admission rates as a percentage of population were 18–24 per cent for countries of the former Soviet Union relative to 16 per cent on average for all OECD countries. About 65–85 per cent of state health budgets was allocated to inpatient care in countries of the former Soviet Union (WHO 2001) compared with 45–50 per cent in OECD countries (OECD 1997).

As in OECD countries, some countries in eastern Europe are examining alternatives to historical budgeting approaches. These approaches generally fall into four categories: (i) payments per day; (ii) payment systems per case or per admission, some with case-mix adjusters; (iii) global budgeting; and (iv) capitation. This chapter examines the adoption and implementation of these approaches in countries of eastern Europe compared with similar systems in western Europe.

The inherited system

Provider payment systems for health services in hospital cannot be separated from larger health care system issues. The health sectors of most countries in eastern Europe are in transition from a centrally planned national health service model to more decentralized systems. (Chapter 2 describes the main features of the Soviet health care model.)

The public system was financed from the general state budget, from enterprise budgets and extra-budgetary funds. Private payments were limited to a few non-essential services as well as some unofficial payments to public providers for preferential treatment.

Funding flowed through a centralized, top-down bureaucratic allocation process, based on national budgets formulated and passed by the central legislative and policy-making bodies. Resources were allocated according to a consolidated national plan. Reserves were allocated according to norms based on the Semashko model: an expert assessment of the number of units of input required for a given population at each level of the system. The norms led to specific budgetary requirements for each health care institution.

Line-item budgets

For a hospital, the number of beds determined the number and type of staff. The total staffing budget was obtained by multiplying staff numbers by the appropriate national pay scale. This reflected the experience of staff, their specialties and some adjustment coefficients. One of the adjustments was for geographical region of working; areas of environmental degradation, such as the area round the Aral Sea or sites of nuclear tests, were considered to justify additional salary. Funding for other line items was based on the facility and population-specific norms. Food expenditure in hospitals (budget line item 9), for example, was based on the number of bed-days in the previous year (Ensor and Langenbrunner 2001) or on the normative number of bed-days. Altogether, there were 18 distinct categories. In an example from the Ukraine, salaries plus payroll tax were the largest category. A capital allocation could be included (budget line item 16) but was perceived as a one-shot allocation and not reflected as annual depreciation. The 'planned' levels at the beginning of the year differed from the 'actual' levels, depending on factors such as inflation and revenues during the budget cycle.

Line-item budgeting was characterized by 'rules of conduct' (Preker and Feachem 1996) as follows.

- The current year's allocation primarily reflected historical budgets plus some inflation factors.
- There was limited or no reallocation across categories or from year to year.
- Salaries, food and medicines took priority under difficult economic constraints.

Line-item budgeting has both positive and negative features. On the positive side, it allows strong central control when management skills in local regions are inadequate, provides predictable levels of budgets and expenses and can mean that minimum standards are met in every facility. On the negative side, however, it means:

- incentives to underprovide or refer out for needed care;
- little flexibility to adapt to local or innovative circumstances;
- no direct incentives for information or management expertise;
- no direct incentives for outputs or outcomes; and
- a tendency to create high levels of fixed resources, as line-item allocations rarely change.

Line-item budgets, especially when tied to resource inputs, have tended to discourage the reduction of excess capacity (building space and personnel), a hallmark of most countries in eastern Europe (Preker and Feachem 1996; Klugman and Schieber 1997; University of York 1998). Second, constrained line-item budgets have encouraged facility managers (and individual providers) to find other sources of funds. This partly explains the widespread use of informal out-of-pocket payments in eastern Europe (Lewis 2002).

The transition

As early as 1987, the Soviet Union began testing new organizational and financing models to improve efficiency. The New Economic Mechanism, for example, picked a number of geographical demonstration areas, reorganized the polyclinics into family practice groups and initiated fundholding arrangements. The objective was to shift the locus of care to less expensive outpatient and primary services. Sheiman (1993) reports that these arrangements in the Russian Federation reduced inpatient admissions by 10–15 per cent and reallocated from approximately 70 : 30 inpatient-to-outpatient spending to levels closer to 50 : 50 (Schieber 1993). Samara, an oblast (region) in the Russian Federation, reported closing 5500 beds. In the Dzhezkazgan region of Kazakhstan, admissions declined by 26 per cent and numbers of beds per capita by 32 per cent (Langenbrunner *et al.* 1994). These demonstration projects did little to upgrade the technology of inpatient payment systems. Fundholders in Dzhezkazgan used only a simple payment system per day with administrative guidelines for admissions and discharges. Average lengths of stay did not drop and case mix did not appear to change over time. The New Economic Mechanism demonstrations ultimately failed when the St Petersburg experiment, which involved a system of budget-holding by primary care organizations, was stopped because of inappropriate declines in referrals to hospitals and underdeveloped quality assurance systems.

Since the early 1990s, the search for a more diverse revenue base in the countries of the former Soviet Union has included: (i) new revenues through small patient co-payments, especially for outpatient pharmaceuticals; (ii) separate employer-based payroll contributions that de-linked revenues from the budgetary process; (iii) private contracting with enterprises; and (iv) a private supplemental insurance sector. These measures have typically been linked with organizational changes such as the enactment of separate, self-sustaining public health insurance trust funds. These funding and organizational changes have catalysed changes in purchasing arrangements, policy on provider payment and organization. Several areas of change typically have emerged, including restructuring of financing, decentralization and local management autonomy and new purchasing arrangements.

- *Restructuring of financing.* Separate dedicated payroll taxes either replace or supplement traditional public budgets for health. Poland is implementing health insurance but uses traditional public health budgets to cover high-end specialized services such as transplants. Some countries of the former Soviet Union use public budgets to cover insurance fund contributions for the non-working population and continue to fund 'specialized' services such as tuberculosis, psychiatry and oncology, as well as 'priority' services such as immunization and AIDS services. Private sources of payment by employers, insurers and individuals also contribute to overall expenditure on care.
- *Decentralization and local management autonomy.* The devolution of decision-making from central committees towards regional and local autonomy varies considerably between countries. In the Russian Federation, relatively autonomous regional insurance funds collect and spend about 85 per cent

of all health expenditure; in other countries, funds are collected centrally and reallocated to regions and local areas. In most of eastern Europe, countries pool and reallocate some funds to improve equity. The 19 regional funds in Poland send 14.2 per cent of revenues to the central fund for reallocation. Decentralization can extend to the provider level, with legal and organizational autonomy for physicians (for example, Croatia, Hungary and Poland) and for inpatient facilities (for example, Kazakhstan and Poland). Most countries in eastern Europe, however, still lack an adequate management and information infrastructure to manage change and risk.

- *New purchasing arrangements.* Purchasers and providers of care are being split. Funds now purchase services through selective contracting (Savas *et al.* 1997) and encourage improved internal efficiency through improved service payment systems. New performance-based or market-oriented hospital payment systems pay for a defined unit of hospital output.

Alternative models of hospital payment

A specification of appropriate units of measurement is an essential precondition for quantifying the relationship between resources and hospital workload. Resource measurement is reasonably straightforward, being specified mostly in monetary terms. Staff resources may be estimated in terms of full-time equivalents or hours worked, or space may be measured in square metres. The quantification of hospital workload is more challenging, however, since alternative units of measurement may include procedure or service, hospital bed-day, hospital discharge, case mix-adjusted discharge units or an aggregate of these units. The option chosen to measure hospital workload is an important constituent of any hospital payment model. These are reviewed briefly here to illustrate the implications associated with a range of alternative hospital payment models.

Payment based on procedure or service

Financing tied to the provision of a specified procedure or service is often referred to as fee for service. The number of procedures or services provided within the specifications agreed between the payer and the service providers determines the level of resources available to the hospital. Factors relevant to the implementation of this approach include:

- This is administratively straightforward for the payer and provider.
- Demands on specificity and timeliness of data may be considerable.
- Specification or quantification of surgical procedures and paraclinical services are more straightforward, which may improve patient access.
- An incentive to perform more procedures may have an adverse effect on quality and overall expenditure.
- There is an incentive to improve efficiency when hospital costs exceed the reimbursement rate but no incentive when the rate exceeds costs.

Payment per day

Financing based on a specified payment per bed-day raises the following issues:

- The data needed are generally available.
- This is administratively straightforward for the payer and provider.
- Incentives exist to maintain long lengths of stay, which may have an adverse effect on access, quality and expenditures.
- The skewed distribution of costs during a hospital stay is not related to the cost of care; costs per day typically follow a bell-shaped curve, increasing on successive days after admission and then decreasing.

Payment per case

There are two basic types of models: per case or per discharge. In the first, a simple discharge-based payment model, hospital financing is based on a specified payment per discharge, regardless of the type of case. Issues arising in the implementation of this model include:

- The data are generally available.
- There is an incentive to increase admissions, especially if payment exceeds costs, which may have an adverse effect on quality.
- The resources allocated may have little relationship to the cost of the care provided.

In the second type, the case mix-adjusted discharge model, financing is based on a specified payment per discharge unit standardized for variations in types of cases or case mix. The most widely used approach internationally is the diagnosis-related group (DRG) system. Using this system, together with estimates of resource use at the patient group level, a case mix index measuring the relative cost of the case mix treated by the hospital can be estimated. The issues arising with the application of this model include:

- This model is somewhat complex administratively and operationally.
- It depends on the availability of relatively consistent and comprehensive activity and cost data.
- It is more equitable, as reimbursement is based on a composite measure of services provided.
- Incentives exist to ensure that costs are limited by service type within payment boundaries.

Global budget

Global budgets for hospitals are aggregate one-line payments fixed in advance to cover expenditures for specified services during a fixed period of time (for example, 1 year). Global budgets constrain the growth in the price and quantity of services while allowing flexibility in the use of resources within budget limits. A budget surplus at the end of the payment period can be kept by the facility for use as it sees fit; spending above the target must be met by the hospital from other sources. Once a budget is established, providers must remain within the budget either by adjusting the price or cost of services or the volume of services. Efficiency improves when global budgets are strictly enforced. The issues arising with the application of this model include:

- The model depends on the availability of more comprehensive activity and cost data.
- Payer complexity generally increases with the complexity of the budget formula and whether it includes only historical budgets (the simplest) or utilization, adjustment for case mix or adjustment for other risks and social equity factors.
- It is somewhat complex administratively and operationally for the provider, so that local management autonomy is critical to reallocate resources efficiently and maintain spending within a fixed budget.
- Incentives ensure a cost profile by service type within payment boundaries, but if revenues are too low, global budgets may contain incentives to lower the quality of care or to ration services.
- Periodic monitoring by the payer may be necessary, as well as an administrative system to enforce the budget and to respond to appeals and special requests.

Capitation

At its simplest, per capita payment is used to provide (i) a specified package of health care services for (ii) a specified population for (iii) a fixed fee per person for (iv) a fixed period of time (for example, 1 year). Per capita payments can be used at a variety of levels in the health sector: to determine regional budgets, to determine budgets for intermediary fundholders within a region or to distribute funds from the payer to a specific health institution or group of institutions.

At the facility level, the capitation amount depends on the types of services included in the benefit package, and the membership group of enrollees must be clearly specified. A fundholder and health institution may choose to provide only some services under a capitation payment (for example, hospital services at a single facility) or all services for an integrated system of facilities (for example, a hospital and its associated polyclinic). The issues arising with the application of this model include:

- Of all the payment systems, this is the one that most depends on the availability of comprehensive data on activities and costs, especially for the provider.
- Payer complexity generally increases with the complexity of the budget formula and whether it includes only historical per capita payments (the simplest) or utilization, adjustment for case mix or adjustment for other risks and social equity factors.

Table 8.1 Rating of selected models of hospital payment against objective criteria

Unit of payment	Efficiency	Access	Quality
Procedure or service	uncertain	surgery positive	uncertain
Bed-day	negative	uncertain	uncertain
Discharge	negative	positive	negative
Case mix-adjusted unit	positive	positive	uncertain
Global budget	positive	uncertain	uncertain
Capitation	positive	uncertain	uncertain

- It is the most complex and risky model for the provider operationally and administratively. The provider manages the entire episode of care, and local management autonomy is critical to reallocating resources efficiently and maintaining spending within a fixed budget.
- Strong incentives exist to ensure a cost profile by service type within the boundaries of revenue limits, but if payment is too low, capitation may contain incentives to lower the quality of care or to ration services.

The models reviewed here can be evaluated against the objectives of efficiency, access and quality care (Table 8.1). None of these models contribute to achieving all the objectives of efficiency, access and quality within a hospital payment system. However, complementary administrative safeguards have been effective in limiting concerns related to access, quality and volume (Coulam and Gaumer 1991).

Early experiences: central and eastern Europe and the former Soviet Union

The most popular approaches in the early years of transition were based on payment per day and per case, which can be viewed as linked. These systems were implemented in some countries in four or five successive stages:

- A specific rate per day based on the historical budget divided by the average number of hospital days, the denominator being based on the hospital, the category of hospital (for example, rural or urban) or a geographical region.
- A specific rate per discharge, regardless of case severity or hospital, which (predictably) encouraged admissions of easy cases relative to severe ones (Wickham 1998).
- A specific rate per discharge, adjusted by type of facility, so that, for example, a specialty hospital was differentiated from a small rural hospital, to proxy both differences in case mix and differences in input costs such as labour costs.
- A specific rate per discharge, adjusted by clinical department across hospitals, with some facility-based adjustments. Real average case costs were calculated for each hospital by each clinical department and averaged across all hospitals, resulting in a unified weighting scale against the average cost of the treated case in the defined region.

Figure 8.1 Case-mix groups: an iterative process

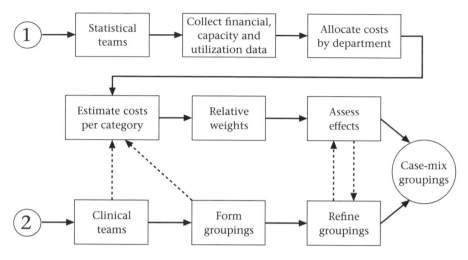

- An iteration process of increasing the number of payment groups from 25–50 to some larger number based on clinical logic and homogeneity of resource use (Figure 8.1).

Countries started at different levels and progressed differently, and typically included only recurrent costs not capital costs or depreciation. Nevertheless, these steps serve as a developmental framework for examining these countries in terms of alternative hospital payment models. Table 8.2 summarizes hospital payment systems in countries in eastern Europe. The following sections illustrate different types of systems with descriptions of how they work in practice.

Fee for service

Czech Republic

One of the first countries to introduce health-sector reform, the Czech Republic initially adopted fees for hospital services, but with very negative results. In 1993, 27 not-for-profit insurance companies were competing for patients in a population of roughly 10 million. They paid providers generally on a fee-for-service basis from price lists of up to 5000 separate services. The volume of services and corresponding expenditures rapidly grew in the early 1990s, from Kcs7112 per capita in 1993 to an estimated Kcs12,744 in 1998. The biggest budget categories were personnel and pharmaceuticals. Health-sector wages mirrored wage growth in the economy at large; pharmaceuticals captured 23 per cent of public expenditures in 1996, well above the OECD average of 11.8 per cent. The new insurance companies began to go bankrupt from 1995, and by 1998 only nine of the original 27 remained, with Kcs2 billion in unpaid debts, especially to hospitals.

Table 8.2 Summary of hospital payment systems in countries in eastern Europe for which information is available

Country	Line item	Per day	Per case	Global budget	Capitation
Albania	X				
Armenia	X		developing		
Azerbaijan	X				
Bosnia and Herzegovina				developing	
Bulgaria			developing	developing	
Croatia		X		developing	
Czech Republic			X	X	
Estonia		X			
Georgia			X		
Hungary			X		
Kazakhstan	X		X		
Kyrgyzstan	X		X		
Latvia		X	developing		
Lithuania			X		
Poland			X		developing
Republic of Moldova	X				
Romania			developing		
Russian Federation	X	X	X	X	uncertain
Slovakia		X			
Slovenia		X			
Tajikistan	X				
Turkey	X				
Turkmenistan	X		X		
Ukraine	X				
Uzbekistan	X				

The remaining insurers have shifted to new payment systems. By 1998, general practitioners were paid on a capitated basis for all basic outpatient services; specialists were paid on a point system; hospital payment is evolving and represents the biggest source of overspending. Budgetary financing based on historical allocation was introduced in 1997, and some pilot hospitals have a mixed arrangement, receiving a budget adjusted for the prospective case mix. The earlier incentives led to a rise in the cost structure of hospitals, and the insurance bankruptcies and new payment caps brought about accumulating debts. Ministry of Health hospitals have the largest outstanding debt at over Kcs400 million. Municipal and private hospitals (about 25 per cent of the total) have less debt, partly because there is greater accountability and less access to discretionary funds from the Ministry of Health (Fidler 1999).

Per day

A summary of the per day systems across countries is provided in Table 8.3.

Table 8.3 Features of systems of payment per day for hospital services across selected countries in eastern Europe

Country	Case-mix adjuster	Hospital adjuster	Overall expenditure cap	Other features
Croatia		X	X (1999)	Point system for providers
Estonia	X		X	Fee-for-service for some procedures
Slovakia		X		
Slovenia	X (high cost cases)		X	

Croatia

Facilities are paid for services according to a three-tier system of bed-days (adjusted for level of hospital), a separate payment for physicians using a medical work point system, plus reimbursement for specific material inputs such as food and drugs. Bed-day payments are adjusted according to three levels of hospital facility specialization: general, regional and university. The medical work point system is based on the staff skill mix and an estimated time for each procedure. There is an exhaustive list of more than 90,000 procedures and their point values. These arrangements have severely distorted incentives in cost-increasing ways (for example, unnecessary bed-days and excessive drug use). The costs of inpatient care increased by 70 per cent in real terms over 5 years (1994–98) and by 26 per cent from 1997 to 1998 alone. This led to a recent cap on inpatient spending. The hospital share of total health care spending dropped slightly to about 50 per cent in 1997. Admissions and the hospital share of total spending also increased during the early to mid-1990s, despite national efforts to develop primary care, which had the unintended effect of encouraging referral to specialists and hospitals. The Ministry of Health still allocates the budget for specialized services and capital investments. Health spending as a share of gross domestic product in Croatia has climbed to somewhere between 10 and 12 per cent by some estimates (World Bank 1999a).

Slovak Republic

Health care is 96 per cent covered through health insurance and 4 per cent through other resources. The six health insurance agencies are public-service institutions; the General Health Insurance Agency is the largest, with 62 per cent of the insured people. About 45 per cent of health expenditure goes to hospitals. In 1998, hospitals were reimbursed based on the number of days per bed, with payment adjusted by type of hospitals according to three categories: regional (four departments), district (greater range of departmental specialties) and highly specialized institutions mostly associated with university medical schools. The medical staff are salaried.

The average length of stay was 11 days in 1997. A World Bank analysis in March 1999 found relatively little variation by type of hospital; for example, the uniform length of stay in maternity cases was 7.5 days. Anecdotal evidence suggests that, to keep hospitals full, and consequently receive payments, patients were admitted over a weekend, thus increasing their length of stay by 2 days. Hospitals were said to admit patients with less severe conditions and keep them longer than necessary rather than admit more severe cases for whom they would receive the same compensation. In 1999, the government took a number of measures intended to control the costs of the insurance-based system, including a proposed move from a system of payment per day to a global budget system.

Slovenia

Hospitals are paid by the number of prospectively contracted bed-days, which control the overall hospital expenditure envelope. Nevertheless, this input-based budget does not include any latitude to reallocate potential savings through reduced average length of stay or other efficiencies. Savings cannot, for example, be used for staff bonuses or to purchase new equipment. Staff are paid on a salary basis. Some exceptions have been introduced such as incentive payments for maintaining empty beds and flat-rate payments per admission for high-cost cases such as heart surgery, transplants and dialysis. The World Bank is to fund a project costing US$11.3 million to develop a national health information system from 2000, which will assist in providing a statistical baseline for moving to a more output-based hospital budget.

Latvia

The country has consolidated 33 local sickness funds into eight regional funds. Specialized and tertiary services remain under a separate budget-financed state programme but later will merge with the regional sickness funds. The hospital sector is characterized by excess capacity (10.3 beds per 1000) and inefficiency. Government-run tertiary hospitals are still paid on the basis of inputs such as beds and personnel. The Sickness Funds pay on the basis of bed-days, although DRG payment pilots have begun in some regions. A new World Bank project of US$42 million includes a long-term strategy to restructure health services (World Bank 1998).

Estonia

The country has implemented a health insurance system that pays for inpatient services by bed-days. The bed-day calculation includes adjustments for specialty ward and the number of beds as a proxy for complexity. The payment level is further adjusted for 57 types of cases, which differ on a range of areas, including diagnosis, treatment, nursing, food, simple medical procedures, laboratory tests and pharmaceuticals. Some additional procedures, such as physiotherapy, can be billed separately on a fee-for-service basis according to price lists. There is an overall cap, however, on inpatient services. The health insurance fund may move to a less complex system with more bundled payments. There is a relatively *ad hoc* approach to reimbursement for capital, although facilities in

Table 8.4 Features of systems of payment per case for hospital services across selected countries in eastern Europe

Country	Payment categories	Payment rate basis	Facility adjustments	Outlier payment feature	Overall spending cap
Georgia	30	Historical budget and throughput norms			
Hungary	758	Historical costs	X	X	X
Kazakhstan	55	Historical budgets	X		
Kyrgyzstan	154	Historical budgets	X	X	
Lithuania	50	Historical bed-days		X	
Poland	9–29	Estimated payroll tax revenues			
Russian Federation	Up to 10,000	Varies	X		

Estonia, Latvia and Lithuania often lease equipment through private vendors (International Finance Corporation 1999).

Per case

Table 8.4 summarizes the characteristics of systems of payment per case in selected countries.

Lithuania

A Territorial Patient Fund pays for inpatient services on a case-mix system, using medical profiles with attached prices. The price is based on historical bed-day costs by specialty and covers salaries, laboratory tests and part of depreciation. Prices for the 50 categories vary by a factor of 12. Secondary inpatient services are divided into 14 disease groups for adults and nine for children. In tertiary care (university level), there are 17 groups for adults and 10 for children. Payment is per bed-day if the length of stay is less than 4 days. There are supplemental payments for outlier cases that surpass a cost threshold of 130 per cent and supplemental payments for six categories of diagnostic tests and treatments (for example, computed tomographic scan, angiography and lithotripsy).

Capital costs are mainly reimbursed on an *ad hoc* basis through municipal budgets and Ministry of Finance allocations, but accounting systems fail to incorporate depreciation (International Finance Corporation 1999). The average length of stay (10 days in 1996) and average number of beds per capita have been dropping. The mix of incentives (primary care capitation) and payment per case may be responsible for admissions steadily increasing in the 1990s (Heijnen and Schneider 1999). Volume limits for inpatient care may be needed. The World Bank is financing a new US$37 million project to support, among other things, information systems and health services restructuring, which may contribute to new refinements in the payment system.

Poland

The 19 regional insurance funds began implementing a new system from January 1999. Most regional funds have chosen a simple case-mix payment system composed of 9–29 categories, with efforts underway to refine the groupings, supported by a World Bank loan. The payment system is for recurrent costs only and, until facilities receive independent juridical status, managers are constrained by national labour codes and an inability to make decisions on capital investments. Budget allocations are still made for specialized services and capital investments. The funds are paying claims for inpatient admissions that are running up to 30 per cent higher than last year. There also are anecdotal reports of a lack of access for difficult cases and cream-skimming through admissions of easy cases.

Russian Federation

The country is difficult to characterize, although discharge systems per case appear to dominate. Some regions use payments per day, typically adjusted by level of hospital, and cap payments through length-of-stay norms for each disease category. The Russian Federation is an agglomeration of 89 regions tied together loosely by the old federal Ministry of Health and regional administrative structure and the new health insurance system funded by a 3.6 per cent payroll tax paid by employers. Local budgets also make corresponding contributions to the health insurance fund on behalf of the non-working population. In some regions, money pooled at the health insurance fund level is then administered by intermediate-level insurance companies, which are both public and private. These companies selectively contract with providers for some population group and also may sell private, supplemental insurance policies. However, local government contributions are not always forthcoming, and local budgets and mandatory insurance funds are often separated. The traditional budget covers programmes of social importance, non-working population groups and municipal health.

The 1991 and 1993 laws were vague on provider payment mechanisms and each regional fund has chosen its own approach. A recent Federal Fund survey shows that the regions use a mix of payment systems for inpatient care (Figure 8.2). Most use some form of system using bed-days or payment per case. In the Kemerovo oblast and the Chuvash Republic, for example, the health insurance fund pays according to a complex formula of completed inpatient case and per outpatient visit. The categories of payment are adjusted by International Classification of Diseases (ICD) diagnostic codes (approximately 10,000) and by five levels of care (level of hospital mostly). This produces over 50,000 possible inpatient rates and over 10,000 outpatient rates. The rates are updated for inflation periodically in a crude percentage update across the board. Kemerovo recently abandoned this system due to severe upcoding of claims and is moving to a simpler system of under 100 categories. High volumes of

Figure 8.2 Inpatient payment systems in the Russian Federation according to the number of regions

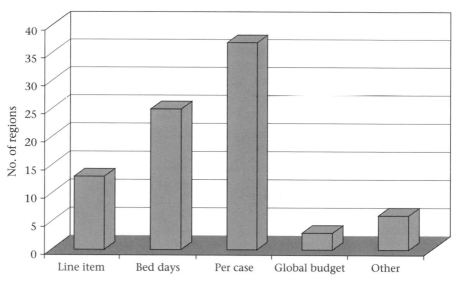

admissions have been reported in a number of oblasts over the past few years, the response being to cap overall spending.

The payments per day and per case typically cover salaries, medicines and food. Capital and maintenance costs are covered through a number of pockets at the administrative levels in the oblasts, cities and rayons. The flow of funds typically is fragmented, via separate administrative levels and programmes, while multiple and often *ad hoc* pots of funds dilute payment reforms. The national and oblast hospitals continue to receive budgets on the line-item model.

Georgia

A new health system introduced a case-mix payment system of 30 disease categories for payment to hospitals in 1995. Weights were calculated using measurable direct costs per stay plus averages per day for indirect costs (maintenance, administration and laundry) times the average length of stay. There are complications, since salary costs assume standard admissions and occupancy, but dropping throughput has cut the real levels of payment. Categories are revised each year to adjust for input costs (Rhodes *et al.* 1999). The incentives in this or any system, however, are blunted by the levels of out-of-pocket payments, currently estimated at a huge 87 per cent of all spending (Lewis 2002). A similar case-mix system is under development in Armenia.

Kazakhstan

The geographical regions have begun to pilot a relatively simple case-based payment system consisting of 55 different clinical groups, which vary by diagnosis, treatment department, whether the patient had surgery and whether the patient was admitted to the intensive care unit. The new insurance funds, in regions such as Semipalatinsk and Dzhezkazgan, have moved from payments per day in the mid-1990s to one payment level per case to more sophisticated case-mix systems of 55 categories. The changes coincided with other organizational reforms. In Dzhezkazgan, the number of hospitals declined from 55 to 22 from 1994 to 1997 and the number of beds from 6225 to 2919 (Horst 1998). At the same time, the reductions in beds and facilities have been 40–50 per cent nationally (Kulzhanov and Healy 1999). At the beginning of 1999, the government of Kazakhstan abolished the insurance fund, replacing it with oblast purchasing centres independent from the oblast health administrations. The centres are supposed to contract with health facilities for services for the population on an open-tender basis, which could, in theory, mean that the most efficient facilities gain through additional funding.

Kyrgyzstan

After pilots in several regions, the health insurance fund went from the traditional system to 55 and, most recently, to 154 categories. The health insurance fund cannot pay the full cost per case, only for staff, drugs, supplies and food, altogether less than 30 per cent of total case costs. The health insurance fund initially contracted with general hospitals (oblast, city, central rayon and a few national hospitals), not dispensaries, specialty hospitals or small rural hospitals. Hospitals targeted for closure in rationalization plans also were excluded. The health insurance fund now has a database of over 300,000 cases for analysis, which provides a good opportunity to track the effects of change (O'Dougherty 1999). Preliminary results show drops in average length of stay from 14.3 days to 13.2 days, although case mix had not changed significantly (Samushkin 1998). Changes in hospital payments have not apparently driven structural reforms as few, if any, wards and hospitals have been merged or shut. Fixed costs will be addressed simultaneously with rationalization and changes in flow of funds over the next few years (O'Dougherty 1999).

Hungary

This country has been developing a sophisticated system of payment per case since the early 1990s, after the establishment of a universal compulsory employment-based health insurance scheme. Since 1993, the national Health Insurance Fund Administration has entered into performance-based contracts with providers. The Fund pays primary care on an adjusted capitation basis; outpatient services are paid on a point system similar to that in Germany; acute hospital care is paid through homogeneous disease groups, adapted from DRGs in the United States. Importantly, the three areas (primary care, outpatient care and inpatient care) each have expenditure caps. The initial relative shares determined in 1992 have remained much the same. Most health professionals are salaried public servants, most general hospitals are owned by local government (county and municipality), while national institutes and medical universities are run by central government. Homogeneous disease group payments cover salaries and other variable costs but not capital costs or depreciation. The latter costs are the responsibility of the institution's owners, subsidized from the central health budget, which is determined jointly by the Ministries of Finance, Health, and Internal Affairs (OECD 1999).

The current 758 homogeneous disease group categories stem from 26 main diagnosis categories, with splits for additional diagnosis, procedures and the age of the patient. The weight (relative cost) of each of the 758 categories is also adjusted for lengths of stay. Once an upper day limit is reached, cases are paid per day according to a national formula for chronic care patients, and until 1998 types of hospital-specific adjustments were based more on historical cost structure (OECD 1999). The national cap on hospital spending means that, as volume changes, the base payment fluctuates, thus changing the relative payment for a homogeneous disease group. The weights were initially based on 28 pilot hospitals, selected as having better information systems and motivated managers. The homogeneous disease group system was extended to all of Hungary in 1993 and has undergone several structural modifications since then (National Economic Research Associates 1998). Day patients are paid on an average per day based on homogeneous disease group multiplied by a coefficient of 0.7. Inpatient long-stay cases are reimbursed per day. Expensive services such as transplantation, provided only in regional or national institutions, are paid on a fee-for-service basis and financed separately by the central government.

The impact of the homogeneous disease group system has been mixed. Discharges have grown considerably as lengths of stay decreased from 9.9 to 8.0 days in the 1990s and beds per capita decreased. But these trends, except for beds per capita, predate the new payment incentives. Orosz and Hollo (2001) report that the expenditure cap helped avoid the collapse of health care finances.

Hospital admissions per 100 rose from 21.8 to 24.2 between 1990 and 1996, however, suggesting that the new payment system and reduction in hospital beds did not stop increasing hospitalization. In addition, there is no incentive to improve quality or shift services to outpatient settings, as similar services are reimbursed at a higher rate as inpatient care. Software has proliferated for upcoding claim forms, resulting in code creep (Dorotinsky 1998; Orosz 1999), so that the national case-mix index increased from 0.97 in 1993 to 1.10 in 1996 (Orosz *et al.* 1997). In consequence, payments per case fell by 22 per cent in real terms between 1994 and 1997 (OECD 1999).

Excess hospital capacity has become even more apparent, but the system of payment per case failed to trigger significant structural changes. The government has tried and failed three times since 1995 to close public wards and hospitals. Some hospitals outsource services such as laundry and food to cut costs and generate some revenue through private services (National Economic Research Associates 1998). The elimination of hospital beds was not followed by a proportional reduction in personnel. The number of physicians increased by 27 per cent between 1990 and 1996 and specialists by 12 per cent, despite high physician : patient ratios. Although employment in the whole economy fell by 20 per cent between 1991 and 1997, employment in the health care sector declined by only 2 per cent (National Economic Research Associates

1998; Orosz and Hollo, in press). Health workers enjoy special status under the Public Servants Act and Civil Servants Act (OECD 1999).

Transitional payment systems

Bosnia and Herzegovina, Bulgaria and Romania are in the early stages of transition to new health insurance systems, with legislation passed in 1997 and 1998. Little has been published so far on new payment systems to providers (Adeyi *et al.* 1998/1999; Balabanova 1998/1999). Romania has proposed payments per case or per day (World Bank 1999b), with the elimination of staffing caps and increased flexibility for negotiating salaries. In Bulgaria, policymakers have expressed interest in payments per case or perhaps global budgets (unpublished data, Health Insurance Commission, Australia 1999). In Bosnia and Herzegovina, payments per case or budget caps have been discussed. In each case, a new project financed by the World Bank will provide support for developing the payment system. This legislation does not address capital investment issues. In Romania, the new health insurance law stipulates that buildings and expensive equipment will continue to be financed from the central budget, but only 3 per cent of the budget goes to capital investment, forcing hospitals to raise other revenues. Azerbaijan, the Republic of Moldova and Ukraine have maintained the traditional line-item approach for hospital payment. Some central Asia republics (Tajikistan, Turkmenistan and Uzbekistan) and Turkey continue with traditional line-item budget reimbursement.

Towards global budgets and capitation?

Several countries in eastern Europe see global budgets and capitation as the next generation beyond systems of payment per day and per case and have begun by instituting simple caps on hospital expenditure. Most of the current global-budget activity is in the Russian Federation, with capitation pilots in some other countries. Much of this activity is in response to volume problems under systems of payment per day and per admission.

Global budgets

The Czech Republic has moved to hospital budget caps to stem the recent increases in expenditure. Albania retained historical budgets but has aggregated several line items, essentially a global budget arrangement. A World Bank project of US$17 million will finance the restructuring of overall health services. In Croatia, the runaway costs for inpatient care were capped recently, and global budget methods introduced in pilot sites may use case-mix adjustments.

Turkmenistan has attempted to introduce pilot global hospital budgets instead of traditional line items and input norms. Some hospitals in Ashkhabad permit some expenditure flexibility, and the Tejen district hospital has a global hospital budget as part of a World Bank pilot. Without a computerized information system, it would be administratively costly to introduce a more complex payment system. Government administrators in the central Asian republics initially opposed a global budget model, seeing it as a licence to defraud; the assumption was that the money was handed to chief physicians to spend as they wish, rather than according to a business plan agreed with the Ministry of Health (University of York 1998). A global budget plan usually states how the hospital will meet its main objectives through planned activities, resource reallocation and expenditure by line item, with its progress monitored and incorporated in the planning process (Ensor and Langenbrunner 2002).

Russian Federation

At least two oblasts (Tver and Kaluga) are instituting global budgets in response to growing volume problems resulting from payment systems per day and per case. In Kaluga, global budgets are part of the broader reform of health-sector payments. The new provider payment plan incorporated pooling of funds to include emergency care, pharmaceuticals for special population groups and outpatient care. A partial fundholding model was developed, with capitation payments going to outpatient providers. The global budget to hospitals is allocated as a monthly lump-sum, giving managers more autonomy. One polyclinic reported quick results, with drops in patient unit costs, referrals to hospitals and specialists, and cuts in district hospital beds and staff. Within the global budgets, hospitals will institute a 10 per cent withholding fund for staff bonuses, to be based on measurable indicators of volume and quality.

In Tver oblast, global budget payment models were initiated in six pilot sites in 1996, calculated on historical allocations with age and sex adjustments phased in. The model was extended oblast-wide to 67 hospitals from early 1997. Each rayon (district) now receives a per capita amount to allocate as global budgets to facilities. In rural rayons, the central rayon hospital holds and distributes the funds. Early results are encouraging, with drops in admission by 5–20 per cent by catchment area and a downsizing of inpatient capacity for the region from 23,000 to 15,000 hospital beds. Part of the downsizing has been a reallocation to day care beds, which now number about 3000. Lengths of stay have dropped slightly, by 5–10 per cent. Some funds have been reallocated to outpatient care. Utilization management techniques have taken hold, mostly for surgical admissions. Despite these gains, a recent law by the Russian Federation central government calls for line 3 of this old line-item budget to be the responsibility of the founder of the facility, in virtually all cases the local rayon, municipal or oblast government. This decree has blunted the Fund's ability to develop a true global budget, as these costs are about 20–30 per cent of all facility costs.

Capitation

Croatia, Hungary and Poland have expressed interest in integrated care delivery organizations, while in the Russian Federation, Tula and Kemerovo oblasts have reported developing a managed care organization, although no assessment is available. For the most part, capitation is used in regional allocation. Insurance funds use the principle of per capita payment to reallocate across regions, adjustments for local variation in need (however measured) and input costs (Carr-Hill *et al.* 1994).

In some geographical regions, the health sector receives per capita payments as a kind of at-risk arrangement. For example, in the Novgorod oblast of the Russian Federation, the insurance fund payment system has evolved from line-item to activity-related payments; not surprisingly, volume has increased. As a result, in 1999, 21 of 22 rayons received global capitation payments intended to control the overall volume of services. The budgets are based on 5 years of historical patterns of care and were a response to volume problems and to a growing consensus that 30–35 per cent of admissions could be treated on an outpatient basis.

Western European experience

A blend of case-mix adjustment and global budgeting is now applied to many western European countries for the payment of hospital services (Wiley 1998). Case-mix adjustment is used, for example, in Belgium, France, Ireland, Italy, Norway, Portugal and Spain. Whether the adjustment is applied at the national or regional level depends on the structure of the country's health system. The financing of hospital services in countries such as Ireland and Portugal is therefore very centralized, whereas in Spain there is substantial autonomy at the regional level.

Belgium

The country has been revising the hospital system since 1987. The aims are to identify patient needs, reduce costs, improve the quality of care, offer incentives for efficiency and increase equity in resource allocation between hospitals (Closon *et al.* 1996). In 1994, an all-payer DRG was introduced to standardize for morbidity when comparing the length of stay. A hospital running 2–10 per cent over the average length of stay (a standardized national mean) loses 50 per cent of the budget for these extra bed-days; it loses 25 per cent when the observed length of stay exceeds the national average by more than 10 per cent (Closon *et al.* 1996). A substantial reallocation of funds between hospitals may result so that the potential impact on the system may be considerable.

France

A number of hospital rationalization and cost-containment controls have been introduced since the mid-1980s. Public hospitals and private not-for-profit hospitals affiliated to the public sector have been financed based on prospective global budgets since 1984–85. Most notably, since 1997, acute inpatient budgets have been based in part on case mix measured by DRGs (*groupes homogenes de malades*) (Rodrigues *et al.* 1998). Hospital budgets are partly based on hospital-specific costs together with an adjustment for the regional case-mix index. In 1996, *groupes homogenes de malades* determined 0.5 per cent of hospital budgets, which will gradually increase over time. While budgets for public and private for-profit hospitals have been determined separately, in the future all hospitals will be included within the regional budget framework.

Ireland and Portugal

These countries apply a similar case-mix adjustment in the acute hospital global budget model. Initiated in Portugal in 1990, this represented the first application of case mix for budgeting purposes in a European context (Urbano *et al.* 1993). In 1993, the Irish Department of Health and Children built on Portugal's experience. The case-mix adjustment essentially involves estimating the relative costliness of hospital case-mix DRGs (Wiley 1995). In this context, the relative costliness of the hospital's case mix is assumed to indicate relative efficiency. An agreed proportion of the hospital budget is then determined based on the case-mix adjustment. This adjustment may be negative or positive depending on the efficiency of the hospital relative to others in the reference group. The deployment of additional funds gained as a result of this process may be at the discretion of the hospital. In determining the allocation of resources to regional health boards and large hospitals in Ireland, hospitals are stratified according to teaching status (Wiley 1995). Currently, 15 per cent of the case-mix adjustment is based on the cost rating of the peer group hospitals and 85 per cent on the hospital's historical costs. Over time, this ratio will change so that the cost rating of peer hospitals will have a greater effect on the budget adjustment than the hospital's historical costs. In Portugal, more progress has been made towards this objective, with 30 per cent of the case-mix adjustment determined by the peer group hospitals and 70 per cent determined by individual hospital costs (Bentes *et al.* 1996).

Italy

Local health units fund their hospitals directly on a capitation basis. A tariff system was introduced for funding cross-boundary activity and hospitals outside the local health units in 1995. Tariffs based on DRGs are set on a prospective basis within predetermined budget constraints, with some discretion left to the region. For example, a region might choose fee for service or episode of care as the basis for the currency unit. The essential objective, however, is that hospitals are funded on the basis of the volume and quality of services actually delivered. As an additional incentive to promote efficiency, it has been proposed that local area units retain any budget surplus.

Spain

Although each autonomous region of Spain can determine its precise approach, in general hospitals are funded on a global budget basis, determined by historical costs with annual adjustments for such factors as inflation and changes in service delivery. Increasingly, an adjustment for activity is being integrated within the budgeting process (Mossialos and Le Grand 1999). There are several models, with the United States version prevailing in Catalonia, Valencia and the Canary Islands, and all-payer DRGs in the remaining regions. Since 1997–98, several regional systems have incorporated a case-mix adjustment. For example, 30 per cent of the inpatient budget in Catalonia is estimated based on DRGs, whereas Valencia uses a combination of capitation and DRGs. Work is underway to improve cost data for DRGs, which will be required if more extensive application of systems based on case mix is pursued.

The Nordic countries

These countries are also experimenting with case mix. The Nordic DRG is compatible with the DRG system in the United States (version 12) and incorporates ICD-10 diagnosis codes and Nordic procedure codes. Norway, Sweden and Finland are the most advanced, with some experimentation in Denmark and Iceland. The introduction of the DRG system in Norway was associated with reforms directed at reducing hospital waiting lists and improving efficiency. However, case-mix applications in the other countries were intended to address a range of objectives, including an improved basis for costing and pricing, resource allocation and contracting for hospital services. Norway's pilot scheme introduced in 1991 progressively tested a combination of fixed grants with a payment scheme based on DRGs and patients. Hospitals continue to be jointly funded by the government and the county administration, but the most recent financial reform increased the government allocation. In 1997, the government funded 30 per cent of average patient treatment costs on a DRG basis, which is intended to increase to 45 per cent. As waiting lists continue to attract a high political priority, this reform is intended to increase capacity for patient treatment (Lundgren *et al.* 1998).

Overall, the changes in western European spending patterns for inpatient care over the last two decades are positive. Table 8.5 shows some interesting divergences in these trends for 15 countries. In general, only a minority of countries reduced the share of DRGs devoted to total health expenditure between 1980 and 1995, whereas most reduced the proportion of total health expenditure allocated to public expenditure on inpatient care. The nine European Union countries showing this decline in the period 1980–85 increased to 12 in the late 1980s. Over the 1980s as a whole, the European Union countries that showed an overall reduction in the proportion of total health expenditure devoted to public expenditure on inpatient care were Belgium, Denmark, France, Italy, the Netherlands, Spain and the United Kingdom. By 1990–95, this trend was beginning to be reversed, with investment in inpatient care increasing in most European Union countries. Such large-scale changes in complex systems will always be multi-causal, but the introduction of new hospital payment systems are correlated with changes in spending patterns.

Lessons and implications

No single payment model is clearly superior or timeless in its relative utility for achieving sectoral objectives. The choice for a particular health system will

Table 8.5 Percentage change in share of GDP devoted to health (health %) and public expenditure on inpatient care (hospital %) as a proportion of total health expenditure in the 15 countries that are currently in the European Union, 1980–95

	1980–1985		1985–1990		1990–1995	
	Health %	Hospital %	Health %	Hospital %	Health %	Hospital %
Austria	−13.0	20.5	7.5	−10.2	11.1	−6.1
Belgium	12.3	−1.3	2.7	−0.4	5.3	9.3
Denmark	−5.7	−3.1	0.0	−2.4	−2.4	3.5
Finland	12.3	−6.8	9.6	−0.2	−5.0	−12.7
France	11.8	−2.7	4.7	−6.3	11.2	−0.2
Germany	5.7	2.1	−6.4	2.8	19.5	2.3
Greece	11.1	12.7	5.0	18.5	38.1	N.A.
Ireland	−9.2	20.9	−15.2	−6.8	4.5	4.5
Italy	1.4	−0.2	14.1	−3.8	−4.9	−0.7
Luxembourg	−1.6	1.2	8.2	−3.1	1.5	21.1
Netherlands	0.0	−0.6	5.1	−12.5	6.0	5.1
Portugal	8.6	−14.9	3.2	29.4	26.1	13.9
Spain	0.0	3.4	23.2	−6.2	5.8	−1.9
Sweden	−4.3	−22.0	−2.2	−6.7	−3.4	−15.9
United Kingdom	5.4	−13.3	1.7	−6.6	15.0	−4.1

N.A. = not available

be influenced by a wide range of temporal factors, including the priorities and organization of the health and hospital system, available data and techniques together with the level of development throughout the hospital system. Given the dynamic nature of health systems and the continuing pressure on resources, it would be expected that hospital payment models will be subjected to ongoing developments to take account of advances in technology and in information and analytical systems.

Nevertheless, the experience of western Europe suggests where countries in eastern Europe may be headed in terms of payment for hospital services. They are moving away from the traditional line-item approach to more performance-oriented approaches. This is associated with the shift to tax-funded insurance-based systems, as has been the case in western Europe (Saltman and Figueras 1998). Systems of payment per day and per case, from relatively simple to unnecessarily complicated, appear to dominate eastern Europe.

It is not clear to what extent these new approaches have gone beyond stimulating mere activity in provider behaviour. Fortunately, some of the systems of payment per day have expenditure caps (Estonia and Slovenia), but these will be difficult to sustain in a way that promotes efficiency and access, and systems per case, except in Hungary, are in early formative stages. There is little evidence that new performance-based systems have been designed to reflect true costs, improve efficiency or link to health outcomes. Indeed, the early experiences with payments per case and per day are associated with increases in the volume of services, overall costs and administrative games. In addition, these systems require significant investment in management expertise, information systems and administrative oversight (for example, quality assurance and monitoring systems).

Countries in eastern Europe are increasingly borrowing under World Bank-sponsored projects for activity related to payment policies for hospitals. They are now looking more carefully at caps, global budgets and capitation systems. A combination of approaches need not conflict; for example, systems of payment per case coupled with overall caps or global budgets can be complementary. The advantage of a global budget based on past expenditure adjusted for inflation over a norm-based system is that it does not encourage the excessive use of beds. Nevertheless, it could lead to a system with no incentive to deliver health care or an incentive to selectively lower quality and access.

A number of factors blunt the underlying incentives inherent in new payment systems and dilute their effectiveness. One issue is reimbursement for capital and major equipment, since few, if any, countries have addressed the issue of paying for capital. Some capital allocation approaches have been developed in conjunction with World Bank loans, such as in Estonia and the Russian Federation, but payers do not incorporate capital routinely into payment systems. Part of the reason may be related to the broader issue of underfunding, as most countries had less for health in real spending terms in 1995 than in 1990. The short-term response in many countries has been to cut back on capital investment while funding only recurrent costs.

A second and related issue is that the patient-based funding system was introduced alongside rather than instead of the budget system, particularly in the countries of the former Soviet Union. The services financed by the state have been divided between the insurance fund and budget. The budget continues to be allocated along historical (norm-based) lines, and facilities may receive funding from both sources. As a result, if a hospital cuts beds and the length of stay to economize or increase the throughput of patients, it is penalized by the budget but rewarded by the insurance fund (Ensor and Langenbrunner 2002).

A third issue is that funding for care in many countries increasingly relies on consumer out-of-pocket payments, estimated at 29 per cent in Poland (Chawla *et al.* 1998), 42 per cent in Kazakhstan (Sari *et al.* 2000), 52 per cent in the Russian Federation (unpublished data, V.E. Boikov *et al.* 2000) and above 80 per cent in Azerbaijan and Georgia (Mays 1997). The use of unofficial payments, in particular, dilutes or even contradicts incentives to provide care more efficiently and effectively.

A fourth issue is debt and deficit. Most countries in eastern Europe have not been successful at enforcing hard budgets for hospitals (see Chapter 9). Providers have continued to take advantage of soft budgets rather than adjust their behaviour, hospitals in nearly all countries have run up debt and nearly all administrations have bailed them out. Debts are owed to pharmaceutical companies (Albania), utility companies (Croatia and the Czech Republic) and physicians (Albania and Georgia). In Hungary, hospitals accumulate debt every year. Similarly, the system of mutual debt settlement in many countries of the former Soviet Union (such as the state waiving taxes for utilities owed money by hospitals) means that the incentives introduced are more virtual than real.

It is difficult to see how payments can effect real change unless either state guarantees are reduced to a more effective level or revenues are increased (Ensor and Langenbrunner 2001).

Some issues await further analysis. For example, as regions or countries move from payments per day and per case to refined case-mix systems or to global budgets and funding per capita, better information systems and management structures are required. It is not clear whether providers are ready to change staffing mix, capacity, hardware and software or whether regulators and payers are willing to allow such flexibility (Berman 1998). Readiness at the provider level ties closely to the larger issue of whether and how successful payment design can be implemented in coordination with other sectoral elements of reform, such as labour policies, facility autonomy, treatment protocols, quality assurance and improved management capacity and information systems. It is probable that these and other co-determinants are important in successful hospital system reform and implementation, but health sectors do not understand well or appreciate the mix of elements and the overall strategy for coordination.

References

Adeyi, O., Radulescu, S., Huffman, S., Vladu, C. and Florescu, R. (1998/1999) Health sector reform in Romania: balancing needs, resources and values, *Eurohealth*, 4(special issue 6): 29–32.

Balabanova, D. (1998/1999) Health care reforms in Bulgaria: challenges emerging from the 1990's, *Eurohealth*, 4(special issue 6): 33–6.

Bentes, M., do Ceu Mateus, M. and da Luz Gonsalves, M. (1996) DRGs in Portugal: a decade of experience: casemix and change – international perspectives. Paper presented to the *Eighth Casemix Conference*, Sydney, Australia, 19–21 September.

Berman, P. (1998) *National Health Insurance in Poland: A Coach Without Horses?* Boston, MA: Harvard University Press.

Carr-Hill, R.A., Hardman, G., Martin, S. *et al.* (1994) *A Formula for Distributing NHS Revenues Based on Small Area Use of Hospital Beds*, Centre for Health Economics Occasional Paper. York: University of York.

Chawla, M., Berman, P. and Kawiorska, D. (1998) Financing health services in Poland: new evidence on private expenditures, *Health Economics*, 7: 337–46.

Closon, M.C., Azoury, E., Herbeuval, A.F. and Lopez, M. (1996) New financial incentives for acute care hospitals in Belgium. Paper presented to the 12th International Working Conference of Patient Classification Systems/Europe, Sydney, Australia, 19–21 September.

Coulam, R. and Gaumer, G. (1991) Medicare's prospective payment system: a critical appraisal, *Health Care Financing Review*, 13(suppl.): 45–77.

Dorotinsky, W. (1998) *Fine Tuning the Hungarian Health System.* Budapest: Ministry of Finance, Government of Hungary.

Ensor, T. (1997) Options for health sector funding, in S. Witter and T. Ensor (eds) *An Introduction to Health Economics for Eastern Europe and the Former Soviet Union.* Chichester: John Wiley.

Ensor, R. and Langenbrunner, J. (2002) Allocating resources and paying providers, in M. McKee, J. Healy and J. Falkingham (eds) *Health Care in Central Asia.* Buckingham: Open University Press.

Fidler, A. (1999) The challenges of health care reform, in *Country Economic Memorandum*. Washington, DC: World Bank.

Heijnen, S. and Schneider, M. (1999) *Planning of Hospital Restructuring: Lithuania*. Washington, DC: World Bank.

Horst, K. (1998) Implementation of health care reform in central Asia: concepts and examples, in *The Experience from Dzheskasgan Oblast, Kazakhstan*. Almaty, Kazakhstan: Abt Associates.

International Finance Corporation (1999) *Interim Report: Health Sectors of Baltic Countries*. Washington, DC: World Bank.

Klugman, J. and Schieber, G. (1996) *Reforming Health Systems in Central Asia*. Washington, DC: World Bank.

Klugman, J. and Schieber, G. (1997) A survey of health reform in central Asia, in Z. Feachem, M. Henscher and L. Rose (eds) *Implementing Health Sector Reform in Central Asia*, EDI Learning Resources Series. Washington, DC: World Bank.

Kulzhanov, M. and Healy, J. (1999) *Health Care Systems in Transition: Kazakhstan*. Copenhagen: European Observatory on Health Care Systems.

Langenbrunner, J., Sheiman, I., Zaman, S. *et al.* (1994) *Evaluation of Health Insurance Demonstrations in Kazakhstan: Dzheskasgan and South Kazakhstan Oblasts*, Technical Report No. 14, Health Financing and Sustainability Project. Bethesda, MD: Abt Associates.

Lewis, M. (2002) Informal health payments in eastern Europe: issues, trends and policy implications, in E. Mossialos, A. Dixon, J. Figueras and J. Kutzin (eds) *Funding Health Care: Options for Europe*. Buckingham: Open University Press.

Lundgren, S., Kindseth, O. and Magnussen, J. (1998) New financial reform of hospital stays payment in Norwegian hospitals: preliminary experience after six months of use. Paper presented to the *14th International Working Conference of Patient Classification Systems*, Manchester, England, 1–3 October.

Mays, J. (1997) *World Bank Mission to Georgia, Estimating Health Spending*. Washington, DC: World Bank.

Mossialos, E. and Le Grand, J. (1999) Cost containment in the EU: an overview, in E. Mossialos and J. Le Grand (eds) *Health Care and Cost Containment in the European Union*. Aldershot: Ashgate.

National Economic Research Associates (1998) *The Health Care System in Hungary*, Financing Health Care Series, No. 25. White Plains, NY: National Economic Research Associates.

O'Dougherty, S. (1999) *Health Financing Reforms in Kyrgyzstan: Progress Report*. Almaty, Kazakhstan: Abt Associates.

OECD (1997) *Health Systems and Comparative Statistics: Facts and Trends*. Paris: Organisation for Economic Co-operation and Development.

OECD (1999) *OECD Economic Surveys: Hungary*. Paris: Organisation for Economic Co-operation and Development.

Orosz, E. (1999) The health care system, in *OECD Economic Surveys: Hungary*. Paris: Organisation for Economic Co-operation and Development.

Orosz, E. and Hollo, I. (in press) Hospitals in Hungary: the story of stalled reforms, *Eurohealth*.

Orosz, E., Ellena, G. and Jakab, M. (1997) *The Hungarian Health System in Transition: The Unfinished Agenda*. Budapest: World Bank.

Poullier, J.P., Schieber, G. and Greenwald, L. (1994) Health system performance in OECD countries, *Health Affairs (Millwood)*, 13(4): 100–12.

Preker, A.S. and Feachem, R.G.A. (1996) *Market Mechanisms and the Health Sector in Central and Eastern Europe*, World Bank Technical Paper No. 293. Washington, DC: World Bank.

Rhodes, G., Schaapveld, K. and Iliev, D. (1999) *The Use of Case-mix Indicators in Georgia and Armenia*. Washington, DC: World Bank.

Rodrigues, J.M., Coca, E., Trombert-Paviot, B. and Abrial, V. (1998) How to use case mix to reduce inequities and inefficiencies among French hospitals. Paper presented to the 14th International Working Conference of Patient Classification Systems, Manchester, England, 1–3 October.

Saltman, R.B. and Figueras, J. (1998) Analysing the evidence on European health care reforms, *Health Affairs (Millwood)*, 17: 85–108.

Samushkin, Z. (1998) *Hospital Database Analysis: MHI Fund Kyrgyzstan 1997–1998*, Technical Note. Bishkek, Kyrgyzstan: Abt Associates.

Sandier, S. (1989) Health services utilization and physician income trends, *Health Care Financing Review*, 11(suppl.): 33–48.

Sari, N., Langenbrunner, J. and Lewis, M. (2000) Affording out-of-pocket payments for health services: evidence from Kazakhstan, *Eurohealth*, 6(special issue 2): 37–9.

Savas, S., Sheiman, I., Tragakes, E. and Maarse, H. (1997) Contracting models and provider competition, in R.B. Saltman, J. Figueras and C. Sakellarides (eds) *Critical Challenges for Health Care Reform in Europe*. Buckingham: Open University Press.

Schieber, G. (1993) Health care financing reform in Russia and Ukraine, *Health Affairs (Millwood)*, 12(suppl.): 294–9.

Sheiman, I. (1993) New methods of finance and management of health care in the Russian Federation. Paper presented to the Health Sector Reform in Developing Countries Conference, Durham, New Hampshire, 10–13 September.

University of York (1998) *Projection Preparation for the Kazakhstan Health Sector Project: Final Report*. Almaty, Kazakhstan: Ministry of Education, Culture and Health and Fund for Compulsory Health Insurance.

Urbano, J., Bentes, B. and Vertrees, J. (1993) Portugal: national commitment and the implementation of DRGs, in J.R. Kimberley and G. de Pouvourville (eds) *The Migration of Managerial Innovation*. San Francisco, CA: Jossey-Bass.

WHO (2001) *WHO European Health for All Database*. Copenhagen: WHO Regional Office for Europe.

Wickham, C. (1998) *Kazakhstan Health Mission Trip Report*. Almaty, Kazakhstan: World Bank.

Wiley, M.M. (1995) Budgeting for acute hospital services in Ireland: the case-mix adjustment, *Journal of the Irish Colleges of Physicians and Surgeons*, 24(4): 283–90.

Wiley, M.M. (1998) Financing operating costs for acute hospital services, in R.B. Saltman, J. Figueras and C. Sakellarides (eds) *Critical Challenges for Health Care Reform in Europe*. Buckingham: Open University Press.

World Bank (1998) *Project Appraisal Document: Latvia Health Project*, Report No. 18448 LV. Washington, DC: World Bank.

World Bank (1999a) *Project Appraisal Document: Georgia Health Project*. Washington, DC: World Bank.

World Bank (1999b) *Romania: Health Sector Support Strategy*, Report No. 18410-RO. Washington, DC: World Bank.

chapter nine

Linking organizational structure to the external environment: experiences from hospital reform in transition economies

Melitta Jakab, Alexander Preker and April Harding

Introduction

The transition countries of eastern Europe have been the settings for a series of natural experiments that offer important insights into the susceptibility of hospital systems to different levers for change. In many countries, general taxation has been replaced with, or supplemented by, social insurance based on payroll taxes, hospital ownership has been transferred to local governments, new performance-based payment mechanisms have been adopted and input supply markets have been partly or fully privatized and deregulated. This contrasts markedly with the situation that existed during the communist era. Hospitals then functioned under the direct hierarchical supervision of a Ministry of Health and received input-based budget allocations, and inputs were heavily regulated and supplied by public monopolies (Ensor 1993; Goldstein *et al.* 1996; Klugman and Schieber 1997; Saltman and Figueras 1997).

These external changes were expected to trigger changes in hospital behaviour and to improve performance. In particular, the move to social insurance and the implementation of performance-based provider payment mechanisms were expected to automatically reduce excess hospital capacity, reduce reliance on inpatient care and improve service quality. The transfer of hospital ownership to local governments was regarded as an instrument to improve responsiveness to the needs and expectations of local communities. These envisioned behavioural changes have not occurred, however, and transition economies have to contend with the same weaknesses in hospital performance as a decade ago: excess capacity, inefficiency and poor responsiveness to patient expectations (Goldstein *et al.* 1996; Staines 1999; Ho (in press)).

This chapter explores why hospitals have not responded as expected to changes in the external environment, drawing on the experiences of 11 countries in central and eastern Europe and the former Soviet Union: Albania, Croatia, the Czech Republic, Estonia, Georgia, Hungary, Kazakhstan, Latvia, Lithuania, Poland and Romania. For convenience, this chapter refers to these countries collectively as eastern Europe. The main finding is that performance has not improved because the organizational structure of hospitals has not been systematically redesigned to ensure synergies with external incentives. In particular, rigidity in terms of input use (labour and capital) inherited from the era of central planning has remained and, as a result, hospital management still has limited autonomy to influence the hospital production function. Furthermore, the persisting practice of soft budgets, lack of accountability measures and lack of formal market exposure have weakened the efficiency pressures of the new mechanisms for provider payment. Overall, this has created an inconsistent incentive environment: on the one hand, the external incentives link rewards and sanctions to performance; on the other, the organizational structure reflects an input-oriented central planning approach in which rewards and sanctions are unrelated to performance. This has prevented the expected gains from provider payment reform and decentralization from materializing.

This chapter demonstrates how the current structure of hospitals in central and eastern Europe and the former Soviet Union undermines the potential of hospitals to improve efficiency and quality. First, the conceptual framework is presented. This is followed by a brief description of the changes that have taken place in the environment of hospitals, including the establishment of social insurance and decentralization. The next section analyses the organizational structure of hospitals in this region based on a sample of 11 countries. The final section discusses the interaction between external incentives and organizational structure and their impact on improving performance.

As the organizational structure of hospitals is not well documented in the countries in this region, this study is based on a series of structured interviews conducted in summer 1999. The interviewees included government officials in ministries of health, health insurance funds, members of academic institutions, professionals at World Bank resident missions and hospital-based physicians in the 11 countries. The countries were selected based on the availability both of requested information and contact people. Thus, the sample is not representative for all countries in central and eastern Europe and the former Soviet Union. In fact, it over-represents higher-income countries that have established social insurance systems, undertaken provider payment reform and decentralized the ownership of hospital facilities to local governments. As a result, the conclusions of the study cannot necessarily be generalized to lower-income countries in which the reforms are less advanced, but some lessons are relevant to both middle- and high-income countries.

Figure 9.1 Determinants of hospital behaviour

Owners

External incentives

Government

Governance

Stewardship

Organizational
structure

Autonomy

Accountability

Market exposure

Social functions

Policy-driven
purchasing

Residual claimant status

Market-driven
purchasing

Purchaser(s)

Consumers

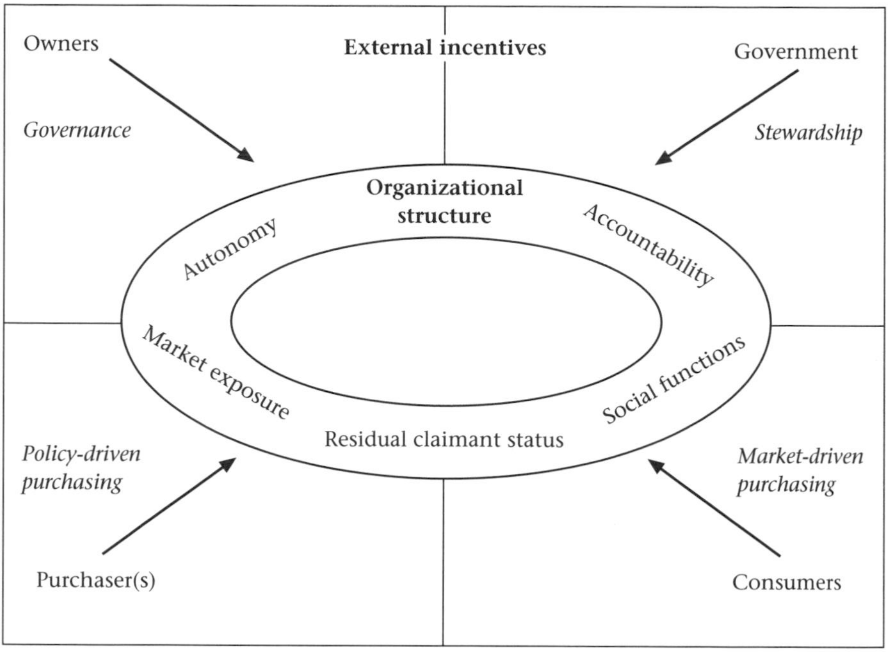

Source: Jakab *et al.* (2001)

Determinants of hospital behaviour

The organizational structure of hospitals is increasingly recognized as a significant determinant of hospital behaviour. Previous literature on hospital performance mostly focused on the impact of incentives emanating from the external
environment. In particular, payment mechanisms and competitive pressures
were much explored (Wiley 1992; Wiley 1995; Maynard and Bloor 1999).
Focusing on external incentives alone, however, assumes that hospital behaviour
is the result of a rational adaptation process to external determinants. This
approach ignores the possibility that the organizational structure of hospitals
might mitigate any pressures emerging from the external environment.

This chapter argues that the behaviour of hospitals is determined by the
interaction of external incentives and organizational structure (Figure 9.1).
In this framework, hospital behaviour is changed positively by introducing
complementary and synergetic reforms to both the external environment and
the organizational structure of hospitals or hospital networks. Alone, neither
is sufficient to change the behaviour of organizations. If the external environment does not generate performance pressures, hospitals will have no reason
to strive for high performance. However, even with a well-structured external
environment, the direction and magnitude of hospital behavioural change
might be moderated by the organizational structure of the hospital. Thus,

synergistic design between the external environment and the organizational structure of hospitals together create the incentives hospitals face, and hence their alignment is critical to successfully change organizational performance.

External environment

The external environment of hospitals can be conceptualized in terms of four functional relationships producing four sources of performance pressure: collective purchasing, market-driven purchasing, stewardship and governance. First, the relationship of hospitals with purchasers (policy-driven purchasing) determines the performance pressures embedded in the payment mechanisms, and the competitive pressures to which hospitals are subjected by organized collective purchasers. The link between hospital performance and various provider payment mechanisms is well documented and is thought to be the key incentive for improving hospital performance. Second, the relationship of hospitals with consumers (market-driven purchasing) determines the extent of competitive pressures on the hospital from unorganized individual consumers. Third, the relationship of the hospital with the government (stewardship) subjects the hospital to various pressures from government rules and regulations. Finally, the relationship of the hospital with its owner determines supervisory arrangements and distributes decision-making authority and rights to revenue between the hospital and the owner. Residual rights refer to the right to make decisions over the use of an asset that is not explicitly assigned by law or contract to another party. Residual returns refer to income from an asset or business that remains after all fixed obligations are met (Milgrom and Roberts 1992). The function related to ownership arrangements is termed 'governance'. These four functional relationships do not necessarily coincide with four distinct external organizations. Depending on the health system, several of these functions can be subsumed by the same organization.

Organizational structure

The organizational structure of hospitals mediates the pressures present in the external environment. Many elements of organizational structure are important in different ways and at different times. The reforms taking place in transition countries are increasingly subjecting hospitals to market-type pressures through performance-based payments. Harding and Preker (2001) argue that the key dimensions of the organizational structure of such reforms (sometimes termed 'marketizing reforms') include: (i) autonomy, (ii) market exposure, (iii) residual claimant status, (iv) accountability and (v) social functions. With these five dimensions, organizations can be characterized as to their location on the continuum between the core public bureaucracy and the market.

- *Autonomy*. The degree of autonomy (decision rights) hospitals retain in relation to their owner, organized purchasers, the government and consumers provides the first key organizational dimension. In the context of hospitals, critical decision rights include control over input mix and level, outputs and scope of activities, financial management, clinical and non-clinical administration, strategic management (formulation of institutional objectives), market strategy and sales.

- *Market exposure.* Market exposure refers to the extent to which hospitals are at risk for their financial and professional performance. Greater exposure to markets is expected to act as a disciplinary force on hospitals by rewarding good performers and penalizing poor performers. Organizational reform can be characterized by the extent to which it exposes hospitals to market forces in the product, factor and equity markets. In the product market, the proportion of hospital revenues collected from user fees determines the degree of market exposure: the greater the proportion of revenue from user fees, the greater the financial incentive for a hospital to attract patients.
- *Residual claimant status.* The organization's residual claimant status reflects its degree of financial responsibility. This refers both to the ability to keep savings and responsibility for financial losses (debt). In hospitals operated by ministries of health financed through line-item budgets, the public purse is often the residual claimant: if hospitals generate extra revenues, save or cannot spend their budgeted allocation, the funds are withdrawn from hospitals and reallocated within the health-sector budget. At the same time, budgets are soft so that when hospitals overspend, the public purse steps in to bail them out. Residual claimant status is jointly determined by explicit regulations regarding surplus funds and debt and the nature of the provider payment mechanism.
- *Accountability.* As the autonomy of providers increases, the ability of a ministry of health to assert direct accountability through the hierarchy is diminished. Alternative accountability instruments need to be put in place through indirect mechanisms such as contracts and regulations combined with consistent monitoring and enforcement. This requires new functions and roles from the purchasers, the Ministry of Health and other, potentially new, regulatory agencies in the health sector.
- *Social functions.* The final factor characterizing organizational structure is the extent to which social functions delivered by the hospital, such as care for dependent people, are implicit and unfunded versus specified and directly funded. Successful strategies require a strong complementary oversight function (stewardship) and complementary reforms in health care financing, including subsidies for poor people.

Provider organizations can be characterized along these five dimensions in terms of whether they display characteristics of a budgetary department within the core public bureaucracy at one extreme or of a private organization operating in a market context at the other extreme (Table 9.1). In a simplified way, budgetary organizations of the core public bureaucracy have limited autonomy and no financial risk for performance, with accountability imposed by the government bureaucracy. In contrast, privately owned organizations have full decision rights and incur financial risk for their performance. For such organizations, non-market-based objectives can be ensured through indirect

Table 9.1 Scaling of the organizational structure of hospitals

	Core public bureaucracy		Private organization
Autonomy	Few decision rights	X	Full autonomy
Market exposure	None	X	At full risk for performance
Residual claimant	Public purse	X	Organization
Accountability	Hierarchical direct control	X	Regulation and contracting
Social functions	Unfunded mandate	X	Funded explicit mandate

accountability mechanisms such as contracts, regulations and performance monitoring, as well as through explicitly funding social functions.

Each of the five dimensions can be assessed on a continuum between budgetary units and private organizations. For the first three dimensions (decision rights, market exposure and residual claimant status), moving to the right on the scale implies a change in the nature of the incentive element (for example, accountability enforced by direct hierarchical control versus through contracts and regulations). It also implies an increase in magnitude (for example, greater residual claims for the hospital). For the fourth and fifth dimensions (accountability and social functions), a move to the right implies a change in the nature of the structures for pursuing these objectives, but not any necessary increase in accountability or delivery of social functions.

The external environment in central and eastern Europe and the former Soviet Union

Applying the above conceptualization of the external environment to transition economies, the emerging theme is increasing separation of the four external functions into distinct and separate organizational arrangements.

The inheritance

For the present purposes, the key features of the Soviet health care system (described in Chapter 2) were as follows. In the pre-transition era, the Ministry of Health was the predominant actor in the environment of hospitals. The Ministry of Health was in charge of three of the four functions discussed above: governance, organized purchasing and stewardship (Figure 9.2). All hospitals were state-owned; their governance structure was that of direct budgetary units of the Ministry of Health or its regional arm. Purchasing meant little more than historical, rigid line-item budgeting. The stewardship function consisted of central planning of physical and human resource capacity. As all health care was free of charge to the user and the level of informal payments in the pre-transition era was estimated to be low, the impact of individual choice of providers had little impact on hospital revenue (Ho (in press)).

Figure 9.2 The hospital environment during communism

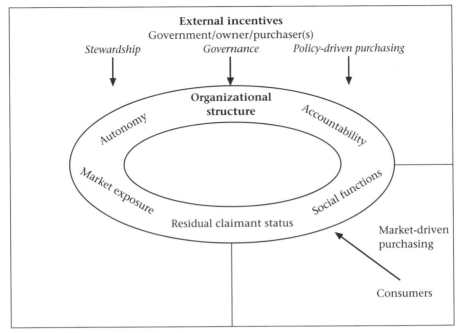

Source: Jakab *et al.* (2001)

Hospital capacity was a key measure of health system performance, and the objective of health policy was to expand the number of facilities, beds and physicians. Hospital budgets were determined from input-based norms such as the number of hospital beds and physicians. Allocations were made for line items often with over a dozen categories, and it was not feasible to transfer resources from one category to another. Initially, this input-based approach contributed to improving access to care for the population. However, over time it created high levels of fixed resources, as line-item allocations rarely changed, it provided incentives for hospital-centred care and allowed little financial flexibility for innovation (Preker and Feachem 1996). This inheritance defined the most egregious problems to be addressed in the reform of service delivery for the transition decade to come: reducing excess capacity and overspecialization, improving micro-efficiency, enhancing responsiveness to users and creating stronger financial management. Provision of health services was overly hospital-centred with weak primary and outpatient care and a lack of rehabilitation facilities and social care.

The transition

The external environment, with its one predominant actor – the Ministry of Health – has fundamentally changed in most countries over the last decade

Figure 9.3 The hospital environment during transition

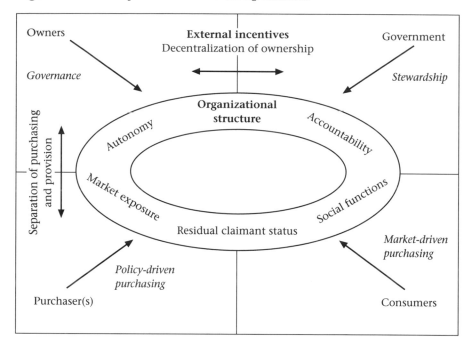

Source: Jakab *et al.* (2001)

(Figure 9.3). This change is characterized by the separation of three external functions of stewardship, purchasing and governance into three distinct organizational arrangements. This separation of functions took place through the establishment of social insurance funds and the decentralization of hospital ownership. The establishment of social insurance meant the transfer of the budget allocation and purchasing functions from the core public bureaucracy (Ministry of Health) to newly created quasi-public organizations. Decentralization is characterized by the separation of the stewardship and governance functions, which meant that the core public-sector bureaucracy transferred its ownership of hospital facilities to local governments. Both developments resulted in the entry of new organizations into the health sector, creating a pluralistic hospital environment and thereby a new set of external incentives and pressures.

From the perspective of hospitals, the key change that accompanied the establishment of social insurance was the implementation of performance-based payment mechanisms and the introduction of explicit contracting with providers. Chapter 8 discusses in detail the new payment mechanisms in countries in central and eastern Europe and the former Soviet Union. Most countries reviewed here have either fully introduced or at least experimented with payment mechanisms that link hospital revenues, fully or in part, to some aspect of their output. The adopted provider payment mechanisms range from sophisticated payment mechanisms based on diagnosis-related groups

(DRGs) with over 700 categories in Hungary to simple case-based payment with 30 categories in Georgia, but also include other performance-based systems such as payments per day, fee-for-service or mixed systems. Many expectations were attached to these new payment mechanisms. Although some of these may have been misguided based on international experience, the most important expectation was that output-based payment would make excess hospital capacity obvious and costly for hospitals to maintain. Thus, it was hoped that hospitals would respond to change in the provider payment mechanism by downsizing their physical and human resource infrastructure.

The second key change from the perspective of hospitals was the transfer of the ownership of general hospitals from the core public bureaucracy to municipalities. Teaching and tertiary hospitals remained under the control of the Ministries of Health and Education (Table 9.2). As hospitals became local political assets as a result of ownership transfer, it was expected that local governments would provide a layer of local accountability over hospital behaviour both in the financial and professional sense. Local governments, being more sensitive to the needs of local populations than the central core bureaucracy (Ministry of Health), were expected to pressure hospitals to be more responsive to users.

The assumption underlying this reform was that, through the local electoral process, communities would be able to convey their preferences to local authorities and directly exercise their voice in matters of hospital performance. Voters' ability to appoint and remove elected officials was key in holding local government officials accountable. In turn, this required that local government officials should hold hospitals accountable for their performance in line with community expectations (Schiavo-Campo 1994; Saltman and Figueras 1997).

The establishment of social insurance and decentralization both reflected the transition ideals of reducing the centralized powers of the former monolithic state bureaucracy and removed key functions from the Ministry of Health. This has required massive institutional adjustments to move away from the former command-and-control approach to governing the health sector and to redefine its new roles and functions. Ministries of Health, the new social insurance organizations and local governments had to build new capacity and expertise in contracting, performance monitoring, formulating health-sector strategy and regulating the health sector.

Changes in the organizational structure of hospitals during transition

In contrast to the systematic changes in the environment of hospitals, changes in the organizational structure of hospitals have been minimal and *ad hoc* in nature and often emerged as side-effects of other reforms. This section tracks the changes in the organizational structure of hospitals in terms of hospital autonomy, market exposure, residual claimant status, accountability structures and societal functions.

Table 9.2 Ownership and legal organizational status of hospitals in 11 selected countries

Country	Organized purchaser of hospital care	Ownership of hospitals		Hospital governance status and relevant legal regulation
		Central state ownership	Local government ownership	
Albania	Ministry of Health	X		Budgetary unit
Croatia	Single-payer national health insurance fund since 1993		X	Separate legal entity
Czech Republic	Competing health insurance funds since 1993		X	Not-for-profit institutions: act not yet drafted
Estonia	Single-payer regional health funds		X	Three types of non-tertiary hospitals: • municipal not-for-profit • joint-stock company law • trust form
Georgia	Part Ministry of Health and single-payer national health insurance (State Medical Insurance Company)		X	Treasury enterprises (self-financing state enterprises) as separate legal entity governed by Law on Enterprises
Hungary	Single-payer national health insurance fund since 1992		X	Separate legal entity that can enter into contractual arrangements, also budgetary unit subject to public finance law
Kazakhstan	Central and oblast budgets and part health insurance		X	Some hospitals are health enterprises: legal entities responsible for raising most revenues from user fees
Latvia	Single-payer regional funds		X	Two types of non-tertiary hospitals: municipal institutions and joint stock company law
Lithuania	Single-payer regional health insurance funds		X	Not-for-profit institutions under Law on Health Care Institutions from June 1996
Poland	Ministry of Health since 1999, single-payer regional health insurance funds established in 1999		X	Budgetary units; legislation passed on 'independent units'
Romania	Ministry of Health until 1999, single-payer regional health insurance funds established in 1999	X		Extra-budgetary units governed by the Public Finance Law from 1998

Autonomy

Autonomy is the extent to which hospitals have decision rights over various aspects of the service production process. Decision rights over six aspects are reviewed: labour input, capital input, other inputs, output level and mix, pricing towards the purchaser and management processes.

Decision rights over labour input

In the communist era, physicians (like all employees) were employees of the state and were paid on a salary basis. Overall staffing and salary levels were centrally planned and regulated, including the number of employees, appointments, remuneration levels and firing of staff. This meant that hospitals had little autonomy over personnel decisions.

During transition, the central planning of human resource capacity has been de-emphasized and certain decision rights over employment of staff have been transferred to hospitals (Table 9.3). In most countries, the state has ceased to be the direct employer of physicians and hospitals contract directly with their employees. In principle, decision rights over hiring, firing and remuneration have been transferred to hospital directors. In practice, however, this autonomy is constrained through still rigid labour markets, political pressures and financial constraints.

- *Rigid labour market.* Employment regulations, whether general Employment Acts or Civil Service Acts, create inflexible labour markets by making firing and hiring decisions costly and by making it difficult to differentiate remuneration. For example, hospital staff in Hungary and Poland are civil servants, and rigorous Civil Service Acts afford significant protection to them, such as open-ended contracts and substantial severance payment (Gaal *et al.* 1999; Karski *et al.* 1999). Although Romania does not have a Civil Service Act, the General Employment Act is just as inflexible in requiring open-ended contracts (Havriliuc *et al.* 1996). Furthermore, even though hospitals are the employers of physicians, their pay in nearly all countries is subject to the Act regulating the remuneration of all public-sector employees, even in countries without special status or legislation for civil servants. Estonia, Latvia and Lithuania are an exception, where physicians have been entirely taken off the civil service salary scale (Marga 1996; Cerniauskas and Murauskiene 2000; Jesse 2000).
- *Political pressure.* Hospital directors are mostly appointed through a political process (Table 9.3) based on party affiliation, local political interests and personal networks. This suggests that the actions of hospital directors are influenced by the interest of politicians who appoint them. This limits the range of unpopular measures they are willing to take for the sake of greater efficiency. The autonomy of hospital managers is also limited by health-sector labour unions, which are typically powerful and engage in fierce salary negotiations with the government. These negotiations define an across-the-board pay for all staff that is binding for all hospitals. This leaves little room for managers to reward individual performance.

Table 9.3 Decision rights regarding labour input, selected countries

Country	Employer of physician	Relevant legal regulation	Physician payments	Appointment of hospital director
Albania	Hospital	General employment law (civil service status does not exist)	Salary – controlled by Ministry of Finance during annual budget negotiations	Minister of Health
Croatia	Hospital	General employment law	Salary subject to national uniform wage structure	Mayor of owning municipality
Czech Republic	Hospital	General employment law (civil service status does not exist)	Salary subject to Act No. 143 of 1992, regulating remuneration of all public-sector employees	Mayor of municipality
Estonia	Hospital	General employment law	Salary – off civil service pay scale	Tertiary facilities: Minister for Health Municipal institutions: mayor Joint-stock companies: board Trusts: board
Georgia	Hospital	General employment law (civil service status does not exist)	Salary plus some fee for service based on the number and severity of cases	Minister for Health
Hungary	Hospital	Civil Service Act	Salary regulated by Civil Service Act	Municipality (municipal assembly or mayor)
Latvia	Hospital	General employment law	Salary – off civil service pay scale	Tertiary facilities: Minister for Health Municipal institutions: mayor Joint-stock companies: board
Lithuania	Hospital	General employment law	Salary – off civil service pay scale	Owning local government
Poland	Hospital	Civil Service Act	Salary	Owning level of government
Romania	Hospital	General employment law (civil service status does not exist)	Salary subject to Law No. 154 of 1998, regulating the remuneration of all public-sector employees	Advertised, selection and appointment by the district health authority based on Ministry of Health criteria

- *Financial constraint.* With a significant decline in hospital budgets, many hospitals have problems funding severance pay and other benefits required on dismissal.

Decision rights over assets and capital input

In contrast to labour inputs, hospitals do not have decision rights over physical assets and capital investment decisions. Decision rights over assets are vested with the owners: the central state or the local government. Thus, although hospitals have incentives to downsize facilities to become more efficient, they do not have decision rights to do so. Owners, on the other hand, do have decision rights, but for political reasons have no incentives to sell their assets. This misalignment of incentives and decision rights is at the heart of the difficulties experienced with downsizing the hospital sector. Even in Estonia, where hospitals can form trusts under foundation law and own assets, by-laws restrict the trust's autonomy to liquidate assets. If the trust decides to divest its physical assets, the money goes back to the founding owners.

Not only do hospitals have no decision rights over the sale of assets, they also have no instruments to ensure that their assets retain their value. The new provider payment mechanisms do not contain depreciation costs, and all capital investment continues to be financed from general tax revenues in most countries. Allocations of capital investment continue to resemble the communist central planning process. Rational medium-term planning criteria are not applied, and decisions are often *ad hoc* and ultimately determined by personal and political networks. Medium-term planning is more likely to occur where international donor assistance is the major source of financing for capital investment and where donors require medium-term plans, as in Albania. Exceptions are Croatia, where the Health Insurance Institute procures and distributes all equipment, and the Czech Republic, where insurance payments to hospitals contain a depreciation allowance (Struk 1996; Vulic and Healy 1999; World Bank 1999).

Capital expenditures in all transition economies have declined significantly and generally are below the replacement rate. As a result, the condition of physical assets has deteriorated considerably. Despite decentralization of ownership, municipalities are not explicitly required to maintain the value of their assets. Furthermore, their ability to do so is constrained by their lack of revenue rights. In other words, transfer of ownership, and with it the implicit responsibility to finance asset maintenance and new investments, has not been matched with revenue-raising authority. This implies a contradictory arrangement for maintaining the asset value.

Decision rights over other inputs

Nearly all countries have extended full autonomy to hospitals to purchase other inputs than labour and capital, such as pharmaceuticals and appliances. This is a considerable departure from the pre-transition era, with centralized procurement of pharmaceuticals and other supplies through the Ministry of Health. To regulate procurement processes, most countries have passed public procurement laws that regulate hospital procurement practices and attempt to introduce transparency.

Little is known about how hospitals have actually used their increased autonomy to procure and manage pharmaceuticals. However, anecdotal evidence suggests consistent problems across the region. In Croatia and Hungary, hospital managers often complain that physicians have no incentives to economize on drugs, because the more drugs patients get, the more likely they are to reward their physicians with gratuities. Fraud and corruption are also often mentioned, such as staff selling the hospital's drugs and pocketing the money.

Decision rights over output mix and level

Within their budgets, hospitals have full autonomy in determining output mix and level. This autonomy already existed, since central planning under communism was oriented towards input and not output. With the purchaser–provider split, purchasers are supposed to shift the emphasis from specifying inputs to specifying outputs both in terms of mix and level in their purchase agreements. Most countries, however, have not been successful in moving away from the inherited central planning approach and continue to focus on inputs. In Hungary, contracts between the Health Insurance Fund and hospitals still specify inputs, including the number of hospital beds, number of staff, supplied physician hours and types of hospital departments. Outputs are only mentioned as aggregate service categories of inpatient or outpatient care. This is all the more puzzling, since payment from insurance funds is formally related to outputs and not inputs. In Romania, for example, the District Health Insurance House signs an agreement with individual hospitals without specifying outputs and without any binding legal force. This lack of focus on outputs in the contracting process is a generic problem across the countries in central and eastern Europe and the former Soviet Union.

An exception is the Czech Republic, where contracts between insurers and hospitals specify the volume and type of services, reimbursement method, data provision requirements, termination conditions and period of effectiveness. This is based on an overall list of services, the Schedule of Procedures, which specifies 5000 procedures. Hospitals can decide what services to provide but are reimbursed only for those in the contract.

Decision rights over pricing towards organized purchasers

By and large, hospitals have little autonomy over payments that are exogenous to hospitals and uniform for the entire country. This is the case in Croatia, Estonia, Georgia, Hungary, Lithuania and Romania. Prices are set not by the payer but by the Ministry of Health or an appointed committee made up of various interests (typically physicians). In Estonia, regional sickness funds pay hospitals by a combination of bed-days and fee-for-service based on a price list generated by the Health Care Services and Investigations Price Committee housed in the Ministry of Health. Although hospitals are allowed in theory to offer services at a price 25 per cent lower than on the price list, this rarely happens. In Hungary, relative DRG weights are estimated and updated by Gyogyinfok, an institute of the Ministry of Health. Final approval, however, is by a committee of physicians appointed by the Ministry of Health where medical specialties bargain and lobby. In Georgia, the prices of services in the state benefit package are set by the Committee on Medical Standards under the Ministry of Health and approved by Parliament. In a few countries, payment rates are set by negotiation between payers and hospitals, which gives hospitals some influence over pricing. This group of countries includes the Czech Republic, Georgia and Poland.

Decision rights over management processes

An interesting issue is how the transfer of decision rights to hospitals has affected decision-making processes and management practices within hospitals. In most countries, hospital directors and department heads enjoy considerable power by using the management instruments inherited from the past. Historically, there was relatively strong control and accountability for use of inputs in accordance with the plan, but virtually no scrutiny or accountability for the actual operation of the hospital or the quality of care or the delivery of outputs. For example, in Romania, one observer noted that hospital directors are like 'feudal lords' with full authority over many processes. Because hospital directors are appointed in a political process (municipal and/or national), the incumbent directors enjoy the support of the political establishment, which often motivates their actions and protects them from further scrutiny by staff, patients or representatives of the local government or community at large.

Some countries attempted to enhance managerial professionalism and transparency by creating a management team to run the hospital. In Hungary, a three-member management team was initially appointed with a general director, a nursing director and a finance director, but this system was quickly abolished because it proved ineffective as a decision-making mechanism.

Other initiatives to improve internal processes include increasing the participation of hospital managers and physicians in management training programmes. Some independent schools of public health and health service management have been established (the Czech Republic, Hungary and Poland), but numerous courses and diploma programmes and professional networks increasingly draw attention to the importance of improving internal management practices.

Market exposure

Market exposure determines to what extent hospitals are at risk for their performance: whether they lose revenues as they treat fewer patients or, conversely, whether they gain revenues as they treat more patients. The level of hospital exposure to the disciplining force of the market is jointly determined by the provider payment mechanism and by the level of direct out-of-pocket charges from patients (Harding and Preker 2001). In the countries in central and eastern Europe and the former Soviet Union, the formal market exposure of hospitals is low because the proportion of hospital revenues from user charges is small. Nevertheless, the widespread practice of informal gratuity payments creates significant effective market exposure.

During the communist era, all health care, including hospital care, was free of charge for users. During the transition, a few countries have imposed user charges for hospital use. For example, in Croatia, patients are charged 15 per cent of hotel costs and a fixed flat amount set centrally. In Latvia, co-payment levels are determined centrally as part of the health insurance benefit package. In Georgia, hospitals are allowed to charge co-payment for services in the municipal benefit package. The proposed co-payment levels must be submitted annually to the Ministry of Health for approval. The price list must be posted in a visible place in the hospital. In most cases, however, user fees affect marginal areas of hospital admissions. For example, in Hungary, hospitals can charge patients who arrive without appropriate referral and/or insurance coverage and can set the level.

Formal user charges, however, and their (potential) impact on hospital performance have to be evaluated in light of the practice of informal payments. Lewis (2002) defines informal payments as 'payments to individual and institutional providers in-kind or cash that are outside official payment channels, or are purchases that are meant to be covered by the health care system'. Formal user charges are crowded out by the practice of informal payments. This trend clearly threatens the financial health of hospitals, since official co-payments contribute to the overall hospital budget, whereas physicians and other staff retain gratuity payments. As a result, the upgrading of medical equipment, innovations requiring up-front investment, cost-effective medical protocols, raising nursing standards and other elements of a functioning health care system lack appropriate funding.

Ministries of Finance and international donors often argue that the introduction of official co-payments will automatically drive out informal gratuities. Current experience shows, however, that with low physician salaries and in the absence of enforcement, physicians forgo charging official co-payments for lower informal gratuities: a win–win situation for physicians and patients, while hospitals lose out.

Informal user fees make physicians directly accountable to patients and allow patients to obtain higher-quality services than they could purchase officially. In this sense, informal user charges create direct incentives for physicians to improve the responsiveness of their service provision. However, informal payments create many distortions. For one, the purported improvement in responsiveness takes place only for those who can pay. Furthermore, out-of-pocket payments, formal or informal, restrict access for those who cannot pay, and payment levels are usually quite arbitrary. In this sense, informal payment is a less desirable form of out-of-pocket payment than formal payment, in that it is impossible to protect patients from the financial loss resulting from an illness episode. Finally, the more widespread the practice, the less physicians are committed to reforming the public health care system, because they have the best of both worlds: their own private business run within the safety of the public system (Lewis 2002).

The relative weight of the informal payment to public funding differs markedly in the systems we reviewed. The highest proportion in our sample was in Georgia, where about 70–80 per cent of hospital revenues derived from informal payments. This is in marked contrast to Croatia, Estonia, Hungary, Latvia and Lithuania, where estimates suggest that informal payments do not exceed 10–20 per cent of total hospital revenues (Lewis 2002; Preker *et al.* 2002). The market exposure of hospitals and resulting expectations for their behaviour vary with the relative weight of public to private payments. The impact of informal payments on hospital and physician behaviour is expected to be much greater in the low-income countries in central and eastern Europe and the former Soviet Union, where public financing collapsed, than in the early reformer countries with higher incomes.

Residual claimant status

The organization's residual claimant status reflects its degree of financial re-sponsibility. This refers both to the ability to keep savings and responsibility for financial losses (debt). The residual claimant status of a hospital is a key incentive to generate savings and efficiency gains. In the communist era, the central budget was the residual claimant: resources that remained unspent by hospitals were taken back by the Ministry of Health and reallocated. Since hospitals had no residual claims on revenue flows, coupled with input-based line-item budgets (often with over 30 line items), they had no incentive to generate savings and efficiency gains.

During transition, the public purse has ceased to be a residual claimant, as new payment mechanisms have been introduced. As most countries are moving towards output-based payment systems (see Chapter 8), hospitals are auto-matically becoming residual claimants. Moreover, hospitals are increasingly able to generate and keep their own revenue (in addition to the purchaser or central budget) through four main mechanisms: charging co-payments, renting out facilities, collecting donations and offering corporate services to private companies (for example, health screening).

The other aspect of the residual claimant status is the hardness of the budget. Hospitals are not held liable for their deficit, as most countries have not been successful in enforcing hard budgets. This has weakened incentives to achieve savings and efficiency gains. Hospitals in nearly all countries have run up debt, and nearly all administrations have responded by a centrally arranged bail-out, repeatedly in many cases. Debt was accumulated towards different parties, most typically to pharmaceutical companies that have not been fully privatized (for example, Albania), utility companies (Croatia and the Czech Republic) and physicians (Albania and Georgia). In Hungary, hospitals accumulated debt every single year from 1995. Initially, few hospital directors were replaced and loss-making hospitals continued to receive interest-free loans from central budget resources that were not paid back. To stop the process, the Public Finance Act was amended in 1998, making owners explicitly responsible for financial losses of hospitals, and bankruptcy commissioners have been appointed to oversee problem hospitals.

The Czech Republic has been an exception in its handling of hospital debt in line with its more market-oriented health-sector strategy. Only two hospitals were offered interest-free loans from the state-owned Consolidation Bank; the others were required to pay back from their own future savings. Estonia, Latvia and Lithuania are also exceptions in that hospitals have not incurred any debt, primarily because inpatient care expenditure in real terms has actually increased over the past years. It is questionable whether this financial discipline will be maintained as the health sector is being subjected to tighter budgets.

Accountability

In the socialist era, accountability was ensured by hierarchical direct administrative control exercised by the Ministry of Health or its regional offices. This control consisted of, for example, financial inspections to ensure that resources were spent according to the budget line items. Thus accountability, as in other aspects of socialist health systems, focused heavily on inputs.

With health-sector reform, the Ministry of Health has been divesting its functions, including its powers to exercise direct supervision and control. The new organizations that are the recipients of these functions (local governments and social insurance organizations), however, have been unable to develop appropriate accountability arrangements. This has created an accountability vacuum in the region.

Accountability towards owners

As hospital owners, municipalities lack the incentives, instruments and capacity to hold hospitals accountable for their performance, both financial performance and service quality. The idea behind decentralized ownership was that responsibility for service delivery would be transferred closer to the people, who through the local electoral process would assert their expectations for hospital services. This seems to be working in most countries. However, since local governments do not finance health services and have little control over capital investment, they lack instruments to influence the behaviour of hospitals. Thus, their response to the complaints of their local electorate consists of putting the blame for dissatisfactory service provision on the central government and the purchasers for not providing adequate funding for hospitals.

For example, in Hungary, as hospitals are independent legal entities and receive their budget from the Health Insurance Fund, the municipalities as owners have no legal right to supervise and monitor internal hospital processes. Hospitals refuse to allow local governments to look into their activities and account books. This problem became acute in 1999 when municipalities were made legally responsible for the financial losses of hospitals.

Some countries have been attempting to strengthen hospital accountability towards owners by creating governance boards (the Czech Republic, Estonia and Latvia). Whether these boards can create a meaningful link between the organization and its owner is questionable. In the Czech Republic, for instance, the Minister of Health appoints board members, but hospital directors also nominate people. Furthermore, the boards work based on overall impressions and not hard data provided by the hospital. In Latvia, the boards of joint-stock company hospitals consist of only three people. Given the general lack of functioning accountability structures for hospitals throughout the countries in central and eastern Europe and the former Soviet Union, research on the actual effectiveness of boards in enhancing accountability is clearly needed.

Accountability towards purchasers

Similar issues arise regarding accountability structures towards payers. There is ample evidence that underscores the need to improve accountability towards purchasers: all countries that moved to performance-based financing are encountering fraud in performance reporting and in up-coding co-morbidity (DRG creep). Although social insurance organizations could rely on contracts as new accountability mechanisms in principle, contracts are not used as instruments. The contracting process is not performance-oriented: performance measures, targets and benchmarks are not relied on, and there is no selective contracting with providers. In most countries, purchasers are required to contract with all publicly owned facilities.

Hungary is an example of the weak use of contracts as purchasing and accountability instruments. These contracts contain the capacity of the contracted hospital in terms of the number of hospital beds and physician hours provided but remain silent on any aspect of volume, service mix and quality, even though hospitals are paid on the basis of their output (DRGs).

Even the more market-oriented reformers have shied away from relying on performance pressure through the purchasers. In the Czech Republic, insurers were required initially to contract with any hospitals that applied for a contract. Since 1995, selective contracting has been allowed in theory. In practice, however, contracting decisions are made not by insurers but by a committee. These include representatives of health insurance funds, the Ministry of Health, the Chamber of Physicians and the Hospital Association. No contracts have been withdrawn or refused, and only some marginal shifting of services has occurred. How the new legislation will translate into practice in Romania will be interesting to see, because it explicitly allows selective contracting and attempts to ensure sector neutrality by allowing health insurance houses to contract with private as well as public providers. Hungary had difficulty implementing sector neutrality for lack of any clear guidelines on contracting with private-sector providers.

Such inconsistencies result from the difficulty in moving from central planning of inputs to proactive purchasing based on outputs and performance targets. This requires institutional adjustments in rules and regulations, capacity-building and eventually a change in public-sector culture and norms.

Accountability towards the Ministry of Health

Quality assurance and minimum standards are in the early stages. Although these have become buzz-words, most countries are unsure how to use such instruments. In Hungary, physicians defined the minimum standards, but most hospitals and departments did not meet them in the first inspection. Since it would be too costly to upgrade all to the defined standards (equipment, access to laboratories and so on), the issue has been temporarily taken off the agenda.

Accountability towards patients

Accountability structures towards patients are lacking, since there are no accessible formal procedures for patients to complain. The exception again is the Czech Republic, where one of the main new tasks of the Ministry of Health is to deal with the increased number of patient complaints.

Societal functions

Societal functions in the communist era were unfunded and implicit. These societal functions included hospitalizing non-medical cases, such as dependent elderly people. With increased financial pressure, these traditional functions are gradually disappearing, but unfunded and implicit societal functions are appearing in new forms. For example, although health insurance is compulsory in most countries, many people fall through the social safety net. Their number may be small, but there is no information on what happens to them. In the Czech Republic, hospitals incur the cost of treating people without insurance. In Romania, the recent insurance legislation assumes that everyone is covered, but this is not the case. Hospitals in lower-income countries bear the cost of societal functions in a different way: hospital budgets are often delayed for months and physicians continue to work without pay. In some sense, in these consistently underfunded systems, all hospital services have become social services, with volumes unspecified and services delivered at the discretion of staff.

Summary of organizational structure

As Table 9.4 attempts to illustrate, most hospitals in the these countries no longer function as direct budgetary units of the core public-sector bureaucracy. Their organizational structure has changed somewhat on the five key elements. However, the current organizational structure of these hospitals cannot be clearly labelled because there is no consistency in their five key organizational features. The resulting inconsistency of their overall incentive regime has contributed to their limited success in improving performance.

Although hospital autonomy has increased in various decision areas, additional regulations or political pressures in practice have limited the decision rights of hospital managers. Societal functions also have changed little as hospitals continue to provide unfunded societal functions. In contrast, residual claimant status, market exposure and accountability structures have undergone significant changes. The public purse has ceased to be the residual claimant of savings, unspent allocations and efficiency gains, at least under the new

Table 9.4 Internal hospital incentive environment during transition

	Core public bureaucracy	→			Private organization
Autonomy	Few decision rights	Albania	Croatia, Czech Republic, Estonia (municipal), Georgia, Hungary, Kazakhstan (enterprise), Poland, Romania	Estonia company and trust	Full autonomy
Market exposure	None		Albania, Croatia, Czech Republic, Estonia (municipal, company and trust), Hungary, Poland, Romania	Georgia, Kazakhstan (state and enterprise)	At full financial risk for performance
Residual claimant	Public purse		Albania, Croatia, Czech Republic, Georgia, Hungary, Estonia (municipal, company and trust), Kazakhstan (state and enterprise), Poland, Romania		Organization
Accountability	Hierarchical direct control	Albania	Czech Republic		Regulation and contracting
Societal functions	Unfunded mandate	Albania, Estonia (municipal), Croatia, Hungary, Georgia, Poland, Romania	Czech Republic, Kazakhstan (enterprise)		Funded explicit mandate

Note: Estonia (municipal): hospitals operated as municipal institutions; Estonia (company): hospitals operated under joint-stock company law; Estonia (trust): hospitals operated as trusts; Kazakhstan (state): operated by the state; Kazakhstan (enterprise): operated as a health enterprise.

payment mechanisms. The practice of informal payments has created an effect-ive market exposure with its distorted incentives.

Perhaps the most striking feature of the current organizational structure is the lack of effective accountability mechanisms. As the nearly empty account-ability row in Table 9.4 suggests, most countries do not enforce direct account-ability through the hierarchy or through explicit regulations and contracting. The changes in the external environment removed several decision rights from the Ministry of Health, including its powers to exercise direct supervision and control. The new organizations that are the recipients of these decision rights have been unable to develop appropriate accountability arrangements.

Discussion: implications for hospital behaviour and performance

The changed external environment created new pressures for hospitals to adapt their behaviour. Reduced real budgets and new provider payment mechanisms were expected to trigger greater efficiency, and decentralized governance was expected to improve responsiveness to community needs and user expectations. However, organizational structure was inconsistent with the external environ-ment, which resulted in weak and contradictory incentives for behaviour change and loss of potential synergies.

The incoherence between internal and external incentive environments has had three manifestations. First, decentralization created unclear governance structures. The operational meaning of local government ownership and govern-ance has remained unclear in systems funded by social insurance. In terms of funding hospitals, local governments have played a small role, as hospitals' operational expenditure comes from social insurance receipts and capital invest-ment allocations come partly from the central budget and only to a limited extent from local government budgets. Thus, in terms of financial responsib-ility, local governments are limited in their ability to play an important role in the strategic development of hospitals.

A further issue with local government ownership is the resulting legal status of hospitals. When social insurance organizations were established and required to contract with hospitals, the hospitals needed to be granted legally inde-pendent status to sign binding contracts and to act as legally recognizable contracting partners. At the beginning of transition, they did not have this independence as budgetary units of the core government bureaucracy. This dilemma over the meaning and enforceability of contracts between two public bodies provided the opportunity to systematically rethink the organizational form and governance structure of hospitals. Nevertheless, few countries gave attention to this issue, and most did not develop new legal regulations regard-ing the governance of hospitals. Instead, the issue was quickly addressed under already existing laws designed for the governance of general not-for-profit organizations and state-owned companies. As a result, hospitals were turned into such entities as extra-budgetary funds, not-for-profit institutions and state-owned enterprises, regardless of whether these forms and existing regulations were appropriate for the health sector.

The second manifestation of incoherent external incentives and organizational structure is the misalignment between incentives and decision rights. Decision rights were not transferred to the organizational level that would benefit from introducing behaviour change: hospitals had incentives to change their behaviour but not the instruments. Anticipation of greater (technical) efficiency was based on the expectation that hospitals would respond to new payment incentives and financial pressure by reducing excess physical and human resource capacity. These two inputs are the most significant for savings and efficiency gains. Personnel expenditure comprises 60 per cent of all health care costs in the middle-income countries in central and eastern Europe and the former Soviet Union, and physical capacity determines most fixed costs. Given that hospitals had no decision rights over physical capacity and were limited in their decision rights over human resources, the expectation that hospitals would reduce their inputs to produce the same level of output was overestimated.

In contrast to hospitals, local governments do have decision rights over physical assets, but they lack incentives to divest or manage them well. Closure of a local hospital appears to the local electorate as a loss of community assets and as a failure of local government to fulfil its legal (and sometimes even constitutional) mandate. As a result, previous patterns of input use remain despite changes in external structures and increasing financial pressure.

Finally, hospitals did not incur risk for their lack of behavioural and performance adjustment. The interaction between the lack of market exposure and lacking accountability structures created an incentive environment that did not penalize poor hospital behaviour and performance. The repeated bailout of loss-making hospitals by government, a lack of monitoring of financial and non-financial performance, a lack of reporting requirements and no threat of exit made it cost-free for hospitals to continue their previous patterns of behaviour. Although hospitals were rewarded for improved performance, in that they could keep savings and efficiency gains, they were not penalized in the absence of behaviour adjustment. As a result, an improvement in behaviour depended on the drive and entrepreneurial spirit of hospital managers.

Conclusion

This chapter has offered an initial analysis of the organizational structure of hospitals in transition economies. It is suggested that the expected hospital behaviour change did not materialize because the external environment and the organizational structure of hospitals were not in synergy. In particular, hospitals continue to have limited autonomy over key input factors, which has been a significant obstacle to downsizing. Soft budgets undermine efficiency incentives by rewarding financially imprudent behaviour, while accountability structures lack checks and balances on hospital financial and professional behaviour.

As performance has fallen short of expectations, several countries have returned or are contemplating a return to old ways of delivering and financing hospital services. The hospital sector has another reform alternative to abandoning the implemented reforms: redesigning the organizational structure of hospitals to strengthen the efficiency and quality incentives embedded in the already implemented external incentives. This would mean aligning incentives and decision rights, enforcing hard budgets and introducing new accountability mechanisms through more effective use of contracts, quality assurance and performance monitoring. This will necessitate clarifying the future role of local government owners and completing the transition to a more proactive model of purchasing health services. Finally, reorienting the capacities of the Ministries of Health to undertake a stewardship function is essential for the success of any kind of health reform in the countries in central and eastern Europe and the former Soviet Union.

References

Cerniauskas, G. and Murauskiene, L. (2000) *Health Care Systems in Transition: Lithuania.* Copenhagen: European Observatory on Health Care Systems.

Ensor, T. (1993) Health system reform in former socialist countries of Europe, *International Journal of Health Planning and Management,* 8: 169–87.

Gaal, P., Rekassy, B. and Healy, J. (1999) *Health Care Systems in Transition: Hungary.* Copenhagen: European Observatory on Health Care Systems.

Goldstein, E., Preker, A.S., Adeyi, O. and Chellaraj, G. (1996) *Trends in Health Status, Service and Finance: The Transition in Central and Eastern Europe,* World Bank Technical Paper No. 341, Social Challenges of Transition Series. Washington, DC: World Bank.

Harding, A. and Preker, A.S. (2001) A conceptual framework for organizational reforms of hospitals, in A.S. Preker and A. Harding (eds) *Innovations in Health Care Delivery: The Corporatization of Public Hospitals.* Baltimore, MD: Johns Hopkins University Press.

Havriliuc, C., Scintee, S. and Marc, A. (1996) *Health Care Systems in Transition: Romania.* Copenhagen: WHO Regional Office for Europe.

Ho, T. (in press) Eastern European hospitals in transition, *Eurohealth.*

Jakab, M., Preker, A.S. and Harding, A. (2001) Hospital organizational structure in Central Eastern Europe and the former Soviet Union, in A.S. Preker and A. Harding (eds) *Innovations in Health Care Delivery: The Corporatization of Public Hospitals.* Baltimore, MD: Johns Hopkins University Press.

Jesse, M. (2000) *Health Care Systems in Transition: Estonia.* Copenhagen: European Observatory on Health Care Systems.

Karski, J.B., Koronkiewicz, A. and Healy, J. (1999) *Health Care Systems in Transition: Poland.* Copenhagen: European Observatory on Health Care Systems.

Klugman, J. and Schieber, G. (1997) A survey of health reform in central Asia, in Z. Feachem, M. Henscher and L. Rose (eds) *Implementing Health Sector Reform in Central Asia,* EDI Learning Resources Series. Washington, DC: World Bank.

Lewis, M. (2002) Informal health payments in eastern Europe: issues, trends and policy implications, in E. Mossialos, A. Dixon, J. Figueras and J. Kutzin (eds) *Funding Health Care: Options for Europe.* Buckingham: Open University Press.

Marga, I. (1996) *Health Care Systems in Transition: Latvia.* Copenhagen: WHO Regional Office for Europe.

Maynard, A. and Bloor, K. (1999) *Payment Contracting and Regulation of Providers: Flagship Course Material on Health Sector Reform and Sustainable Financing.* Washington, DC: World Bank.

Milgrom, P. and Roberts, J. (1992) *Economics, Organization and Management.* Englewood Cliffs, NJ: Prentice-Hall.

Preker, A.S. and Feachem, R.G.A. (1996) *Market Mechanisms and the Health Sector in Central and Eastern Europe*, World Bank Technical Paper No. 293. Washington, DC: World Bank.

Preker, A., Jakab, M. and Schneider, M. (2002) Health financing reform in transition economies, in E. Mossialos, A. Dixon, J. Figueras and J. Kutzin (eds) *Funding Health Care: Options for Europe*. Buckingham: Open University Press.

Saltman, R.B. and Figueras, J. (1997) *European Health Care Reform: Analysis of Current Strategies*, WHO Regional Publications, European Series, No. 72. Copenhagen: WHO Regional Office for Europe.

Schiavo-Campo, S. (1994) *Institutional Change and the Public Sector in Transitional Economies*, World Bank Discussion Papers, No. 241. Washington, DC: World Bank.

Staines, V.S. (1999) *A Health Sector Strategy for the Europe and Central Asia Region*. Washington, DC: World Bank.

Struk, P. (1996) *Health Care Systems in Transition: Czech Republic*. Copenhagen: WHO Regional Office for Europe.

Vulic, S. and Healy, J. (1999) *Health Care Systems in Transition: Croatia*. Copenhagen: European Observatory on Health Care Systems.

Wiley, M.H. (1992) Hospital financing reform and case-mix measurement: an international review, *Health Care Financing Review*, 13(4): 119–33.

Wiley, M.M. (1995) *Hospital Financing and Payment Systems: A Review of Selected OECD Countries*. Paris: Organisation for Economic Co-operation and Development.

World Bank (1999) *Health Policy Note: Croatia*. Washington, DC: Europe and Central Asia Department, Human Development Unit, World Bank.

part three

Internal strategies for change

chapter ten

Improving performance within the hospital

Judith Healy and Martin McKee

Introduction

This chapter examines how the people working within a hospital, whether clinicians, managers or others, can optimize the quality of the patient care provided. The prerequisites for high-quality care were identified in Chapter 7 as facilities, people and knowledge; it was also noted that social capital, as manifest by a supportive culture, is increasingly being recognized as a valuable input in its own right. Within the hospital these contribute to the more traditional elements (Figure 10.1): place (the facilities within which the hospital operates), people (the human resources available to it) and tools (encompassing not just equipment but also the knowledge required to use it effectively). In this model, social capital, or culture, is considered as an overarching input, interacting with each of the others. Here we identify examples of how hospital

Figure 10.1 Improving health care from inside the hospital

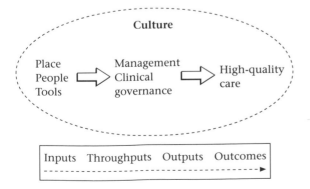

management can encourage a culture that supports staff and patients. The chapter concludes by examining how these elements can be brought together within a coherent overall programme through strategies such as clinical governance. The overall questions that this chapter addresses are: What strategies are hospitals adopting to improve patient care? What is the evidence that these strategies are successful?

Hospital inputs

We begin by considering the inputs that are available within the hospital and associated strategies that can be used to improve hospital performance. Chapter 7 discussed how external agencies harness such inputs to influence hospital activities. This chapter shifts to an internal perspective. Since there are many other textbooks on staff and budgetary management, we concentrate here on three types of inputs – the place (the building and its internal design), the people (the health care staff), the tools (the technology) – as well as the hospital working environment (a supportive culture).

The place

Across the world, many different types of buildings are used as hospitals: medieval monasteries, purpose-built skyscrapers, converted factories and even tents in zones of conflict such as the Balkans. Once the essentials are in place, such as a roof, heating, lighting and running water, does it matter what the building looks like? How important is design to the operation of a hospital? As discussed in Chapter 4, the current configuration of hospitals reflects their historical origins and subsequent development. Thus, understanding why hospitals look the way they do today requires reflecting on how they have evolved over time.

The design of hospitals has been influenced by several sets of ideas (Figure 10.2). These include ideas about society and people (such as religious beliefs and political views on how much to spend on hospitals), ideas about architecture and building, ideas from medicine and nursing (such as germ

Figure 10.2 Factors influencing hospital design

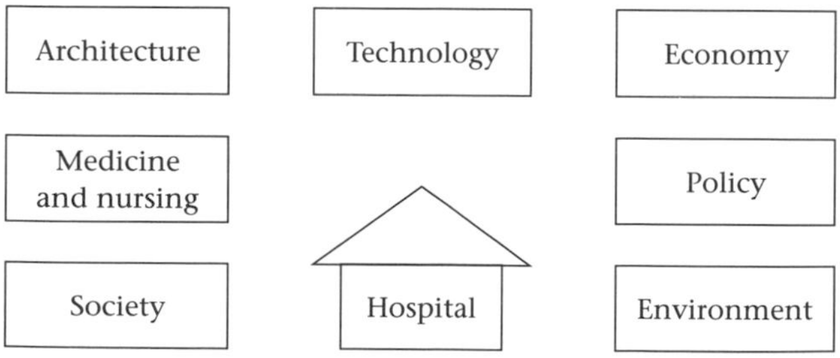

Figure 10.3 Various types of hospital design

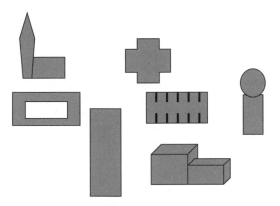

theory) and ideas from health care policy (Francis *et al.* 1999). Ideas about society and architecture were dominant in earlier centuries, whereas ideas from medicine and health policy became more important in the twentieth century, as did the more recent concern about the environment.

People's expectations of a hospital have changed over the centuries. Until the nineteenth century, the appropriate place to be ill was at home. Only those who could not afford to pay for physicians and nurses to care for them at home went into a hospital. Hospitals were associated with death, and the term 'patient' emerged as a description of those who were waiting patiently to meet their maker (James and Tatton-Brown 1986). Figure 10.3 suggests different types of hospital design. Since hospitals in western Europe originally were attached to religious institutions and medical treatment was of limited effectiveness, communication with God was more important than with a physician. The hospital was designed in such a way that the sick could see the altar at the end of the ward, thus giving rise to the cruciform design. This hospital design emerged by the mid-fifteenth century in Italy, consisting of four wards radiating from a central altar. The cruciform plan was taken up across Europe in the sixteenth and seventeenth centuries (Pevsner 1976) and, especially for asylums, continued into the nineteenth century. The radial plan of the seventeenth and eighteenth centuries suggested an octagonal church at the centre of eight radiating wards.

The next type of hospital design had detached pavilions on either side of a courtyard, with a church at its end. Some pavilion buildings, most notably French hospitals, were based also on the geometric designs of the Boullée–Ledoux–Durand school of architecture. The later advantage of cruciform and radial plans was that they made it easier for staff to monitor patients from a central point.

Medical and nursing needs and health beliefs played little part in hospital design until the mid-nineteenth century. Beliefs about miasma then became influential and miasma theory saw the chief enemy of the sick as stale air. The views of Florence Nightingale on hospital design and nursing practices in her

Notes on Nursing (Nightingale 1860) were based on miasma theory, which supported the building of hospitals based on an airy pavilion design, with patients lying in neat rows of beds along the ward.

Hospital design changed radically in the late nineteenth century, reflecting the ascent of germ theory. Good plumbing, hand-washing by physicians and nurses and the separation of infectious patients then became more important than vigorous ventilation. Hospitals were designed to promote antiseptic and aseptic practices. For example, staff treating patients must be able to scrub their hands under running water with chlorine or carbolic soap. Hospitals were designed, furnished and equipped to minimize the transmission of infectious diseases. These measures, combined with the introduction of anaesthesia and later X-rays, fundamentally changed the nature of surgery. By the 1880s, operating theatres and hospitals were becoming hygienic and well equipped.

Hospital design now revolved around the requirements of medical and nursing care and, increasingly, the demands of new technology. The function of hospitals shifted from custodial care to active intervention. The presence of an operating theatre came to define a hospital. The number of beds increased with patient demand as hospitals offered safer and more successful inpatient treatment. The middle classes increasingly came to hospital for the best health care and also expected good facilities and polite service. These trends all produced a massive increase both in the complexity and size of hospitals. This can be illustrated by the doubling of space per bed in hospitals in the United Kingdom, from 20 m^2 to 40 m^2 in the first half of the twentieth century (James and Tatton-Brown 1986).

By the latter half of the twentieth century, many countries were using standard hospital designs based on pre-fabricated components, a model applied equally to schools, apartment blocks and supermarkets. This led to the construction of compact many-storey buildings, which brought significant savings in construction costs (Martinez 1986). Within such a purpose-built building, hospital design aimed to produce a fully functional and integrated organization. This design was based on the relationships between the nursing area (where patients spend their stay in hospital), the clinical zone (diagnostic and treatment facilities) and the support zone (facilities that support the running of the hospital) (James and Tatton-Brown 1986).

Building strategies can be classified into two groups: vertical and horizontal (James and Noakes 1994). In vertical strategies, the zones are arranged one above the other so that the movement is mainly vertical. Models vary from the single tower-on-podium to articulated slabs-on-podium and vertical monoliths. In horizontal strategies, the zones are linked together laterally, so that the movement is mainly horizontal. This includes the nucleus strategy that was developed in response to the need for growth and change, whereby a hospital is built in stages, the first stage being a 300-bed nucleus, capable of expansion in stages to 600 beds.

The high vertical building, a response to the need for a large hospital on a small urban site, has rarely been a success. The high-rise block building based on industrial conveyer-belt principles did not offer a therapeutic environment for patients or a functional work environment for staff (James and Noakes 1994).

Many hospitals in Europe, however, are not purpose-built but have as their core an old building around which later additions are built. The sites of old, prestigious hospitals in inner cities are often architectural nightmares left over from the building dreams of earlier decades.

The continuing design challenge is how a hospital building can adapt to changes in its internal and external environment. An optimal design is one that inhibits change of function least rather than one that fits a specific function best. This strategy aims to combat obsolescence; the perennial problem for the hospital planner is that, by the time a new hospital is designed and built, it is already out of date. The key issue, therefore, is flexibility. The second challenge is that, despite some common features, there is no one standard hospital model. Hospitals must be designed to fit the requirements of different countries and localities: the population health needs, the building budget, the particular site, the climate and the cultures. To this we should add the more recent concern about the environment, such as the environmental footprint the hospital makes on its surroundings in terms of energy use and waste disposal. The hospitals participating in the WHO Regional Office for Europe network Hospitals for Health are discussing some of these issues.

A therapeutic design?

An important issue is whether hospital design can, itself, have a therapeutic value. This concept was much debated in the twentieth century (and unsuccessfully applied) in relation to psychiatric hospitals (Scull 1979). More recently, the therapeutic potential of hospital design gained credence following a study of patients undergoing cholecystectomy in a Pennsylvania hospital. Twenty-three surgical patients assigned to rooms with windows looking out on greenery had shorter post-operative hospital stays and required less pain relief than 23 matched patients in similar rooms with windows facing a brick building wall (Ulrich 1984). Although it is less researched, many health professionals have argued that the use of art in a hospital brings therapeutic benefits (Glanville 1996).

These ideas have been developed most extensively in the United States using the Planetree model (Blank *et al.* 1995). This model also has been adopted in Sweden, where some recent hospital designs put patient-focused care principles at the centre of hospital planning, with the aim of making the hospital a supportive environment for patients and staff (Dilani 2000). Patient-friendly hospital design, which pays attention to colour, shape and furnishings as well as to easier interactions with staff, can be a tool for empowering patients. Furthermore, it has been shown to provide higher levels of patient satisfaction than conventional designs (Martin *et al.* 1998). Similar interventions, in Norway and the United Kingdom, also suggest higher levels of patient satisfaction, lower use of potent analgesia and earlier discharge from hospital (Lawson and Phiri 2000).

Considerable efforts have been made to adapt the hospital environment and its procedures to the needs of children (Pletinckx 2000). The research evidence on the psychological and therapeutic effects of a stay in hospital has been

---

Box 10.1 The model Children's Charter of the Department of Health of England

- Your child to be cared for in a children's ward under the supervision of a specialist paediatrician
- Your child to have a qualified, named children's nurse responsible for his or her nursing care
- To be able to stay in the hospital with your child
- If your child is having an operation and where circumstances permit, you can expect to accompany them into the anaesthetic room and be present until they go to sleep
- To be told what pain relief will be given to your child
- The health system to respect your child's privacy, dignity and religious or cultural beliefs
- Your child to be offered a choice of children's menus
- To have facilities to breastfeed your child
- Your child to wear his or her own clothes, and have personal possessions
- The hospital to be clean, safe and suitably furnished for children and young people
- You can expect all the staff you meet to wear name badges, so that you know who everyone is, and for security
- Your child to have the opportunity for play and meet other children
- Your child has the right to receive suitable education

Source: Department of Health (1996)

---

taken up more readily in relation to children than adults. For example, some hospitals have adapted variations on a children's charter: a statement of what children and their care-givers can legitimately expect from a hospital (Box 10.1).

Generalizing from these human aspects of hospital design is difficult, because of the relative lack of research and because factors may vary between cultures. Nevertheless, these studies demonstrate the potential for relatively simple interventions (Scher 1996). For example, focus group discussions at one hospital highlighted the importance of the view from the bed, especially among bedridden patients, the quality of washing facilities, privacy and the ability to control noise levels (Lawson and Phiri 2000). A study in Germany identified specific colour preferences for rooms, furnishings and bed linen: beige, white, green and pink (Schuschke and Christiansen 1994). Other cultures might have other colour preferences, but hospital interior design does matter to patients. The main message, however, is that patients should be consulted on hospital design, not just to increase patient satisfaction but to achieve better therapeutic outcomes.

A second issue that is often overlooked is access to the hospital by patients, most of whom are elderly, disabled or temporarily incapacitated. For example, a study in the United Kingdom found that most hospital lifts were inaccessible to those with limited mobility or with visual or hearing impairments (Brown *et al.* 1997). Research involving people using wheelchairs identified various frustrations: issues of independence, the attitudes and lack of understanding by others and lack of involvement of people with disabilities when facilities are designed (Pierce 1998). These were similar to issues emerging from a study of the childbirth experiences of mothers with physical disabilities (Thomas and Curtis 1997).

Although some hospitals have done much to adapt to the needs of people with disabilities (Moore 1997) and considerable evidence-based guidance is available (Jones and Tamari 1997), many hospitals remain essentially inaccessible or unresponsive to those who need them most. Although well recognized by disabled people and their care-givers, this issue has received rather less attention in the scientific literature. Policy-makers should ensure that hospitals are accessible to people with disabilities and should also address the wider issue of disempowerment that prevents such views being taken into account (Fawcett *et al.* 1994).

A third issue is the need to ensure that hospital design reduces, rather than increases, the risks of infection (discussed in Chapter 3). This vast topic encompasses the need to design cooling systems that do not spread *Legionella* bacteria as well as promoting hygienic practices in hospital kitchens to reduce the risk of food poisoning among staff and patients. Despite the threats posed by the growth of hospital-acquired infections, including antibiotic-resistant bacteria, many hospitals still have inadequate or inaccessible hand-washing facilities (Fox 1997; Kesevan 1999). Some physicians still fail to wash their hands between patients even where there is a clear risk of cross-infection (Daniels and Rees 1999). Poor design also can negate hygienic efforts. For example, in one study, 60 per cent of surgeons had to re-scrub because their hands had desterilized through insufficient scrub room space (Morgan-Jones *et al.* 1997). Hospital patients also are at risk from injuries from poor design. Again, relatively simple measures can reduce risks. In one study of falls among elderly patients, only 17 per cent of those falling on a carpeted floor sustained injuries compared with 46 per cent of those who fell on vinyl (Healey 1994).

Finally, although this chapter focuses primarily on the needs of patients, we should not overlook the needs of staff, many of whom live on hospital premises or spend long working hours in the hospital. Their legitimate expectations must also be taken into account in the provision of high-quality residential accommodation.

Looking to the future, trends in four rapidly developing areas of health technology have implications for the built environment: the miniaturization of diagnostic equipment, developments in remote diagnostic imaging, minimally invasive surgical procedures and therapeutic interventions whereby drugs are targeted to an organ or a specific cell (MARU 1996). These new techniques and equipment mean not only that diagnosis is made easier and safer for patients in a more compact environment, but also that the patient and specialist do not have to be in the same location. The challenge facing policy-makers is to ensure that hospitals adapt to these changing circumstances while continuing to provide welcoming environments that are conducive to physical and mental healing (Francis *et al.* 1999).

The people

Hospitals are labour-intensive enterprises that depend on their staff to achieve cost-effective outcomes for patients. Staff management, therefore, is a major challenge for hospital managers. The hospital workforce in industrialized countries is highly professionalized and contains a multiplicity of occupational groups, who are stratified vertically (according to occupation) and horizontally (in terms of hierarchical levels). Getting the levels and mix of hospital staff right involves two main considerations: first, ensuring that the hospital has the appropriate mix of skills for the tasks that need to be undertaken and, second, ensuring that those employed are well trained and highly motivated.

This implies that the hospital workforce should be managed actively within a strategic framework. This can range from an incremental approach, putting in place the appropriate policies and working gradually towards defined goals, or it can involve a fundamental re-engineering of the hospital workforce (see Chapter 11). Chapter 14 explains that process re-engineering 'redesigns job responsibilities and determines who does the work, where the work is located and by what processes or patterns the work will be done'. Re-engineering covers a miscellany of approaches as follows: grouping patients in terms of care requirements, creating multidisciplinary teams, matching skill and function, downsizing the workforce, developing work protocols, setting performance standards, decentralizing services such as laboratory tests, redesigning the physical environment, implementing total quality management and offering performance incentives such as recognition, promotion, cash or other in-kind rewards. Re-engineering has been advocated enthusiastically, but rigorous evaluation so far has found few clear benefits (Walston and Kimberley 1997), while some doubt that the costs and practices prevailing in the United States can translate to a European setting (Hurst 1995). The huge literature on personnel management (Armstrong 1991) and the many rapidly changing management fads are beyond the scope of this chapter, so here we select two issues of particular relevance to hospital managers: skill mix and good employment practices.

Skill mix

Those managing a hospital must decide on the right mix of staff to deliver effective care. The scope for multiskilling and task delegation in a western European hospital depends largely on whether certain activities are the statutory responsibility of specific professional groups. Professions such as physicians and nurses retain exclusive jurisdiction over certain tasks, which in some countries are protected by statute. The history of professions in industrialized countries is characterized by competition over work jurisdictions (Abbott 1988). The classic comparison is between the United States and United Kingdom. In some states of the United States, physicians have a monopoly on delivering babies but nurses can give some anaesthetics; in the United Kingdom, midwives deliver most babies and anaesthesia is exclusively a medical responsibility. This is primarily because, in the United States, delivering a baby attracts a fee, and the presence of a medical anaesthetist would oblige the surgeon to hand over a larger proportion of the fee for the operation.

The potential for substitution between hospital staff is a key element of re-engineering and has attracted much attention, both to produce better services and, more often, to cut costs. Traditionally, hospitals have very rigid demarcations as to which staff can undertake which tasks. Efforts to introduce more flexibility in service delivery through staff substitution have been facilitated in some countries by a move away from historical professional demarcations towards a competence approach. This first defines the task and then asks who could perform it most cost-effectively (Armstrong 1991); in effect, an emphasis on competence rather than credentials and making it possible to break the link between a job and a particular professional jurisdiction. The substitution debate has centred around three main types of initiatives:

- substitute less expensive and less highly trained staff;
- expand the task jurisdictions of existing staff; and
- develop new occupational groups.

Substitution
The main thrust is to substitute less expensive and lesser trained staff. This has progressed most at the interface between medicine and nursing (see Chapter 11). In the countries where nursing is highly professionalized, there is considerable evidence that qualified nurses often achieve better results than physicians at some tasks, partly because they spend more time with patients (Shum *et al.* 2000). The second area is the substitution of nursing assistants for certified nurses, as noted later. There is a large literature on nursing skill mix, but as Chapter 11 indicates, there is no unanimity on whether cost savings result from substituting less highly trained nurses for more highly trained ones. Another area is the interface between medicine and pharmacy, with pharmacists taking responsibility for tasks such as monitoring anticoagulation therapy.

Substituting tasks between professionals is not, however, simply a technical exercise. Delegation tasks that involve supervision is usually more acceptable, whereas transferring responsibility is more problematic. Such transfers involve shifts in professional power and may therefore be strongly contested, especially since this may mean considerable change in the roles of the groups involved.

Some argue that the process of delegation to less intensively trained staff in the United States has harmed the quality of care. For example, cost-containment strategies in the United States in the 1990s led to many registered nurses being replaced by health care assistants (Brannon 1996). Chapter 14 notes some possible adverse consequences: units and hospitals with more and better-trained nurses achieve better patient outcomes.

The expected cost-efficiency does not always follow. A nurse-led service may not be any cheaper (Venning *et al.* 2000), as nurses then demand greater rewards for their additional skills and responsibilities and their extended role may lead to additional services being provided (Richardson *et al.* 1998). Furthermore, professional groups taking on tasks that were previously the responsibility of physicians may, reasonably, expect a level of discretion and decision-making power similar to that of physicians. Thus, there may be sound reasons, based on effectiveness, to give professionals other than physicians an enhanced role in the provision of care, but this may not save money in the long term.

Expansion

The second strategy is to expand the jurisdiction of existing occupational groups. In some countries, nurses take much greater responsibility for delivering care to patients with chronic illnesses, often running clinics and prescribing within guidelines for patients with conditions such as asthma and hypertension. Nurses have altered their work jurisdiction in three areas, which often brings them into conflict with other occupational groups: technical tasks have been delegated from medicine; routine nursing tasks are increasingly delegated to aides; and psychosocial assessment of patient needs competes with social workers (Gardner and McCoppin 1989).

New cadres

The third strategy is to develop new occupations. Occupational groups in the medical workforce continue to proliferate. For example, many practical tasks are being delegated by professional groups to new groups, such as taking blood samples, now undertaken by specially trained phlebotomists in many countries (McKee and Black 1993). New technical specialties have arisen as the technical content of clinical care has become more sophisticated. Thus, this third strategy in many ways runs counter to the multiskilling trend that encourages more flexibility, whereby occupational groups undertake some agreed tasks (especially in an emergency) that otherwise by convention fall within another occupational jurisdiction.

Good employment practices

Several employment practices can be identified that aim to recruit and maintain a high-quality and well-motivated workforce. These are the sort of policies and practices that constitute good staff management in large organizations, including hospitals, in many high-income countries (Table 10.1). Good staff management involves ensuring that jobs offer high levels of staff satisfaction. This

Table 10.1 Good employment practices

Skill mix	Achieve the right numbers and mix of staff
Staff development	Training and development based on life-long learning
Retention	Policies addressing staff turnover
Equal opportunities	Policies on recruitment and harassment
	Family-friendly policies
Healthy workplaces	Policies on sickness absence
	Policies on workplace accidents
	Occupational health services
Staff involvement	Involve staff in policy decisions
	Encourage staff to identify problems and solutions

Source: Department of Health (1998)

calls for ensuring that staff are empowered to participate in decision-making, are fairly rewarded, have equality of opportunity, are enabled to develop their skills through a process of life-long learning, have employment security and have a satisfactory work environment. We discuss some policies of particular relevance to hospitals, as follows.

Staff development
In the past, a basic professional qualification was considered sufficient to allow one to practise until retirement. The rapidly changing nature of health care means that hospital staff need to engage in life-long learning, not least to retain a basic level of clinical competence. This is necessary to ensure high-quality patient care. It is also in the financial interests of hospitals, since, as discussed in Chapter 7, hospital employers increasingly are subject to grievance complaints from patients as well as malpractice suits. Hospitals have a clear responsibility to monitor the care provided by those who work within their walls and to put in place mechanisms to deal with staff who fail to meet such standards. Importantly, continuing training can also enhance job satisfaction and improve staff retention rates. These issues are discussed later in this chapter under the heading of 'Clinical governance'.

Retention
Poor management of staff contributes to a downward cycle of low morale and stress, often apparent in high rates of short-term sickness absence and high staff turnover. Salary levels, working conditions and job security are important in both retaining and motivating staff. Grindle and Hildebrand (1995: 441) argue that a pay packet is not the only motivator, however, even in low-income countries: 'We . . . found that effective public management performance is more often driven by strong organizational cultures, good management practices, and effective communication networks than it is by rules and regulations or procedures and pay scales'. Although this study refers to public-sector management in general, it has particular relevance to the staff who work in hospitals. People want to feel that the organization has an important and clear mission and that they are part of this endeavour. Job satisfaction is important in that people should enjoy the work they do and feel it worthwhile. People should regard themselves as part of a well-regarded profession or occupation that has social status in society. People want recognition and respect from peers and managers for the tasks that they do well. These findings are important, since they suggest that, even where financial resources are very constrained, staff retention and performance can be improved through efforts to create effective organizational cultures. For example, in hospital intensive care units, the best predictors of better patient outcomes were organizational factors such as a patient-centred culture, strong professional leadership, effective collaboration between staff and an open approach to problem-solving (Zimmerman *et al.* 1993).

Equal opportunity
Many hospitals now describe themselves as an equal opportunity employer, paying attention in their recruitment, management and promotion practices

to avoiding discrimination based on any or all of the grounds of ethnic origin, national origin, religion, disability, age, gender and sexual preference. For example, the United Kingdom National Health Service set up a women's unit in the 1990s to promote equal opportunities for women and to develop more women-friendly working practices, crucial in a sector where the majority of the workforce are women (Adams 1994). The shortage of qualified nurses in the European Union has focused attention on strategies for retaining women in the workforce (Versieck *et al.* 1995). Hospital employers, like other employers, should also ensure that they have in place policies and procedures to deal with sexual harassment in the workplace (Davidhizar *et al.* 1998). The issue of age discrimination recently has come to the fore in the United States in terms of which staff are made redundant during hospital restructuring (Fiesta 1997).

Offering a range of family-friendly work practices (Forth *et al.* 1997) is especially important for the hospital workforce, most of whom are women. Such practices include part-time work, flexible working hours, parental leave, compassionate leave, telephone access and child care. Thirty-two countries have ratified the Workers with Family Responsibilities Convention of the International Labour Organization. The European Union has urged its member countries to promote family-friendly workplaces and has signalled a new directive on the reconciliation of work and family responsibilities. Such a reconciliation will not be easy. The organizational culture generally frowns on the family intruding on work (Wolcott and Glezer 1995). A business case, however, can be made for providing benefits that improve staff retention, especially when these staff are highly trained workers, and where recruitment and induction costs are considerable (Galinsky *et al.* 1991). Some countries in eastern Europe previously had family-friendly workplaces, such as Hungary, which had generous maternity benefits, although it has also been argued that the provision of child care at the workplace tended to deny mothers the option of remaining at home. The problem is that many of these benefits and practices have been dismantled in a bid to make enterprises more efficient. In contrast, many western European firms, especially those with highly skilled women workers, such as hospitals, are looking for ways to retain women with children in the workforce; the shortage of qualified nurses in many European Union countries is an example.

The tools

Hospitals have developed in part because they are the repositories of much health care technology (knowledge, skills and equipment). Technology has transformed the design and functions of hospitals (as discussed in Chapter 3), plays a crucial role in improving the performance of hospitals, influences the skill mix in the hospital workforce and has enormous cost implications.

The stock of technology varies enormously across industrialized countries (Banta 1995). An example is the number of magnetic resonance imaging scanners, with 18.8 per million population in Japan in 1996 (the highest rate), 2.5 in France and 1.1 in the Czech Republic (OECD 1999). Another major item of expenditure for hospitals is the installation of a new information and communication technology system. This can handle a complex range of tasks: staff communications within the hospital, computerized patient records, patient monitoring, the ordering of clinical tests, stock control and telemedicine (van Bemmel and Musen 1997). Many countries now involve national or even cross-national bodies in technology planning, as discussed in Chapter 7, and their deliberations potentially guide technology decisions made by individual hospitals.

Chapter 12 explores the adoption of technology within hospitals and notes the array of factors that influence such decisions. In case studies in hospital trusts in the United Kingdom, clinicians made decisions on adopting technology, with hospital managers involved only in big-ticket items or when departmental budgets were exceeded. There was little evidence that decisions were based on good evidence of clinical effectiveness. The issue, therefore, is how to provide the information that hospitals need when investing in new technology. There is a large and growing body of evidence on the efficacy and cost-effectiveness of health technology, but the extent to which hospital managers use this varies.

A supportive culture

Policy-makers have paid relatively little attention to the final prerequisite for high-quality health care: the culture of the hospital. Its significance has emerged from a growing body of research on the relationship between organizational culture and quality of care. Many studies have found tangible benefits to patients from a supportive culture among clinical staff (Shortell *et al.* 1995). Such research helps explain why some hospitals perform better than others (discussed in Chapter 14). We now describe two international programmes that seek to develop hospital cultures that support staff and patients.

The Health Promoting Hospitals programme was developed by the World Health Organization based on the principles of the Ottawa Charter on Health Promotion (WHO 1986) and the Ljubljana Charter on Reforming Health Care (WHO 1996). A workshop in Vienna in 1997 agreed on key principles and set up the WHO International Network of Health Promoting Hospitals for participating hospitals. The programme seeks to foster participation by patients, staff and others outside the hospital, to improve communication with other levels of the health care system, to offer information and education, to reorient hospitals towards health promotion and to encourage learning from experience (WHO 1997).

The Baby-Friendly Hospital Initiative, developed by UNICEF and the World Health Organization, urges hospitals to promote breastfeeding, which could save the lives of 1.5 million babies each year (UNICEF 1996, 1999). In 1990, 31 governments agreed to the Innocenti Declaration on the Promotion, Protection and Support of Breastfeeding. This set out operational targets for all countries to achieve by 1995 in four areas: a national breastfeeding committee, the certification of hospitals as baby-friendly, regulations on the marketing of breastmilk substitutes and the right to paid maternity leave and breastfeeding breaks at work (UNICEF 1995). A hospital is designated

---

Box 10.2 Baby-Friendly Hospital Initiative: ten steps to successful breastfeeding

Every facility providing maternity services and care for newborn infants should:

- Have a written breastfeeding policy that is routinely communicated to all health care staff
- Train all health care staff in skills necessary to implement this policy
- Inform all pregnant women about the benefits and management of breastfeeding
- Help mothers initiate breastfeeding within one half-hour of birth
- Show mothers how to breastfeed and how to maintain lactation even if they should be separated from their infants
- Give newborn infants no food and drink other than breastmilk, unless *medically* indicated
- Practise rooming in – that is, allow mothers and infants to remain together 24 hours a day
- Encourage breastfeeding on demand
- Give no artificial teats or pacifiers (also called dummies or soothers) to breast-feeding infants
- Foster the establishment of breastfeeding support groups and refer mothers to them on discharge from the hospital or clinic

A Baby-Friendly Hospital does not accept free or low-cost breastmilk substitutes, feeding bottles or teats, and implements these 'Ten Steps' to support breastfeeding.

Source: Adapted from UNICEF (1999: 6)

---

baby-friendly when it has agreed not to accept free or low-cost breastmilk sub-stitutes, feeding bottles or teats and implements ten specific steps to support breastfeeding (Box 10.2). Since the initiative began, nearly 15,000 hospitals in 128 countries have been awarded baby-friendly status. Information for hos-pitals wishing to participate in the network is available at http://www.who.dk/WHO-Euro/about/babies.htm

The next section considers how hospital management might bring the various resources together in the most effective way. We focus on clinical governance as an emerging concept in health care management. This is an approach that brings the hospital back to its primary goal, that of caring for patients, by ensur-ing that managers and health care professionals work together to optimize the care provided.

From management to clinical governance

Public-sector management underwent a major transformation in some countries during the mid-1980s. The new managerialism emerged from a private-sector paradigm. The emphasis was on producing a measurable product, devolving power to technocratic managers, achieving specific goals and harnessing the organization to broad government policies (Considine 1988). The discourse of management had become the dominant language in the public-service culture by the early 1990s in countries such as Australia and the United Kingdom (Pusey 1991; Gray and Jenkins 1993). This managerialist culture aimed to transform spenders into managers, make managers more accountable, flatten previously hierarchical management structures, engineer competition to produce greater efficiency, link inputs to results and set performance indicators against which to assess staff compliance and productivity (Healy 1998). These management techniques were applied later in hospitals than in the rest of the public sector, given the complexity of health care and the greater power of physicians.

One aim in transforming hospitals from budgetary units of government to autonomous public-sector organizations was to enable the managers to manage. Hospital managers, however, often are subjected to conflicting behavioural incentives arising from both the external and internal environment of their hospital (Chapter 9). For example, hospitals are expected to both balance the budget and invest in staff training.

Hospital management has also become a more political process, especially where ownership has been devolved to autonomous boards that include a range of stakeholders. Furthermore, the respective responsibilities of hospital managers and board members are sometimes blurred, while other external stakeholders such as purchasers (as discussed in Chapter 7) now have considerable say over internal hospital activities (Shamian 1998; Hoek 1999). The people who manage hospitals have changed in some countries, with responsibility for management shifting from physicians to clinical teams, and by the mid-1980s to professional managers (Harrison and Pollitt 1994). In many European countries, however, hospital directors are often physicians with little management training (Hansen 2000).

In the context of these more complex ownership and management arrangements, managerial strategies in some countries aim explicitly to enhance the quality of care and not just achieve financial targets. These approaches include medical and clinical auditing (the latter distinguished from the former by its involvement of several professional groups), as well as more wide-ranging programmes such as continuous quality improvement and total quality management (Berwick *et al.* 1992)

The essential elements of quality assurance are: defining criteria against which clinical practice can be assessed; developing standards that should be attained for each of these criteria; monitoring progress towards attainment; improving changing clinical practice; and revisiting the initial standards to determine whether they should be relaxed or enhanced (Black 1992). Such a cyclical and continuing process should involve everyone who can provide input into patient care, including the patient. Many texts address this extremely large topic (Morrell and Harvey 1999).

Total quality management is a concept developed in Japan after 1945 as a means of enabling Japanese industry to compete with the then-dominant United States manufacturers. Its key features are shown in Box 10.3. It is a means for hospitals to accentuate their focus on the patient and reduce what is increasingly being recognized as a relatively high rate of errors occurring in modern health care (Berwick and Leape 1999). It takes a whole-system approach, which will be increasingly important as the provision of health care becomes more complex and multidisciplinary.

Box 10.3 Key elements of total quality management

- Making customers' needs a priority for everyone
- Defining quality in terms of customers' needs
- Recognizing the existence of internal customers and suppliers
- Examining the process of production rather than individual performance for explanations of flaws or poor quality
- Using sound methods of measurement to understand how to improve quality
- Removing barriers between staff and promoting effective team work
- Promoting training for everyone
- Involving the whole workforce in the task of improving quality
- Understanding that quality improvement is a continuous process

Source: Adapted from Moss and Garside (1995)

The challenges involved in implementing quality assurance programmes have often been underestimated (Black and Thompson 1993) and, although attitudes have changed greatly in recent years, in some countries health professionals remain apathetic or suspicious. High-quality care depends on a supportive organizational context. Factors that have been found to support the development of quality assurance activities include fostering a culture of quality, ensuring that staff are able to participate; strengthening interpersonal skills; the use of quality assurance facilitators to gather and analyse data; assurance of confidentiality; involvement of all relevant staff; and evaluation of the overall process (Johnston *et al.* 2000).

Patient-focused care

This increased emphasis on quality assurance has run in parallel with more attention to the concept of patient-focused care. Although it is self-evident that care should be focused on the needs of the patient, in reality many hospitals are run more for the convenience of the staff. Thus, in the traditional model, patients are admitted under individual specialist clinicians, who either 'own' them or transfer them to the care of another clinician. Junior medical staff and ward nursing staff manage patients, and the progress of a patient through a hospital and its many procedures is often inefficient and disorganized. The patient-focused concept attempts to address such problems through a range of methods (Chapter 11). Some of these issues are discussed in the following paragraphs.

Multidisciplinary care
The traditional single-specialty organizing principle of hospital structures and patient management is increasingly outdated. A patient in an acute care hospital today is likely to be older and sicker and to have more co-morbidity (for example, heart disease, hypertension and chronic lung disease related to smoking). Surgery on older and sicker patients runs a greater risk of multiple-organ

failure post-operatively, thus requiring intensive post-surgical monitoring (Hillman 1999). This suggests that, in some cases, patients should be defined less by the condition or body system being treated than by the severity of their overall condition, with management by a multidisciplinary team.

Systems to detect iatrogenic illness
Deaths in hospital, either from medical errors or hospital-acquired infections, have increasingly been recognized as a serious issue in most industrialized countries (Brennan *et al.* 1991). Furthermore, for every preventable death, there are many preventable serious complications. Drawing on the analogy of the system in use to report near-misses by aircraft, the National Health Service in England is setting up a mandatory reporting system for logging all errors and near-misses (Donaldson Report 2000). Initial work pointed to more than 850,000 adverse health events each year at huge cost; an example of persistent failure to learn lessons is that 13 patients have died or been paralysed since 1985 because a drug has been wrongly administered by spinal injection.

Enhancing continuity of care
Whereas in the past (as noted in Chapter 2) patients undergoing a complex series of investigations were admitted for a lengthy stay, they are now more likely to have a series of short admissions and outpatient visits. This requires a higher level of coordination. Importantly, it has been shown that patients undergoing non-urgent surgery have better outcomes under a system of co-ordinated care than a matched group (Caplan *et al.* 1998). Such coordinated care involved pre-admission assessment, patient education, admission to hospital on the day of surgery and post-acute care after discharge. This resulted in shorter lengths of stay, a reduced risk of wound infection and a higher level of patient satisfaction.

Clinical governance

The parallel tracks of managerialism and quality assurance began to converge in the late 1990s, not least because real improvements in quality often require shifts in resources. This concept has been termed 'clinical governance', since it requires a hospital to integrate financial control, service performance and clinical quality (Scally and Donaldson 1998). Clinical governance within the hospital, therefore, encompasses a large range of activities, including improving information systems, implementing continuing professional development programmes and developing peer review systems. It builds on many of the elements developed earlier within the framework of total quality management.

This has been taken forward in the United Kingdom, where the government has placed a statutory duty on all health care organizations to seek quality improvement through clinical governance (Secretary of State for Health 1997). In particular, the chief executive of a National Health Service trust is ultimately responsible for assessing the quality of services provided by the trust (NHS Executive 1998). This presents a major challenge for hospital managers, who must set up a structure to oversee and monitor the many staff and many activities involved in a clinical governance process (Edwards and Packham 1999). Hospital chief executives are required to submit annual quality assurance statements on clinical governance arrangements in place in their trusts.

Lessons and implications

Effective hospital care requires a combination of inputs. Facilities should be designed to be safe, be a pleasant environment in which to visit or work and be sufficiently adaptable to respond to changing needs and expectations. The workforce must be trained, highly motivated and participate in programmes of life-long learning. In addition, evidence is growing that a supportive environment not only makes a hospital a better place to work but improves patient outcomes. Concepts such as the WHO International Network of Health Promoting Hospitals offer many examples of good practice.

These inputs must be combined effectively. This requires new ways of working for both managers and health professionals. Management and quality assurance activities have often proceeded along two parallel but separate trajectories. The concept of clinical governance requires that these activities converge. This calls for involvement by all those working in the hospital in improving the quality of care, within a wider framework for optimizing the achievements of the health care system.

References

Abbott, A. (1988) *The System of Professions: An Essay on the Division of Expert Labour.* Chicago, IL: University of Chicago Press.

Adams, J. (1994) Career development: opportunities 2000, *Nursing Times*, 90(16): 31–2.

Armstrong, M. (1991) *A Handbook of Personnel Management.* London: Kogan Page.

Banta, D. (1995) *An Approach to the Social Control of Hospital Technologies*, Current Concerns SHS Paper No. 10. Geneva: World Health Organization.

Berwick, D.M. and Leape, L.L. (1999) Reducing errors in medicine, *British Medical Journal*, 319: 136–7.

Berwick, D.M., Enthoven, A. and Bunker, J.P. (1992) Quality management in the NHS: the doctor's role, part 1, *British Medical Journal*, 302: 235–9.

Black, N. (1992) The relationship between evaluative research and audit, *Journal of Public Health Medicine*, 14: 361–6.

Black, N. and Thompson, E. (1993) Obstacles to medical audit: British doctors speak, *Social Science and Medicine*, 36: 849–56.

Blank, A.E., Horowitz, S. and Matza, D. (1995) Quality with a human face? The Samuels Planetree model hospital unit, *Joint Commission Journal of Quality Improvement*, 21: 289–99.

Brannon, R.L. (1996) Restructuring hospital nursing: reversing the trend toward a professional work force, *International Journal of Health Services*, 26(4): 643–54.

Brennan, T.A., Leape, L.L., Laird, N. *et al.* (1991) Incidence of adverse events and negligence in hospitalized patients: results of the Harvard medical practice study, *New England Journal of Medicine*, 324: 370–6.

Brown, A.R., Sutherland, J. and Mulley, G.P. (1997) An uplifting experience? Hospital passenger lifts and their suitability for disabled people, *Disability and Rehabilitation*, 19: 117–19.

Caplan, G., Brown, A., Crowe, P., Yap, S. and Noble, S. (1998) Re-engineering the elective surgical service of a tertiary hospital: a historical controlled trial, *Medical Journal of Australia*, 169(5): 247–51.

Considine, M. (1988) The corporate management framework as administrative science: a critique, *Australian Journal of Public Administration*, 47(1): 4–18.

Daniels, I.R. and Rees, B.I. (1999) Handwashing: simple, but effective, *Annals of the Royal College of Surgeons*, 81(2): 117–18.

Davidhizar, R., Erdel, S. and Dowd, S. (1998) Sexual harassment: where to draw the line, *Nurse Management*, 29(2): 40–4.

Department of Health (1996) *The Children's Charter*. London: Department of Health.

Department of Health (1998) *Working Together: Securing a Quality Workforce for the NHS*. London: Department of Health.

Dilani, A. (2000) Healthcare buildings as supportive environments, *World Hospitals and Health Services*, 36(1): 20–6.

Donaldson Report (2000) *An Organisation with a Memory*. London: Department of Health.

Edwards, J. and Packham, R. (1999) A model for the practical implementation of clinical governance, *Journal of Clinical Excellence*, 1: 13–18.

Fawcett, S.B., White, G.W., Balcazar, F.E. *et al.* (1994) A contextual-behavioral model of empowerment: case studies involving people with physical disabilities, *American Journal of Community Psychology*, 22(4): 471–96.

Fiesta, J. (1997) Labor law update: part 4, *Nurse Management*, 28(9): 12–13.

Forth, J., Lissenburgh, S., Callender, C. and Millward, N. (1997) *Family-friendly Working Arrangements in Britain, 1996*. London: Department for Education and Employment.

Fox, N.J. (1997) Space, sterility and surgery: circuits of hygiene in the operating theatre, *Social Science and Medicine*, 45(5): 649–57.

Francis, S., Glanville, R., Noble, A. and Scher, P. (1999) *50 Years of Ideas in Health Care Buildings*. London: The Nuffield Trust.

Galinsky, E., Friedman, D. and Hernandez, C. (1991) *The Corporate Guide to Work-Family Programs*. New York: The Families and Work Institute.

Gardner, H. and McCoppin, B. (1989) Emerging militancy? The politicisation of Australian allied health professionals, in H. Gardner (ed) *The Politics of Health: The Australian Experience*. Melbourne: Churchill Livingstone.

Glanville, R. (1996) Northern exposure, *Hospital Development*, 27(10): 17–18.

Gray, A. and Jenkins, B. (1993) Markets, managers and the public service: the changing of a culture, in P. Taylor-Gooby and R. Lawson (eds) *Markets and Managers*. Buckingham: Open University Press.

Grindle, M. and Hildebrand, M. (1995) Building sustainable capacity in the public sector: what can be done?, *Public Administration and Development*, 15: 441–63.

Hansen, A. (2000) Organisation and management structures of hospitals and hospital departments, *Hospital*, 2(1): 18–20.

Harrison, S. and Pollitt, C. (1994) *Controlling Health Professionals: The Future of Work and Organization in the NHS*. Buckingham: Open University Press.

Healey, F. (1994) Does flooring type affect risk of injury in older in-patients?, *Nursing Times*, 27(6–12 July): 40–1.

Healy, J. (1998) *Welfare Options: Delivering Social Services*. Sydney: Allen & Unwin.

Hillman, K. (1999) The changing role for acute care hospitals, *Medical Journal of Australia*, 170(7): 325–9.

Hoek, H. (1999) The art of governance of Dutch hospitals, *World Hospitals and Health Services*, 35(3): 5–7.

Hurst, K. (1995) *Progress with Patient Focused Care in the United Kingdom*. Leeds: NHS Executive.

James, P. and Noakes, T. (1994) *Hospital Architecture*. Essex: Longman.

James, W.P. and Tatton-Brown, W. (1986) *Hospitals: Design and Development*. London: Architectural Press.

Johnston, G., Crombie, L.K., Davies, H.T.O., Alder, E.M. and Millard, A. (2000) Reviewing audit: barriers and facilitating factors for effective clinical audit, *Quality in Health Care*, 9: 23–36.

Jones, K.E. and Tamari, I.E. (1997) Making our offices universally accessible: guidelines for physicians, *Canadian Medicine Association Journal*, 156: 647–56.

Kesevan, S. (1999) Handwashing facilities are inadequate, *British Medical Journal*, 319: 518–19.

Larkin, P. (1972) The building, in P. Larkin (ed.) *High Windows*. London: Faber & Faber.

Lawson, B. and Phiri, M. (2000) Room for improvement, *Health Service Journal*, 110 (20 January): 24–6.

Martin, D.P., Diehr, P., Conrad, D.A. *et al.* (1998) Randomized trial of a patient-centred hospital unit, *Patient, Education and Counselling*, 34(2): 125–33.

Martinez, E. (1986) Modular buildings cut costs of adding office space, *Hospitals*, 58(8): 74, 76.

MARU (1996) *Scanning the Spectrum of Healthcare from Hospital to Home in the UK*, in MARU viewpoints seminar programme 1996. London, Medical Architecture Research Unit.

McKee, M. and Black, N. (1993) Junior doctors' work at night: what is done and how much is appropriate, *Journal of Public Health Medicine*, 15: 16–24.

Moore, G. (1997) Improving health access: it's about attitude, *Nursing in British Columbia*, 29(3): 27–30.

Morgan-Jones, R.L., Buckley, S. and Carmichael, I. (1997) An audit of theatre scrubrooms in a district general hospital, *Annals of the Royal College of Surgeons of England*, 79(4): 296–8.

Morrell, C. and Harvey, G. (1999) *The Clinical Audit Handbook: Improving the Quality of Healthcare*. London: Balliére Tindall.

Moss, F. and Garside, P. (1995) Management for doctors: the importance of quality: sharing responsibility for patient care, *British Medical Journal*, 310: 996–9.

NHS Executive (1998) *A First Class Service: Quality in the New NHS*. London: The Stationery Office.

Nightingale, F. (1860/1969) *Notes on Nursing: What It Is and What It Is Not*. New York: Dover.

OECD (1999) *OECD Health Data 99: A Comparative Analysis of 29 Countries*. Paris: Organisation for Economic Co-operation and Development.

Pevsner, N. (1976) *A History of Building Types*. London: Thames & Hudson.

Pierce, L.L. (1998) Barriers to access: frustrations of people who use a wheelchair for full-time mobility, *Rehabilitation and Nursing*, 23(3): 120–5.

Pletinckx, M. (2000) The special nature of children's hospitalisation, *Hospital*, 2(2): 42–3.

Pusey, M. (1991) *Economic Rationalism in Canberra: A Nation Building State Changes its Mind*. Sydney: Cambridge University Press.

Richardson, G., Maynard, A., Cullum, N. and Kindig, D. (1998) Skill mix changes: substitution or service development?, *Health Policy*, 45: 119–32.

Scally, G. and Donaldson, L.J. (1998) Clinical governance and the drive for quality improvement in the new NHS in England, *British Medical Journal*, 317: 61–5.

Scher, P. (1996) *Patient-focused Architecture for Health Care*. Manchester: Manchester Metropolitan University.

Schuschke, G. and Christiansen, H. (1994) Patientenbezogene Farbpräferenz und Farbgestaltung im Krankenhaus, *Zentralblatt für Hygiene und Umweltmedizin*, 195(5–6): 419–31.

Scull, A.T. (1979) *Museums of Madness: The Social Organization of Insanity in Nineteenth-Century England*. London: Allen Lane.

Secretary of State for Health (1997) *The New NHS: Modern, Dependable.* London: The Stationery Office.

Shamian, J. (1998) Quality management: the role of hospital boards, *World Hospitals and Health Services*, 34(2): 4–10.

Shortell, S.M., O'Brien, J.L., Carman, J.M. *et al.* (1995) Assessing the impact of continuous quality improvement/total quality management: concept versus implementation, *Health Services Research*, 30: 377–401.

Shum, C., Humphreys, A., Wheeler, D. *et al.* (2000) Nurse management of patients with minor illnesses in general practice: multicentre, randomised controlled trial, *British Medical Journal*, 320: 1038–43.

Thomas, C. and Curtis, P. (1997) Having a baby: some disabled women's reproductive experiences, *Midwifery*, 13: 202–9.

Ulrich, R.S. (1984) View through a window may influence recovery from surgery, *Science*, 224(4647): 420–1.

UNICEF (1995) *The Progress of Nations 1995.* New York: UNICEF.

UNICEF (1996) *Promise and Progress: Achieving Goals for Children.* New York: UNICEF.

UNICEF (1999) *Breastfeeding: Foundation for a Healthy Future.* New York: UNICEF.

van Bemmel, J. and Musen, M.A. (1997) *Handbook of Medical Informatics.* Heidelberg: Springer-Verlag.

Venning, P., Durie, A., Roland, M., Roberts, C. and Leese, B. (2000) Randomised controlled trial comparing cost effectiveness of general practitioners and nurse practitioners in primary care, *British Medical Journal*, 320: 1048–53.

Versieck, K., Bouten, R. and Pacolet, J. (1995) *Manpower Problems in the Nursing/ Midwifery Profession in the EC.* Leuven: Hoger Instituut voor de Arbeid KU.

Walston, S. and Kimberley, J. (1997) Re-engineering hospitals: experience and analysis from the field, *Hospital and Health Service Administration*, 42: 143–63.

WHO (1986) *Ottawa Charter for Health Promotion*, First International Conference on Health Promotion, Ottawa, Canada, 17–21 November 1986. Copenhagen: WHO Regional Office for Europe.

WHO (1996) *European Health Care Reforms: The Ljubljana Charter on Reforming Health Care, 19 June 1996.* Copenhagen: WHO Regional Office for Europe.

WHO (1997) *The Vienna Recommendations on Health Promoting Hospitals.* Copenhagen: WHO Regional Office for Europe.

Wolcott, I. and Glezer, H. (1995) *Work and Family Life: Achieving Integration.* Melbourne: Australian Institute of Family Studies.

Zimmerman, J.E., Shortell, S.M., Rousseau, D.M. *et al.* (1993) Improving intensive care: observations based on organizational case studies in nine intensive care units: a prospective, multicenter study, *Critical Care Medicine*, 21: 1443–51.

chapter eleven

The changing hospital workforce in Europe

James Buchan and Fiona O'May

Introduction

Health care is a major source of employment, and the hospital represents the most visible concentration of employment in the health sector. This chapter examines trends in employment in the hospital workforce in Europe and reviews the likely impact of significant drivers for change in hospital workforce management.

The health and social care sector employs, on average, one in ten of all employees in the countries of the European Union (Eurostat 1999), and hospital employment accounts for between 2.9 and 5.5 per cent of the working population of the European Union (Verschuren *et al.* 1995). Despite some shift in resource allocation from acute care to primary care, the hospital continues to be the major source of health care employment. For example, hospitals employed more than 50 per cent of the nursing workforce in most European countries in 1997 (WHO 2001).

Health care is also labour-intensive. Even in the relatively capital-intensive acute hospital sector, labour costs normally account for between two-thirds and three-quarters of hospital running costs. The hospital as an organization is sensitive to changes in the external labour market, such as skills shortages and regulation. In turn, the hospital will attempt to change its own internal labour market in response to external pressure by changing staff mix and patterns of deployment.

Two of the main external pressures on hospitals in Europe are cost containment and quality improvement. These pressures arise out of health-sector reform, the transition to market economies in countries in central and eastern Europe and the former Soviet Union (Jackman and Rutkowski 1994) and fiscal constraints in public-sector health systems (Mossialos and Le Grand 1999). In response, performance management mechanisms are being implemented to

Table 11.1 The changing hospital workforce in Europe

Drivers for change	Performance management responses
Cost containment	Decentralization and employment flexibility
Quality improvement	Skill mix and substitution
Shortages of skills	Hospital re-engineering

sustain improvements in productivity while health systems are being decentralized (International Labour Organization and Sectoral Activities Programme 1998).

The third pressure, evident to varying extents for varying groups of employees, relates to shortages of skills and changes in the external labour market. Shortages of skills are stimulating some hospitals to recruit staff from other countries. The Europeanization or globalization of the health labour market is inadequately researched, but greater international mobility of health professionals is likely. Another factor in many industrialized countries is the ageing of the workforce, which has significant implications for working patterns, retirement and replacement of staff and pension provision (OECD 1998). In relation to the management of hospitals and their workforce, these pressures manifest themselves directly and indirectly in a number of ways, as summarized in Table 11.1.

The three main aspects of change in the hospital workforce – employment flexibility, skill mix and substitution and hospital reorganization or re-engineering – are linked and are examined in the following sections.

Decentralization and employment flexibility

Devolving managerial responsibility within hospitals is claimed to allow managers to be more flexible in determining priorities and achieving strategic objectives. Decentralization and greater flexibility in deploying staff are also cited as major elements of health-sector reform. This reflects an increased managerial emphasis on controlling labour costs and meeting targets of productivity and quality by introducing performance management mechanisms (Schut 1995; Hunter 1996; International Labour Organization and Sectoral Activities Programme 1998).

Flexible employment practices are also identified as a key element of a more effective recruitment and retention strategy. This is especially important given increases in the labour force participation rates of women in most countries (Figure 11.1). Family-friendly working practices enable a balance to be achieved between workplace and domestic commitments (Versieck et al. 1995). One major challenge facing most European countries arises from the growth in the proportion of females in the health care workforce (Figure 11.2). Medicine, traditionally a male-dominated profession, will have to adjust its culture and working practices to accommodate the growing number of women physicians.

Medical and nursing staff are the largest cost element in the health care workforce, and these staff are the most involved in 24-hour delivery of patient

Figure 11.1 Proportion of women in the total labour force in 12 western European countries: 1980 (□) and 1997 (■)

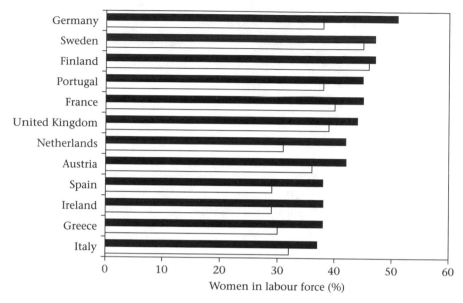

Source: OECD (2000)

Figure 11.2 Female physicians as a percentage of all practising physicians in eight western European countries: 1980 (□) and 1997* or 1998** (■)

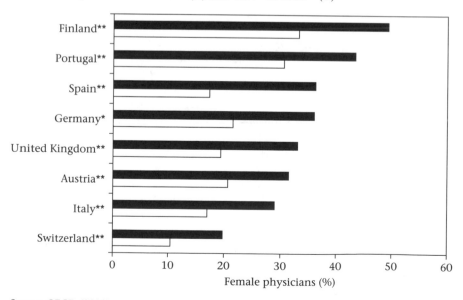

Source: OECD (2000)

care. Some management commentators, therefore, have identified greater flexibility in their deployment as a key requirement in containing costs (Buchan 1998; International Labour Organization and Sectoral Activities Programme 1998). Employment flexibility can cover a number of different aspects (Armstrong 1992):

- contract-based flexibility, such as short-term contracts;
- time-based flexibility, such as altering shift patterns;
- job-based flexibility;
- skills-based flexibility, such as multiskilling;
- organizationally based flexibility, such as contracting out; and
- pay-based flexibility, such as the introduction of performance-related pay (Maisonneuve and Menard 1997; Adinolfi 1998).

Two aspects especially relevant to hospital employment are numerical flexibility and functional flexibility. Numerical flexibility reflects the scope for management to adjust the number of workers to fluctuations in demand; functional flexibility relates to the ease with which the tasks performed by workers can be adjusted to meet changes in the nature of that demand (Atkinson and Meager 1986).

Applying this model of a flexible firm, the core group of permanent employees is supplemented by one or more groups of peripheral workers, who may or may not be employees. The flexible firm deploys these peripheral groups as required to match fluctuations in demand and to achieve numerical flexibility. Peripheral staff may be employed on a casual basis or on short-term contracts or be supplied by an external agency.

The model of the flexible firm, which distinguishes between core and periphery employees, has been influential in shaping assessments of trends in labour flexibility during labour-market restructuring and health-sector reform. It is closely related to the new public management approach to reforming public sectors (Hunter 1996; International Labour Organization and Sectoral Activities Programme 1998). There has been debate about the extent to which the flexible firm is an explanatory model or a management blueprint for change (Pollert 1987) and whether it presents a coherent and strategically focused overview of changing working patterns that are generally fragmented, reactive and uncoordinated in reality.

A second area of debate is employee relations. Does flexibility serve as a blueprint for the casualization of the workforce and for the marginalization or de-recognition of trade unions? Can achieving greater flexibility in working patterns be a win–win outcome of negotiations between employer and employees, or is flexibility a form of organizational change imposed by management as a means of cutting costs and reducing job security?

Employment flexibility in many European labour markets is also significantly constrained by labour market regulations: the Working Time Directive of the European Union (Council of the European Union 1993); the regulation of health professionals; and the rigidity of some national-level pay systems (Fattore 1999). Another constraint is the capacity of management and management systems to facilitate greater flexibility. Although attempts have been made to introduce new styles of management, often following the principles of the

Table 11.2 Trends in the management of the hospital workforce

From:	To:
Oriented towards staff welfare	Oriented towards business
Generalist service	Specialist function
Training	Appraisal and development
Collective relations with staff	Individualized relations
Negotiation	Consultation and communication

Source: Adapted from Buchan and Seccombe (1994)

new public management, and to import private-sector business practices (see Table 11.2), many public-sector health systems remain relatively centralized with limited scope for employment flexibility at the level of the hospital.

Skill mix and skill substitution

Determining the most effective mix of personnel is a major challenge for hospital management. Health care is labour-intensive and, in most hospitals, health system labour costs account for between two-thirds and three-quarters of total operating costs.

Many hospitals in Europe and elsewhere are coming under increasing scrutiny for cost containment and quality improvement, often as a direct or indirect result of health-sector reform. In such circumstances, the level and mix of staff deployed to deliver health care is a central element in the cost of care and a major determinant of the quality of care.

Different countries and health systems report different mixes and levels of staffing. In particular, the mix between physicians and nurses varies markedly, and there is little evidence that this mix has changed significantly over the last 15 years (Figure 11.3). Although there may be general trends in the changing utilization of hospital personnel, there is no common starting point; this limits the potential for transferring the lessons of research on skill mix and highlights the need for more comparison.

Achieving the right personnel is an important strategy for hospitals for several reasons:

- as a guide to management in responding to shortages of skills (Versieck *et al.* 1995; Buchan *et al.* 2000);
- improving the management of labour costs (to reduce costs per unit of output or improve productivity);
- sustaining quality improvements while reducing unit costs;
- as an organizational response to technological innovation; and
- as an organizational response to regulation or legislation on health professionals (Healy and McKee 1997; Irvine 1999).

Altering the personnel mix in a hospital is not the only potential solution to these challenges. Hospital management may also review other options, including improving the utilization of hospital beds, capital equipment and

Figure 11.3 Ratio of certified or registered nurses to all practising physicians in nine western European countries: 1980 (□) and 1997* or 1998** (■). The 1980 data for Germany are for the Federal Republic of Germany.

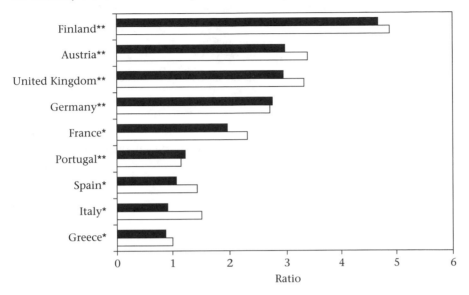

Source: OECD (2000)

other resources; improving staffing patterns in relation to day-to-day fluctuations in workload and patient dependence (see flexibility); and reviewing and altering resource allocation and distribution, for example between tertiary, secondary and primary care.

The two main areas with evidence-based research on hospital staff skill mix and skill substitution are the qualified versus unqualified mix in nursing and the overlap and substitution between physicians and nurses.

Nursing skill mix

Hospitals depend primarily on qualified and unqualified nursing staff to deliver care. Cost-containment strategies have resulted in substitution of less expensive care assistants or aides for more expensive nurses in many countries (Schut 1995; Versieck *et al.* 1995; Buchan *et al.* 1997). However, comparatively few published research studies have examined the implications of this trend for cost and quality and, setting aside methodological and comparability issues, there is no unanimity in results or conclusions. Most studies tend to be single-site before-and-after examinations of the effects of introducing or increasing the use of care assistants.

Drawing on other work (Gardner 1991; Krapohl and Larson 1996; Buchan *et al.* 2000), a typology of approaches to the qualified/unqualified mix in nursing has been developed (see Box 11.1). The typology represents different options

---

Box 11.1 Approaches to skill mix and substitution in nursing

Traditional. Aides, assistants and auxiliaries, mainly trained on the job, performing simple nursing tasks in support of registered nurses

Non-clinical assistant. Clerk or aides role, mainly in non-clinical clerical or house-keeping work (or as a multiskilled support worker)

Technician or nurse technician. Technical assistant or operating department assistant role for complex technological processes, assisting nurses

Primary nursing partner. Nursing assistant paired with nurse to maintain delivery of care by primary nursing

Vocationally trained or qualified care-giver. An addition to the traditional nurses' aide. Training of several weeks or months, in some countries leading to a vocational qualification. Care-giver undertakes nursing care responsibilities under direction of registered nurse

Source: Adapted from Buchan *et al.* (2000)

---

that may be open to hospital management considering skill-mix changes. The key question is whether the aide, support worker or extender is used to supplement, complement or replace or substitute for the work of a qualified nurse.

Buchan *et al.* (2000) suggested that, with the exception of studies conducted in the United States, there is little published evaluation of the costs and benefits of these different approaches to the skill mix of nursing staff. Even in the United States, the findings are not unanimous. Some studies report mainly positive results from skill substitution with identified cost savings (Hesterly and Robinson 1990; Bostrom and Zimmerman 1993). Other studies are more equivocal and highlight problem areas relating to lower quality of care and higher levels of staff absence or turnover (Powers *et al.* 1990; Garfink *et al.* 1991) One study conducted in the United Kingdom (Carr-Hill *et al.* 1995) concluded that investing in additional training and the use of a 'richer' (and more expensive) staff mix in nursing can improve the quality of care.

The United States differs from Europe in staffing patterns, roles and mixes, a much lower level of trade union activity and differences in organizational culture. These factors limit the scope for transferring the lessons to Europe. This does not inherently argue against further developments in skill mix in nursing, but it does highlight the need for further research in a European context to enable informed decisions.

Overlap and substitution between physicians and nurses

The second major focus of published evaluation has been on the scope for extending the role of nursing and midwifery staff, through clinical nurse specialists, nurse practitioners, clinical nurse midwives and nurse anaesthetists.

Several studies and meta-analyses have examined skill substitution and care delivery by nursing and midwifery staff rather than physicians. This is the only area of skill-mix evaluation that has used randomized controlled trials to assess quality and outcome, and the main meta-analysis studies are from North America (for example, Brown and Grimes 1995).

In some areas of health delivery, there is clear evidence (mainly but not exclusively from the United States) of scope for developing advanced nursing and midwifery roles, while maintaining or reducing costs and maintaining or improving care outcomes. One claim is that 25–70 per cent of physicians' work, depending on the task, could be undertaken by nurses or other professionals (Richardson *et al.* 1998).

In comparative cost evaluations, relying on wages as the cost indicator makes the evaluation highly sensitive to wage differentials between groups of personnel. These differentials can vary markedly between hospitals, health care systems and countries and over time. If a wage ratio between a physician and a nurse is 5 : 1, the potential cost savings of substitution will be much greater than in a system where the wage ratio is 2 : 1.

The extent of scope for substitution or development of alternative models of care delivery in a specific hospital system also has to take account of potential constraints on change, relating to legislation, professional regulation and associated organizational factors.

Hospital reorganization and re-engineering

One aspect of organizational change in hospitals that significantly affects the workforce is hospital merger. Mergers do not always result in improvements (Alexander *et al.* 1996). One issue often underestimated is the transition costs of consolidating separate groups of employees, often with different working practices and different organizational cultures, into a cohesive workforce. Debate is also continuing about the associated impact on job satisfaction and commitment of health care staff during restructuring and merger (Swedish Association of Health Officers 1994; McKee *et al.* 1998; Nolan *et al.* 1999).

The term 'hospital re-engineering' was coined during the restructuring of health care delivery in the United States in the 1980s (see also Chapter 14). The patient-focused hospital concept represents an attempt to redesign or re-engineer the care delivery process. The application of these principles is said to improve quality, increase patient satisfaction, increase job satisfaction for staff and improve efficiency (Booz-Allen and Hamilton 1988; Andersen Consulting 1992). Other commentators (Walston and Kimberley 1997), however, question the scope and magnitude of these claims. Hospital re-engineering is now evident in many European countries, including England (Hurst 1995), the Netherlands (Bainton 1995), Spain (Coulson-Thomas 1996) and Sweden (Brodersen and Thorwid 1997).

In the 1980s, hospitals in the United States were facing increased competition while having to contain costs and cope with more rigorous funding regimes. Some hired management consultants with experience of re-engineering in the manufacturing and electronics industries (Hammer and Champy 1993) and

---

Box 11.2 Main elements of patient-focused care/hospital re-engineering

Clinical protocols, pathways and anticipated recovery paths
Integrated patient records and individual care plans
Patient grouping
Multidisciplinary teams
Multiskilling and cross-training
Decentralized and localized support services

---

commissioned them to re-engineer the hospital as an organization. These consultants identified factors that they claimed contributed to organizational inefficiency in the conventional hospital, including the following:

- excessive steps in routine procedures such as laboratory tests and X-rays;
- a high proportion of the time of direct care staff spent on activities other than direct care;
- excessive centralization of capital-intensive resources in a labour-intensive organization;
- excessive specialization of staff and inefficiencies in staff use resulting from narrow functional areas and professional demarcations;
- a high rate of delay and cancellation in clinical procedures as a result of poor communication between departments and disciplines; and
- excessive management hierarchy and centralized decision-making with management remote from the point of care.

This diagnostic work by management consultants identified claimed inefficiencies and unnecessary complexities in hospital organizations. The term 'patient-focused' reflected the central tenet of the proposed changes: that the structure and processes involved in delivering hospital care should be shaped by the needs of the patients (see Box 11.2). The main implications for the management of the hospital workforce are discussed below.

Principles of patient-focused care and re-engineering

Clinical protocols
Also termed care pathways, or anticipated recovery paths, the clinical protocols for the treatment of specific conditions are developed by a multidisciplinary team that establishes what should be done and how and when it should be done, to achieve the most consistent outcome. The objectives are to develop protocols that underpin the use of an individual care plan for each patient and to support multidisciplinary teamwork.

Integrated patient records
The aims are to develop a single integrated patient record to replace the multiplicity of separate records (often in different formats) held by different departments and disciplines involved in treating the patient. Time spent in

cross-referencing and duplication by staff is reduced. The use of a unitary patient record linked to care protocols also allows exceptions to be reported; that is, the recording of any unanticipated responses to clinical intervention.

Patient grouping or patient aggregation
Patients are aggregated in accordance with care requirements; those with similar service demands as determined by protocols are grouped together. These groups may differ from the traditional specialty-based categorization of patients, since the objectives are to achieve greater homogeneity in terms of patient service requirements, to maximize the use of staff skills and to improve operational efficiency. Patient groupings may be numerically larger than found in conventional hospital wards.

Multidisciplinary care teams
Patient-focused care requires the blurring of perceived traditional boundaries between health care professions. Cooperation and collaboration are required to facilitate the development of clinical and unitary patient records, to reduce the number of staff contacts per patient and to reduce non-productive time.

Multiskilling and cross-training
Maximizing the self-sufficiency and efficiency of care teams in a devolved organizational structure requires redesigning the roles of team members. Significant investment in cross-training and multiskilling is required to introduce patient-focused care. Some research also suggests that this area offers the greatest opportunity for improving the cost–benefit ratio.

Decentralization
Numerous services traditionally centralized in conventional hospitals have been identified as being suitable for decentralization in patient-focused care. These include X-ray, pharmacy, laboratory tests and clerical and administrative support.

Design and redesign of the physical environment
A knock-on effect of implementing patient-focused care is that the physical environment of the hospital may need to be reconstructed or redesigned to support patient aggregation and decentralized services. Principles of patient-focused care may also inform the design phase of a newly built hospital. Claims as to the likely impact of building a new hospital according to these principles include the argument that a re-engineered hospital would require less space overall and less specialized space, leading to a more compact design. This should result in capital cost reduction compared with a conventional hospital and lower operating costs.

Evaluating hospital re-engineering

The main claimed benefits of the hospital re-engineering approach are improved quality and productivity, better management and improved patient and staff satisfaction. There is still little independent evaluation to support or refute these claims, especially in Europe.

Two evaluations of early experiences with patient-focused care in the United Kingdom have been published. One report (NHS Estates 1993) doubted that the scale of improvements claimed for patient-focused care in the United States would be replicable in the United Kingdom, because staffing levels and mix differ and because assumptions about the benefits of decentralization may not be realizable in practice. A second report (Hurst 1995) broadly supported further developments in patient-focused hospitals but concluded that the data are insufficient to support analysis of cost-effectiveness. Since the mid-1990s, the pace of implementation of hospital re-engineering in the United Kingdom has not increased, with the exception of newly built hospitals. This has resulted from a combination of changed political priorities and the high implementation costs of applying re-engineering concepts.

In relation to newly built hospitals, the results are also mixed, partly because there is no standard model of hospital configuration on which costing estimates can be based and because different results will arise depending on the allocation of costs (Rawlinson *et al.* 1993). Reports on new patient-focused hospitals, however, highlight the positive aspects of patient-friendly and staff-friendly design (Glanville 1998). The various elements of hospital re-engineering do not represent a detailed blueprint for change. In practice, many re-engineered hospitals, both in the United States and Europe, have concentrated only on some elements of the approach, such as care protocols.

Practices in managing staff differ between hospitals in the United States and Europe in at least three significant ways that influence the implementation of hospital re-engineering. First, hospital staff in many European countries are heavily unionized, whereas their United States counterparts recognize neither trade unions nor professional organizations. This may limit the scope for radical changes in staffing levels, roles and mixes. Second, hospitals in some European countries have less scope to develop their own reward strategies, which limits the opportunities to use a reward strategy as a lever for change. Third, many European hospitals operate with significantly lower staffing levels than similar hospitals in the United States. As much of the reduction in costs claimed from re-engineering hospitals in the United States relates to the reduction of labour costs by altering skill mix and staffing levels, there may be less potential for change and associated savings in typical European hospitals.

Conclusion

This chapter has examined some key drivers for change in the hospital workforce in Europe and has identified some potential and actual constraints on changes. Table 11.3 summarizes the main issues.

Constraints on change relate in part to limitations in the management capacity of hospitals to initiate significant changes, partly as a result of the limited evidence base. Other external contextual factors include legislative and regulatory constraints on changing the roles of health professionals, opposition from trade unions and professional associations concerned about job security and career opportunities, and more broadly based constraints relating to labour market dynamics and regulation. One demographic and labour-force

Table 11.3 The changing hospital workforce in Europe

Drivers for change	Change	Constraints on change
Cost containment	Decentralization and employment flexibility	Labour market or demographic change
Quality improvement	Skill mix and substitution	Management capacity deficits Training system capacity
Shortages of skills	Hospital reorganization or re-engineering	Regulation of health professionals Opposition by professional association or trade union

factor in many European countries will be the ageing of the hospital workforce, paralleling an ageing of the population. This will have implications for mobility and training of staff and retirement age and pension provision.

Major changes are affecting the hospital workforce in Europe through the three linked features of decentralization and employment flexibility, skill mix and skill substitution, and hospital reorganization. However, the evidence base that could support the direction of change or enable change to be evaluated is weak and fragmented. Change is being driven by organizational and fiscal necessity at a pace that is outstripping the capacity to evaluate its real impact on the hospital workforce.

References

Adinolfi, P. (1998) Performance related pay for health service professionals: the Italian experience, *Health Service Management Research*, 11: 211–20.

Alexander, J.A., Halpern, M.T. and Lee, S.Y. (1996) The short term effects of merger on hospital operations, *Health Services Research*, 30(6): 827–47.

Andersen Consulting (1992) *Patient Centred Care: Reinventing the Hospital*. London: Andersen Consulting.

Armstrong, M. (1992) *Human Resource Management: Strategy on Action*. London: Kogan Page.

Atkinson, J. and Meager, N. (1986) *New Forms of Work Organisation*. Brighton: Institute of Manpower.

Bainton, D. (1995) Building blocks, *Health Service Journal*, 105(23 March): 25–7.

Booz-Allen and Hamilton (1988) *Operational Restructuring: A Recipe for Success*. London: Booz-Allen and Hamilton.

Bostrom, J. and Zimmerman, J. (1993) Restructuring nursing for a competitive health care environment, *Nursing Economics*, 11(1): 35–41, 54.

Brodersen, J. and Thorwid, J. (1997) Enabling sustainable change for healthcare in Stockholm, *British Journal of Healthcare Computing and Information Management*, 14(4): 23–6.

Brown, S. and Grimes, D. (1995) A meta-analysis of nurse practitioners and nurse midwives in primary care, *Nursing Research*, 44(6): 332–9.

Buchan, J. (1998) Further flexing: issues of employment contract flexibility in the UK nursing workforce, *Health Services Management Research*, 11: 148–62.

Buchan, J. and Seccombe, I. (1994) The changing role of the NHS personnel function, in J. Le Grand and R. Robinson (eds) *Evaluating the NHS Reforms*. London: King's Fund.

Buchan, J., Hancock, C. and Rafferty, A. (1997) Health sector reform and trends in the United Kingdom hospital workforce, *Medical Care*, 35(10): OS143–9.

Buchan, J., Ball, J. and O'May, F. (2000) *Determining Skill Mix in the Health Care Workforce: Guidelines for Managers and Health Professionals*. Issues in Health Services Delivery, Discussion Paper No. 3, document WHO/EIP/OSD/00.11. Geneva: World Health Organization.

Carr-Hill, R.A., Dixon, P., Griffiths, M. *et al.* (1995) The impact of nursing grade on the quality and outcome of nursing care, *Health Economics*, 4(1): 57–72.

Council of the European Union (1993) Council Directive 93/104/EC of 23 November 1993 concerning certain aspects of the organization of working time, *Official Journal of the European Communities*, L 307(13/12/1993): 18–24.

Coulson-Thomas, C. (1996) Re-engineering hospitals and health care processes, *British Journal of Health Care Management*, 2(6): 338–42.

Eurostat (1999) *European Labour Force Survey*. Luxembourg: Statistical Office of the European Communities.

Fattore, G. (1999) Cost containment and reforms in the Italian National Health Service, in E. Mossialos and J. Le Grand (eds) *Health Care and Cost Containment in the European Union*. Aldershot: Ashgate.

Gardner, D. (1991) Issues related to the use of nurse extenders, *Journal of Nursing Administration*, 21(10): 40–5.

Garfink, C., Kirby, K., Bachman, S. and Starck, P. (1991) University hospital nurse extender model III: program evaluation, *Journal of Nursing Administration*, 21(3): 21–7.

Glanville, R. (1998) Architecture and design, in K. Schutyser and B. Edwards (eds) *Hospital Healthcare Europe 1998–1999, the Official HOPE Reference Book*. London: Campden Publishing.

Hammer, M. and Champy, J. (1993) *Reengineering the Corporation: A Manifesto for Business Revolution*. New York: Harper Business.

Healy, J. and McKee, M. (1997) Health sector reform in central and eastern Europe: the professional dimension, *Health Policy and Planning*, 12(4): 286–95.

Hesterly, S. and Robinson, M. (1990) Alternative caregivers: cost effective utilisation of RNs, *Nursing Administration Quarterly*, 14(3): 45–57.

Hunter, D. (1996) The changing roles of health care personnel in health and health care management, *Social Science and Medicine*, 43(5): 799–808.

Hurst, K. (1995) *Progress with Patient Focused Care in the United Kingdom*. Leeds: NHS Executive.

International Labour Organization and Sectoral Activities Programme (1998) *Terms of Employment and Working Conditions in Health Sector Reforms*. Geneva: International Labour Office.

Irvine, D. (1999) The performance of doctors: the new professionalism, *Lancet*, 353: 1174–7.

Jackman, R. and Rutkowski, M. (1994) Labour markets, wages and employment, in N. Barr (ed.) *Labour Markets and Social Policy in Central and Eastern Europe*. Oxford: Oxford University Press.

Krapohl, G. and Larson, E. (1996) The impact of unlicensed assistive personnel on nursing care delivery, *Nursing Economics*, 14(2): 99–112.

Maisonneuve, H. and Menard, J. (1997) The Juppé plan, *Lancet*, 349: 792–3.

McKee, M., Aiken, L., Rafferty, A.M. and Sochalski, J. (1998) Organizational change and quality of health care: an evolving international agenda, *Quality in Health Care*, 7(1): 37–41.

Mossialos, E. and Le Grand, J. (eds) (1999) *Health Care and Cost Containment in the European Union*. Aldershot: Ashgate.

NHS Estates (1993) *Health Facilities Notes: Design for Patient Focused Care*. London: HMSO.

Nolan, M., Lundt, U. and Brown, J. (1999) Changing aspects of nurses' work environment: a comparison of perceptions in two hospitals in Sweden and the UK and implications for recruitment and retention of staff, *Nursing Times Research*, 4(3): 221–33.

OECD (1998) *Employment Outlook, June 1998*. Paris: Organisation for Economic Co-operation and Development.

OECD (2000) *OECD Health Data 2000: A Comparative Analysis of 29 Countries*. Paris: Organisation for Economic Co-operation and Development.

Pollert, A. (1987) *The Flexible Firm: A Model in Search of Reality or a Policy in Search of Practice?* Coventry: Industrial Relations Research Unit, University of Warwick.

Powers, P., Dickey, C. and Ford, A. (1990) Evaluating an RN/co-worker model, *Journal of Nursing Administration*, 20(3): 11–15.

Rawlinson, C., Kelly, J. and Whittlestone, P. (1993) *Patient Focused Care: A Suitable Case for Treatment*. London: RKW.

Richardson, G., Maynard, A., Cullum, N. and Kindig, D. (1998) Skill mix changes: substitution or service development?, *Health Policy*, 45: 119–32.

Schut, F. (1995) Health care reform in the Netherlands: balancing corporatism, etatism and market mechanisms, *Journal of Health Politics, Policy and Law*, 20(3): 615–52.

Swedish Association of Health Officers (1994) *How are You Nurse? A Research Report on the Psychosocial Working Environment of Nurses*. Stockholm: Swedish Association of Health Officers.

Verschuren, R., de Groot, B. and Nossent, S. (1995) *Working Conditions in Hospitals in the European Union*. Dublin: European Foundation for the Improvement of Living and Working Conditions.

Versieck, K., Bouten, R. and Pacolet, J. (1995) *Manpower Problems in the Nursing/Midwifery Profession in the EC*. Leuven: Hoger Instituut voor de Arbeid KU.

Walston, S. and Kimberley, J. (1997) Re-engineering hospitals: experience and analysis from the field, *Hospital and Health Service Administration*, 42: 143–63.

WHO (2001) *WHO European Health for All Database*. Copenhagen: WHO Regional Office for Europe.

twelve

Introducing new technologies

Rebecca Rosen

Introduction

The locations in which health care is provided are constantly changing. Developments in medical technology allow selected services, previously provided only in hospitals, to be offered in community clinics, mobile health units and in patients' own homes. Despite this, hospitals still house the majority of high-cost equipment, as well as complex services such as intensive care, organ transplantation and oncology services. This chapter uses case studies from the National Health Service (NHS) in England to examine the role of hospitals in relation to adopting technology, and to study the extent to which adopting technology is linked to evidence of clinical and cost-effectiveness. It considers what might be an appropriate role for hospitals, when multiple new technologies are emerging but health care resources are scarce. This chapter adopts a utilitarian perspective, in which maximizing the health benefits obtained from scarce resources is considered a desirable policy objective. The argument is that decision-making on new technologies should be informed by high-quality research evidence on clinical and cost-effectiveness.

The chapter starts by reviewing the main groups of emerging technologies that may alter the role of hospitals in the future. The case studies are then presented and implications for the role of the hospital are discussed. Questions are raised about the extent to which hospitals should aim to maximize the clinical and cost-effectiveness of the services they offer and the mechanisms they might use to do this.

The US Office of Technology Assessment (1976) broadly defined medical technologies as 'all the drugs, devices and medical and surgical procedures and the organizational and support systems used to provide them'. The problem is to decide what is meant by 'new' in relation to medical technologies: entirely new products or techniques (such as the anti-impotence drug sildenafil citrate (Viagra®)), new applications for well-established techniques (such as using bone marrow transplants for solid tumours) and techniques well established in teaching hospitals that suddenly diffuse more widely (such as diffusing magnetic resonance imaging scanners to general hospitals and clinics). This chapter concentrates on medical technologies from the point they are first used on patients, through the early stages of diffusion into general hospitals.

Emerging technologies and effects on hospitals

Any review of the main groups of emerging medical technologies and their potential effect on the role of the hospital is necessarily speculative, because little research exists on the effect of different types of new medical technology on local health systems.

New health technologies

Major technological advances have been made over the last decade in screening, diagnosis, treatment and palliation through developments in drugs, tests, equipment and surgical techniques. Further advances have been seen in hospital and community support systems, allowing organizational innovations that change how hospitals are used. Emerging technologies can be clustered into broad groups, each of which affects health services differently. The most important of these are as follows.

- *Screening technologies.* Blood or tissue testing (for cystic fibrosis carriers) and image-based screening technologies (ultrasound testing for aortic aneurysms) are applied to populations of well people.
  Testing technologies near the patient. Micro-assay test kits offer on-the-spot screening and diagnosis (for example, cholesterol tests and pregnancy tests).
  Drug delivery technologies. New types of drugs using immunological, pharmacological and biochemical technologies are designed to affect only specifically targeted cells and tissues. In addition, drug delivery equipment such as electronically controlled syringe drivers, trans-dermal delivery systems and implantable drugs allow slow release over longer periods.
- *Drug technologies.* Multiple new drugs, such as ulcer-healing drugs, have replaced the need for hospital-based intervention; others offer treatments supplementary to primary therapy and appear to improve survival (for example, tamoxifen in breast cancer), while others, such as new immunosuppressive drugs for organ transplantation, allow treatment of previously untreatable patients.
- *Gene therapies.* Artificial introduction of genetic material may replace deleted or defective genes. Therapy for cystic fibrosis illustrates the potential for this treatment modality, although progress is being slowed by the hunt for effective delivery systems.
- *Laparoscopic and minimal-access surgical techniques.* These techniques generally result in shorter admissions, more rapid recovery and reduced thresholds for intervention, with consequent increases in numbers treated.

- *Organ transplant technologies.* These use immunological techniques to reduce the rejection of human organs and, increasingly, of animal organs.
- *Imaging technologies and interventional radiology.* Digitized imaging allows image transfer between different clinical centres and increases the use of real-time imaging (ultrasound and angiographic techniques) by interventional radiologists for biopsy and minimal-access treatments such as vascular stenting.
- *Telemedicine links.* Emerging telemedicine services include real-time clinical consultations between distant patients and a central clinician, and data and image transfer between community and hospital settings that allows general practitioners to manage selected patients under the supervision of hospital consultants and allows secondary and tertiary hospitals rapid access to expert advice.
- *Professional role and organizational developments.* Additional specialist training for nurses and other professions allied to medicine (for example, optometrists and physiotherapists) permits assessment and management of selected chronic conditions (for example, asthma, diabetes and glaucoma) in newly established community clinics.

New technologies and the hospital

The clinical roles of the hospital can be classified as screening, diagnosis, treatment, surveillance of chronic conditions and palliation. New screening technologies are emerging for a wide range of genetic conditions, for a range of tumour markers and for other diseases. Many screening tests are conducted on blood or other easily available tissue samples, and acute hospital facilities are not required for specimen collection or for the ensuing patient and/or family counselling. Mobile units can now provide many image-based screening technologies, such as mammography or ultrasound screening for aneurysms. However, the new cases identified through screening may increase the workload of the hospital if the diseases identified require immediate treatment or if the identified genetic traits or disease markers necessitate regular hospital-based surveillance for early detection of overt disease.

The impact of new diagnostic and treatment technologies on acute hospitals also is hard to predict. Minimal-access surgical procedures are replacing selected open surgical interventions, and some simple procedures such as endoscopy and colonoscopy may be provided in clinics away from acute hospitals. Hollingsworth and Barker (1999) describe new forms of tissue-specific gene therapy and new drugs targeted at specific cell receptor sites that could be used to treat cancer and vascular diseases, thus reducing the need for acute hospital-based surgical treatments. Gage (1998) describes emerging forms of cell and tissue therapy in which the implantation of artificially cultured cells and tissues may replace other forms of surgical repair of damaged tissue.

Although these technological developments suggest a reduced role for acute hospitals, other developments in costly equipment may require the sort of complex services typically associated with hospitals. Schwartz (1994) identified a range of imaging technologies for diagnosis and treatment likely to be concentrated in acute hospitals. For example, the rapidly growing specialty of interventional radiology, with its high-technology imaging equipment, is enabling the development of minimal-access techniques, such as tissue embolization, stenting and catheter insertion, which are substituting for open surgery. Harrison and Prentice (1996) point out that forthcoming technologies such as artificial organs also are likely to continue the historical concentration of complex equipment and procedures in hospital settings. On balance, these changes may result in a different rather than a reduced role for acute hospitals.

Advances in telemedicine, patient data transfer and information technology have made community-based surveillance of chronic diseases easier. Until recently, patients with chronic diseases (for example, diabetes or arthritis) or those on toxic drugs (for example, for autoimmune disorders) were monitored in hospital outpatient clinics. However, rapid computerized transfer of results directly to community clinics allows surveillance by primary care clinicians working according to strict protocols, with access to advice from hospital specialists when needed. Combined with developments in nurse training and innovations in service organization, this has resulted in a range of nurse-led primary care clinics that reduce the use of hospital outpatient facilities. This may suggest a reducing role for the hospital, but questions arise about whether additional surveillance work by primary care clinicians might result in more referrals to hospital for illness that clinicians do not have time to investigate and treat.

Finally, in relation to palliative care, advances in nurse and paramedic training, drug delivery systems, service organization and communication and information technologies have resulted in a range of community-based services for patients with terminal illnesses. Although this could reduce the role of the acute hospital in relation to terminal illness, there are strong cultural influences that may limit their use, such as technological developments in clinics and homes.

The effect of new technologies on hospital services

How do new technologies affect hospital services? This question can only be given brief consideration here to illustrate the dynamic nature of technological development, the ripple-effect on hospital and community services and the difficulty of predicting the financial impact of new technologies. Box 12.1 outlines the varied technological developments that have changed the management of peptic ulcers over the last 10–15 years.

The effects of this string of medical technological developments can be considered from several perspectives. From the hospital viewpoint, a complex surgical procedure, usually reserved for patients with severe symptoms, has largely been replaced by minimally invasive diagnostic endoscopy conducted on many patients in day-case centres. However, drug treatment for peptic ulcers is often long term, requiring repeated input from general practitioners with re-referrals to endoscopy clinics and hospital specialists for some patients.

From a financial point of view, the change from occasional complex surgery to frequent endoscopic diagnosis has required hospitals to invest in endoscopy

---

Box 12.1   Technological developments in the management of peptic ulceration

1970s and early 1980s: Open surgery to bowel and/or associated nerve supply was the main treatment.

Mid-1980s: Widespread use of new H_2 antagonist drugs to diminish acid secretion dramatically reduced surgical treatment and increased management by general practitioners.

Mid-1980s: Rapid developments in endoscopy, short-acting anaesthetics and muscle relaxants precipitated a switch of diagnostic technique from X-ray (barium swallow) to gastroscopy or duodenoscopy. Hospitals allowed direct referral for endoscopy by general practitioners without specialist referral, thus increasing numbers of patients and the use of hospital day-case facilities.

Late 1980s and early 1990s: *Helicobacter pylori* was recognized as a common cause of peptic ulceration. Blood tests were developed to identify the organism and the recommended antibiotic therapy, avoiding the need for hospital services in some patients and improving the treatment of those diagnosed through endoscopy.

Mid- to late 1990s: Increasing use of long-term proton-pump inhibitor drugs to control residual symptoms after initial treatment.

---

suites and to train specialist staff. Furthermore, the diagnosis and post-treatment assessment of peptic ulcer disease creates considerable work for pathology services. In addition, the technological developments incur extra costs for general practitioners, whose workload has increased through their greater involvement in diagnosis, eradication therapy and ongoing symptom control. Murphy (1998) has compared the costs of treating peptic ulcer disease using different approaches to diagnosis, treatment and follow-up, concluding that overall costs have increased with the advent of drug treatment. Although comparing the costs of historical and contemporary treatments presents methodological problems and Murphy's study did not apportion costs to hospital and community services, it highlights the difficulties of assessing the financial impact of new technologies on hospitals. Overall, the case of peptic ulcer disease demonstrates how a cluster of technological developments alters the use of hospital and community health services over time. It also highlights how intervention thresholds change when a new technology simplifies diagnosis and treatment, reducing the cost of treating individual patients but, in the absence of narrow patient selection criteria, increasing the number of patients treated and thus overall spending.

The role of the hospital in decision-making

The rapid diffusion of new technologies has long been blamed for increasing health care costs (Altman 1979; Wordsworth *et al.* 1996). A key concern is that widespread diffusion occurs before any evidence of clinical and cost-effectiveness. Studies of technology diffusion across Europe have highlighted the wide range of factors that drive technology diffusion, including clinician enthusiasm, media and public demand, hospital strategy for enhancing reputation and attracting good staff and inducements from manufacturers (Bos 1991; Kirchberger *et al.* 1991). National policies on health care funding and organization were also noted to influence diffusion. For example, countries with global health care hospital budgets had slower technology diffusion, whereas big-ticket technologies diffused more rapidly in countries with large private hospitals.

Research into the effectiveness of new technologies, also known as health technology assessment, ranges from descriptive studies of a small number of patients to large well-designed randomized trials or cohort studies comparing the effects of new and established interventions. It is widely accepted that small, uncontrolled studies are susceptible to bias and may produce misleading results, whereas well-designed randomized trials produce reliable and valid results. Thus, decisions to adopt technology should ideally be based on the results of clinical trials with an associated economic evaluation.

In the case of the United Kingdom, the structure of the health care system could be expected to influence the adoption of technology by hospitals. In the 1990s, the National Health Service was organized into an internal market (also known as a quasi-market and the purchaser–provider split) where hospitals and community health services were provided on the basis of contracts with purchasers (health authorities or groups of fundholding general practitioners). The term 'quasi-market' was used because a tax-funded health system imposed political constraints on the extent to which market forces were allowed to determine available services. As a result, the system was highly regulated and market forces were restricted. Health authorities are statutory bodies responsible for assessing the health needs of a geographically defined population and for ensuring that health services are available to meet identified needs. During the period of the internal market, health authorities used contracts with providers to fulfil their responsibility for providing appropriate health care. Provider income was mainly determined by the content of contracts with purchasers.

This organizational arrangement was important because it created the theoretical possibility that purchasers could create financial incentives to influence the clinical activity of providers. As advocates for the health of the geographically defined population they serve, health authorities aimed to maximize the health improvements obtained from the scarce resources they were allocated. In theory, they could use the contracting system of the internal market to restrict payment for, or allocate funding to, specific new technologies, according to whether available research evidence suggested they were clinically cost-effective.

Case studies of technology adoption

The following case studies illustrate the role of hospitals in decisions about introducing new technologies and examine the extent to which National

Health Service health authorities, as advocates for a utilitarian approach to the adoption of technology linked to evidence of clinical and cost-effectiveness, influence their introduction. The methods have been described elsewhere (Rosen and Mays 1998) and are briefly outlined below.

Methods

The case studies examined the introduction into National Health Service acute hospitals of three contrasting new medical technologies: vascular stents, the triple test (testing for alpha-fetoprotein, human chorionic gonadotropin and unconjugated estriol) and the excimer laser. Stents are small metal tubes that can be inserted by interventional radiologists and used to support arteries after angioplasty, thus avoiding the need for open surgery. The triple test is a pre-natal, three-part screening blood test to assess the risk that a foetus is affected by Down's syndrome. The excimer laser is used for the treatment of short-sightedness and some corneal disorders in the eye. Each technology was studied in three different hospital or health authority sites, including teaching and non-teaching hospitals and adopters and non-adopters of the technologies (nine study sites in total).

Data were collected through 51 semi-structured interviews with clinicians, managers and public health physicians working in the hospitals and their associated health authorities who had been involved in introducing these technologies. In four of the nine study sites, documentary records (archive material, business cases, letters and memos) were made available and were examined for consistency with verbal reports. Data were analysed inductively and used to develop hypotheses about mechanisms for linking the introduction of new technologies to research evidence of clinical and cost-effectiveness.

The type of technology assessment research available to the decision-makers varied, since decisions about adoption were made at different times in each study site. Early decisions about the triple test in one site were based only on assessments by teaching hospitals of the accuracy of the test, whereas later decisions were also informed by community-based studies showing lower detection rates. Research on stenting consisted of multiple case series reports describing outcomes and complications. At the time of the case studies, several randomized trials were underway but had not yet reported. No economic evaluations had been undertaken and a few poor-quality costing studies had been published. Randomized trials of the laser were not ethically possible, but many case series were available describing outcomes and complications. A few poor-quality descriptions of the costs associated with excimer treatment were available.

Key findings from case studies

Findings are presented here from the case studies regarding the involvement of physicians and managers from health authorities and hospitals (that is, purchasers and providers) in decisions on adopting the technologies, and the extent to which they try to promote clinical and cost-effective use. Further data from the case studies are presented elsewhere (Rosen and Mays 1998; Rosen 2000).

Who were the decision-makers?

In six case study sites, different groups of people within the hospitals studied made decisions about introducing these technologies, with minimal involvement of public health physicians or managers from the health authority. In relation to stenting, clinicians made independent decisions for individual patients without reference to senior managers, unless their use of stents was so great as to exceed their departmental budget, in which case hospital managers became involved. In two triple test study sites, clinicians had decided to reject the triple test and introduce an alternative Down's syndrome screening test based on an evaluation of effectiveness. With the excimer laser, staff in two of the health authorities refused to include its use in contracts with the hospitals. They were reluctant partly because they believed that the National Health Service should not provide laser use for cosmetic reasons and partly because studies on longer follow-up were not available. However, both hospital providers decided to use the laser without health authority agreement or funding, to improve the hospital's reputation and attract extra patients, and one site intended to undertake research on effectiveness.

Health authority staff were involved in technology decisions in only three of the nine sites. They were the main advocates for introducing triple test screening in one site, where they argued that early research showed it to be more effective than current practice (for example, the use of amniocentesis) and that an evaluation should be conducted. In the second site, they argued that evidence was insufficient to support routine use of coronary artery stents and that temporary guidelines for patient selection should be developed and modified when trial results were available. In both these cases, health authority work led by public health physicians was based on a review of available research literature. In the third site, the local hospital wished to modify their contract to reflect the growing use of stent technologies, and the administrative response by the health authority made no reference to research evidence.

To what extent were decisions based on evidence?

These stories illustrate the limited involvement of health authorities in deciding on new technologies. Groups of decision-makers within hospitals made most decisions. When health authorities and public health physicians were not involved in adopting technology, research evidence of effectiveness was less used and less predictable. Three clinicians (one excimer site and two stent sites) had thoroughly reviewed available research (albeit small case series studies rather than randomized trials). Four others (one triple test and one stent site and two excimer sites) made decisions based on a brief assessment of selected published papers, verbal recommendation by colleagues and personal enthusiasm.

Hospital decision-making processes

Triggers for health authority involvement in decision-making on new technologies included its high cost, staff with a particular interest, relevance to a local health priority and staff time availability. Within hospitals, clinicians with a particular interest drive new technology.

When introducing the technology would significantly increase departmental spending, clinicians had to involve senior hospital managers. Proposals to introduce the technology were made in the form of business cases presented to hospital executives (chief executive, finance officer and medical director) and/or the hospital board. Clinicians had to briefly summarize how the technology would improve patient health and provide information about the impact of the technology on the hospital itself – that is, on expenditure, patient numbers, contract performance and number of staff. There was no obligation to review the literature on clinical and cost-effectiveness or to propose evidence-based guidelines on how patients would be selected. So long as the new technology was resource-neutral or generated income for the hospital, senior managers supported a proposal and left judgements about clinical appropriateness to the clinicians. The public health physicians, whose role in the health authority was to champion the public health and encourage the provision of clinically and cost-effective services, were not routinely involved in hospital-based decisions.

Discussion

These case studies looked at three contrasting technologies for the treatment or investigation of common health problems. The excimer laser represented the type of high-cost technology that typically attracts the attention of health planners (as seen with magnetic resonance imaging, computed tomography and lithotripsy). The stenting and triple test cases were representative of the hundreds of smaller-scale new technologies that do not require major capital investment and therefore attract less attention from planners but are introduced into clinical practice on a regular basis.

When public health physicians from health authorities were involved in introducing the technologies, their professional commitment to improving population health caused them to emphasize the importance of conducting research comparing the effectiveness of new and established interventions. If necessary, they advocated restricting use of a technology until methodologically rigorous comparative studies (that is, randomized trials or large comparative cohort studies) were available. Although clinicians were clearly committed to assessing the impact of these technologies on patient health, they were less concerned to base technology decisions on rigorous comparative studies but accepted case series that described the outcomes and risks associated with the procedure. Where hospital managers were involved in decision-making, their main objective was to assess how the technology would affect the hospital organization as a whole.

These studies are consistent with the findings of researchers in the United States. Greer (1985) described three different decision systems in relation to adopting technology in community hospitals in the midwestern United States. The individualistic medical system of clinical consultation emphasized promoting patient welfare and reducing risk. The fiscal-managerial decision system at the departmental level focused on how a technology affected the efficient running of the hospital. In the hospital-wide strategic-institutional system, the primary objective of decision-makers was to maintain a hospital's status and competitiveness.

Similar observations were made in studies on the introduction of new technologies in the United States. Studying how technology was acquired at 12 teaching hospitals in the United States, Weingart (1993) noted that many of the people involved in such decisions were general or financial managers who were concerned with the financial and organizational impact of the technologies. Luce and Brown (1995) studied technology assessment processes in hospitals, health maintenance organizations and third-party payers in the United States and concluded that the main focus of the assessment varied between organizations. Hospitals were more interested in assessing their financial impact, whereas health maintenance organizations and payers were more likely to assess clinical effectiveness as well as costs.

Implications

I have argued that most decisions to adopt technology are made within hospitals, with minimal reference to decision-makers, such as public health physicians in health authorities, who take a utilitarian, population perspective and aim to maximize clinical and cost-effectiveness. This raises at least two questions about the appropriate role of the hospital in relation to new technologies. First, should hospital decision-makers routinely take a utilitarian approach and assess whether a proposed technology is clinically effective and cost-effective compared with current practice? If so, through what mechanisms can such a link be strengthened?

The answer to the first question is determined partly by hospital type. One might argue that the only important aim of a private hospital is to maximize profits, regardless of how acquiring technology affects the overall health service; for example, increased insurance premiums or opportunity costs for other services or institutions. However, is a public hospital operating in a tax-funded health system such as Sweden or the United Kingdom obligated to balance the rights of patients to treatment and organizational viability against maximizing health benefit to the taxpaying population? What would happen if public hospitals were to incorporate utilitarian objectives into their decisions to adopt technology, whereas private hospitals were not to, consequently expanding their technology?

These are clearly value judgements, but a number of factors support the incorporation of more utilitarian thinking into hospital decision-making. First, as countries move away from fee-for-service payments and towards global budgets and prospective payment systems (Spibey 1995), hospitals have financial incentives to ensure that new technologies are cost-effective compared with current practice. Second, interest is growing in developing a sounder evidence base for many medical interventions. Third, developments in information technology, databases of trials in progress and on-line access to medical literature make it easier to undertake literature reviews to inform technology adoption decisions. Finally, as all countries face the problem of scarce health care resources, recognition is growing of the opportunity costs associated with acquiring technology that fails to produce the health benefits expected.

These factors support my argument that hospital decision-makers should routinely consider available health technology assessment findings on proposed new technologies and consider delaying acquisition if good-quality studies are not yet available. However, other pressures mitigate against this approach. The risk of being seen as rationing treatments, rather than protecting patients from unproven interventions, may provoke damaging publicity. Legal challenges arguing for patients' rights to receive treatments that may do some good, even if physicians believe that research shows that the potential risks outweigh benefits, have publicly embarrassed hospitals and health authorities.

If hospitals are to incorporate a utilitarian perspective, integrating health technology assessment into decisions to adopt technology becomes important. Several European countries have now established health technology assessment programmes, including Denmark, France, the Netherlands, Spain (in particular Catalonia), Sweden and the United Kingdom (Banta and Oortwijn 1999). Within the United Kingdom, the national programme for health technology assessment is linked to a nationwide dissemination programme (Sheldon and Chalmers 1994) to ensure that the results reach the policy-makers for whom they are intended. As the case studies showed, contract negotiations between health authority purchasers and health care providers are the main mechanism for incorporating health technology assessment into decision-making but appear to be only weakly influential.

In the Netherlands, the 1971 Hospital Act provides national legislative control over a small number of big-ticket technologies and services, and local negotiations take place between sickness funds and hospitals about the use of selected smaller technologies (Bos 1995). France has regional planning on big-ticket technologies based on a *Carte Sanitaire* (health map) informed by assessing population needs and health technology. Selected big-ticket technologies are also planned in Sweden's regionalized health care system (Banta and Oortwijn 1999). The key point about these systems is that they focus on a few highly visible technologies, with much less attention paid to the numerous tests, pieces of equipment, drugs and new operative techniques that regularly creep into routine use. These smaller technologies do not attract attention because of high cost or wizardry, but their costs add up and should be subjected to a routine, critical review of the available research evidence.

A health maintenance organization in the United States, the California Kaiser Permanente group, suggests such a model for health technology assessment. Each clinical department is supported by a systems engineer, trained in the skills of literature review and critical appraisal, who assesses the technology involved in any new intervention or equipment the clinicians wish to introduce (Castaneda and Breivis 1990). Although decisions do not necessarily follow the assessment recommendations, any available research on clinical and cost-effectiveness is routinely considered as part of the decision-making process.

This model could easily be applied within European hospitals to develop the role of the hospital in promoting the prudent use of scarce resources and the effective use of new technologies.

References

Altman, S. (1979) *Medical Technology: The Culprit Behind Health Care Costs?* Washington, DC: US Government Printing Office for the Department of Health, Education and Welfare.

Banta, H.D. and Oortwijn, W. (1999) Health technology assessment in the European Union, *Eurohealth*, 5: 37–9.

Bos, M. (1991) *The Diffusion of Heart and Liver Transplantation across Europe*. London: King's Fund.

Bos, M. (1995) Health care technology in the Netherlands, in H.D. Banta, R.N. Battista, H. Gelband and E. Jonsson (eds) *Health Care Technology and its Assessment in Eight Countries*. Washington, DC: Office of Technology Assessment of the US Congress.

Castaneda, M. and Breivis, J. (1990) Technology assessment, *Health Care Forum Journal*, November/December, pp. 10–11.

Gage, F. (1998) Cell therapy, *Nature*, 392(7): 18–24.

Greer, A. (1985) Adoption of medical technology: the hospital's three decision systems, *International Journal of Technology Assessment in Health Care*, 1: 669–80.

Harrison, A. and Prentice, S. (1996) *Acute Futures*. London: King's Fund.

Hollingsworth, S. and Barker, S. (1999) Gene therapy; into the future of surgery, *Lancet*, 353: 19–20.

Kirchberger, S., Durieux, P., Viens-Bitker, C. *et al.* (1991) *The Diffusion of Two Technologies for Renal Stone Treatment across Europe*. London: King's Fund.

Luce, B. and Brown, R. (1995) The use of technology assessment by hospitals, health maintenance organizations and third-party payers in the United States, *International Journal of Technology Assessment in Health Care*, 11(1): 79–92.

Murphy, S. (1998) Does new technology increase or decrease health care costs? The treatment of peptic ulceration, *Journal of Health Services Research and Policy*, 3: 215–18.

Office of Technology Assessment (1976) *Development of Medical Technology: Opportunities for Assessment*. Washington, DC: US Government Printing Office.

Rosen, R. (2000) Applying research to health care policy and practice: medical and managerial views on effectiveness and the role of research, *Journal of Health Services Research and Policy*, 5: 103–8.

Rosen, R. and Mays, N. (1998) The impact of the UK NHS purchaser–provider split on the 'rational' introduction of new medical technologies, *Health Policy*, 43: 103–23.

Schwartz, E. (1994) In the pipeline: a work of valuable technology, *Health Affairs (Millwood)*, 13(summer): 71–9.

Sheldon, T. and Chalmers, I. (1994) The UK Cochrane Centre and the NHS Centre for Reviews and Dissemination: respective roles within the information system strategy of the NHS R&D programme, coordination and principles underlying collaboration, *Health Economics*, 3: 201–3.

Spibey, J. (1995) Health care technology in the United Kingdom, in H.D. Banta, R.N. Battista, H. Gelband and E. Jonsson (eds) *Health Care Technology and its Assessment in Eight Countries*. Washington, DC: Office of Technology Assessment of the US Congress.

Weingart, S. (1993) Acquiring advanced technology: decision-making strategies at twelve medical centres, *International Journal of Technical Assessment in Health Care*, 9(4): 530–8.

Wordsworth, S., Donaldson, C. and Scott, A. (1996) *Can We Afford the NHS?* London: Institute for Public Policy Research.

thirteen

Optimizing clinical performance

Nick Freemantle

Introduction

It has become increasingly obvious that evidence on the effectiveness and cost-effectiveness of interventions does not automatically translate into appropriate and uniform changes in clinical practice (Freemantle and Bloor 1996). The substantial investment in the development of clinical interventions, their large-scale evaluation and the development of appropriate treatment guidelines cannot produce better patient health outcomes unless the prescribed changes in clinical practice and health care delivery are implemented.

This chapter examines several related areas:

- evidence on suboptimal professional performance and the degree and importance of unexplained variation in the delivery of health care;
- the development of standards in controversial areas of health care;
- the methods used in attempts to change practice and the evidence for their usefulness;
- the failure of some effective and cost-effective interventions to become standard practice; and
- an evaluation of appropriate policy for achieving optimal clinical performance.

Evidence for suboptimal clinical performance

This section considers several key examples of variation in clinical practice and failure to adopt optimal practice.

Variation in the use of interventions in uncertainty: hysterectomy rates in Ticino, Switzerland

In Ticino, the only canton in Switzerland in which most of the population speaks Italian, there were a variety of reasons for the use of hysterectomy that were not related to the evidence for its effectiveness. As Domenighetti *et al.* (1988: 1470) comment:

> International and regional variations in the frequency of hysterectomy and of the most common surgical procedures seem to be best explained by factors such as medical and surgical bed density, insurance and payment systems, professional uncertainty, surgeon's sex, control and review of surgical indications, medical auditing, and second opinion programmes, than by differences in morbidity, mortality, and other sociodemographic characteristics

Given the range of factors that might contribute to the decision to perform a common surgical procedure and the absence of specific direction on the appropriate circumstances in which it is appropriate, substantial variability in rates might be expected. Less clear, however, is an explanation for substantial changes in the overall rate of such an intervention over time, as in Ticino, where rates of hysterectomy were monitored from 1977 to 1986 (Domenighetti *et al.* 1988). The number of hysterectomies in women aged 35–49 years rose from 860 to 1422 per 100,000 women (by 65 per cent) between 1977 and 1982.

Changes of such magnitude in the rate of hysterectomy in the absence of good evidence are disturbing and highlight the importance of establishing appropriate standards of care of commonly used interventions based on evidence of effectiveness and cost-effectiveness. Without such evidence, it is impossible to assess whether the changes that occurred, or the subsequent mass media campaign aimed at mediating the increases, did more good than harm.

Effect of emerging standards of care based on consensus guidelines for a national medical specialty

In the absence of robust standards for care, a range of factors may influence the delivery of health care. Optimal or suboptimal health care are defined through the development of appropriate standards of care. The availability of evidence-based treatment standards is a central tenet of the arguments presented here, since if optimal health care is not defined, neither is suboptimal care.

Lomas *et al.* (1989) evaluated the effect of a national standard on Caesarean section in women in Ontario, Canada. Their study assessed the outcome of the dissemination of national medical specialty consensus guidelines for Caesarean section in circumstances in which, at baseline, Caesarean section was being used substantially outside the guideline indication. The guidelines were disseminated extensively in Canada between March and June 1986 through a mailing to all obstetricians listed with the national specialty society (the Society of Obstetricians and Gynaecologists of Canada), to all hospitals with more than 50 beds, through publication in the national medical journal and bulletin of the Society as well as dissemination through a range of other routes.

So widespread was the dissemination that, 1 year after their distribution, 94 per cent of obstetricians in Ontario indicated that they knew of them. They also appear to have received widespread approval, with over 80 per cent of obstetricians agreeing with recommendations for the management of breech presentation or the management of women who had received a previous Caesarean section. Detailed knowledge of the guidelines was less impressive. Only 3 per cent of respondents identified all four of the recommended actions in the guidelines as well as all four of the actions not recommended. Self-reported performance was more encouraging, although the average overall score was only 67 per cent, and chance alone would suggest a score of 50 per cent. Two years later, about one-third of obstetricians reported changing their personal professional behaviour and one-third also reported that their hospital had changed its policies as a direct result of the practice guidelines.

The self-reported obstetrician response was substantially higher than observed practice rates using interrupted time-series analysis. Such an analysis provides an appropriate quasi-experimental design that may be used to evaluate the effect of an intervention in a population over time with some protection from bias (Wood and Freemantle 1999). Overall, the distribution of national standards reduced the rate of Caesarean section by 0.13 per cent. As Lomas et al. (1989: 1310) commented:

> The limited practical importance of the size of the change detected in observed practice can be highlighted by calculating the number of years it would take for the overall rate of cesarean section in Ontario to be reduced to 10.5%, the approximate rate in England and Wales. Starting from the level of 20.4% seen in the year before the release of the guide-lines and generously assuming that the entire change in rates seen after-wards can be attributed to the guidelines, reaching 10.5% would take more than 30 years.

A similar situation was observed with the distribution of evidence-based recommendations on the use of antidepressants in the United Kingdom, where a small slowing of the rate of increase of use of selective serotonin-reuptake inhibitors was attributed to the guidelines (Mason et al. 1999). The Chief Medical Office distributed a bulletin (NHS Centre for Reviews and Dissemina-tion and Nuffield Institute for Health 1996) to all family practice physicians describing the poor evidence for supporting a switch in clinical practice from older antidepressants to newer, more costly selective serotonin-reuptake inhibitors. At the same time, an Executive Letter directed health authorities to consider action in support of the bulletin recommendations. Several other evaluations of the distribution of guidelines or printed educational materials demonstrate similar results (Freemantle et al. 2000). The dissemination of emerging standards of care, based on the best available evidence, therefore do not appear to be sufficient to achieve appropriate health care delivery.

Interventions with emerging unequivocal evidence of effectiveness

It may not be surprising that clinical practice varies when no consistent standards of care are available or when standards reflect only consensus, albeit based on the best available evidence. How does the situation differ when there is emerging, unequivocal evidence of benefit from large-scale randomized trials? Ketley and Woods (1993) examined the impact of trials of thrombolytic drugs on the treatment of post-myocardial infarction patients in Trent Regional Health Authority, a representative region of England. The publication of the results of several large trials (notably the Second International Study of Infarct Survival (ISIS-2) in 1988 and one by the Gruppo Italiano per lo Studio della Strepochinasi nell'Infarcto Miocardico (GISSI) in 1986) demonstrated that, in a realistic setting, thrombolysis soon after the onset of pain is associated with a reduction in mortality at 5 weeks of about 25 per cent in patients with acute myocardial infarction. Failing to incorporate these findings into routine clinical practice will lead to substantial avoidable mortality.

Not all patients with acute myocardial infarction meet the clinical criteria for thrombolysis, but in the Fourth International Study of Infarct Survival (ISIS-4), 69 per cent of the first 40,000 patients received the intervention, suggesting that at least two-thirds of patients in clinical practice are likely to meet the criteria (Ketley and Woods 1993). During the period immediately after these results were published, variation in rates of patients did decline between districts, from about 6-fold to 2.2-fold. However, Ketley and Woods (1993) identified a practice time lag in that the rate of participation in large trials in the late 1980s (as defined by the percentage of eligible patients randomized) predicted the rates of use of thrombolytic drugs in the early 1990s ($P = 0.003$). Even though reduction in variability in practice declined and rates of appropriate intervention increased, Ketley and Woods estimated that only about 35–50 per cent of eligible patients received thrombolysis in the Trent region in the early 1990s.

A similar situation has been observed for the use of angiotensin-converting enzyme inhibitors, for which there is good evidence of effectiveness and cost-effectiveness. Recent estimates indicate that only about one-third of eligible patients received this treatment in family practice in England (Eccles et al. 1998a; Morgan et al. 1999).

In the short term at least, the availability of good evidence appears to have a positive but limited benefit in optimizing the delivery of health care.

Good evidence available for a long period on intervention effectiveness

How long does evidence take to diffuse into clinical practice? This question was examined in a major evaluation of rates of uptake in the treatment of 186,800 Medicare patients in a national sample across the United States who had experienced an acute myocardial infarction – the Cooperative Cardiovascular Project (O'Connor et al. 1999). In this project, 306 hospital referral regions were identified and patients categorized into those who met the treatment

Table 13.1 Rates of intervention (per cent) among patients in 306 hospital referral regions participating in the Cooperative Cardiovascular Project by type of intervention, among patients meeting clinical criteria for each type of intervention

Intervention	Number of eligible patients	Mean	Range	20th to 80th percentiles
Aspirin during hospitalization	96 246	86.2	67.8–100	82.6–90.1
Aspirin post-hospitalization	60 044	77.8	52.1–96.0	72.5–83.9
Thrombolysis or percutaneous transluminal angioplasty	17 071	67.2	33.0–93.3	59.8–75.1
Beta-blocker on discharge	14 839	49.5	0.0–92.7	35.8–61.5
Angiotensin-converting enzyme inhibitors at discharge	18 114	59.3	6.7–100.0	49.2–69.2
Calcium channel blockers withheld in impaired left ventricular function	9 083	81.9	42.7–100.0	73.6–90.8
Smoking cessation advice given	22 024	41.9	7.3–81.7	32.8–51.3

Source: O'Connor *et al.* (1999)

criteria for specific interventions. The numbers of patients, the mean rates of intervention, range and 20th to 80th percentiles for each intervention are shown in Table 13.1. Thus, only half the patients received beta-blockade at discharge and only six in ten received angiotensin-converting enzyme inhibitors, whereas two-thirds of patients appropriately received thrombolysis or percutaneous transluminal angioplasty.

Beta-blockade in secondary prevention of myocardial infarction has long been associated with substantial benefits (Yusuf *et al.* 1985). Even where interventions are well established and evaluated, their appropriate use varies considerably. Treatment quality, as measured by a specific important intervention, is therefore poor in many hospitals and physician practices, leading to considerable avoidable morbidity, mortality and inefficiency.

Identifying priorities and developing standards for care

Appropriate standards of care, based on the best evidence of effectiveness and cost-effectiveness, are not always available. Indeed, a prerequisite for achieving optimal clinical performance must be the availability of standards that describe optimal care. Given the great many uncertainties on appropriate clinical practice and the nature of available evidence, such standards have necessarily focused on specific groups of patients, such as those with ischaemic heart disease. The evidence available also changes over time. As O'Connor *et al.* (1999: 627) pointed out, 'randomized trials have confirmed the efficacy of some therapies . . . guidelines make it possible to evaluate the processes of care in a meaningful manner and to identify areas for the improvement of the care of patients with acute myocardial infarction'.

Perhaps surprisingly, health policy has only recently begun to systematically develop valid treatment recommendations. In the United States, a major programme for developing guidelines has been set up under the auspices of the US Agency for Healthcare Research and Quality, but as this programme is not linked with any implementation mechanisms, its impact is unclear.

In the United Kingdom, a great deal has been invested in developing systematic reviews of treatment interventions through the Cochrane Collaboration. Considerable progress has been made in developing painstaking reviews of randomized trials, many in areas hitherto unvisited. Priorities have not really been set among review topics and a number of important areas (such as those in cardiovascular disease) have not, as yet, received much attention. More fundamentally, systematic reviews are not the same as evidence-based treatment guidelines. Appreciation of this point is changing, with the introduction of a national framework for the evaluation and development of guidelines for new and existing health care interventions (Department of Health 1998).

To be valid, guidelines need to take into account a range of features not routinely addressed in systematic reviews. These include the following: assessment of the current epidemiology of the condition the intervention is aiming to ameliorate; identification of relevant clinical questions; and an assessment of the effectiveness and cost-effectiveness of different treatment options in the relevant health care system. Optimizing clinical performance requires an assessment of the validity of the clinical standards being used. As Eddy (1992) has commented, considering the amount invested in the development of new technologies, it is remarkable how little effort is devoted to assessing their rational place in practice.

Attempts to change practice

A range of methods has been used in attempts to change practice. Many are essentially behavioural and aim to help clinicians deliver optimal care, such as continuing medical education or computer-generated reminders. Others use financial incentives and penalties, such as co-payments and limited clinician choice in health maintenance organizations, which aim to improve the efficiency of clinical performance by penalizing waste.

Behavioural interventions

Several reviews have analysed the effectiveness of behavioural interventions, defined as 'any attempt to persuade physicians to modify their practice performance by communicating clinical information' (Davis *et al.* 1995). Such interventions include attendance at conferences and other traditional continuing medical intervention activities, but also the less commonly used educational outreach visits (also called academic detailing or counter detailing) and opinion leader interventions (educational influentials). Davis *et al.* (1995) identified 99 randomized trials evaluating 160 interventions that met their inclusion criteria and found little or no benefit associated with conferences and short educational events. Freemantle (1996) found that the distribution of educational materials, examined in 15 studies, was not associated with important changes in clinical practice.

More active interventions, such as educational outreach visits, do appear to affect practice, although the magnitude of this effect is not great (Thomson O'Brien *et al.* 2000a). Studies report various outcomes, but overall it was rare for educational outreach to achieve as much as a 15 per cent change in the behaviour of clinicians, although even this extent of change may be worthwhile.

The audit and feedback approach, used commonly in attempts to change professional behaviour, has a small effect in some circumstances (Thomson O'Brien *et al.* 2000b,c). Similarly, although one trial found the influence of trained opinion leaders to be useful in changing practice (Lomas *et al.* 1991), this finding was not generalized to a further seven studies (Thomson O'Brien *et al.* 2000a). The computer-generated reminder system appears helpful (Johnston *et al.* 1994) but may be limited to routine circumstances in which clinicians agree with the intervention in question but forget to put it into clinical practice. An example is being reminded to prescribe low-dose aspirin when initiating treatment for symptomatic angina (Eccles *et al.* 1998b).

A useful finding from the review by Davis *et al.* (1995) is the apparent dose response for behavioural interventions. Combining several interventions also appears to have a greater effect on clinician behaviour than one used in isolation. This empirical finding has an underlying plausibility: the interventions found to be more effective are not discrete but include a combination of activities. For example, audit and feedback require explicit standards likely to be distributed in printed form; similarly, educational outreach visits probably include printed standards of care and a review of clinical performance. Adding further interventions may increase the likely effect of a behavioural programme but may also increase the costs. The cost-effectiveness of an intervention depends on the size of the effect in practice and the context (Mason *et al.* 1999). Achieving a relatively small change in rates of use of a highly cost-effective intervention may itself be cost-effective, whereas quite large changes in an intervention that is marginally cost-effective may not be cost-effective overall.

A review on the effectiveness of different forms of formal continuing medical education (Davis *et al.* 1999) found that traditional didactic teaching techniques did not affect practice, whereas focused interactive teaching did have an effect. Although the findings were preliminary, this does suggest a need to change the format of much activity aimed at keeping clinicians up to date with clinical practice.

In summary, while of considerable interest, behavioural approaches that aim to persuade clinicians to use interventions appropriately appear to have only limited effect. Although there may be further scope for improvement, these methods alone do not seem to provide an answer to the problem of ensuring optimal clinical performance.

Financial and organizational interventions

Many health systems explicitly attempt to use incentives or organizational structures to influence practice (Bloor and Freemantle 1996; Freemantle and

Bloor 1996). This is a complex area of study, but the limited number of experimental and quasi-experimental studies available do provide a remarkably consistent (and plausible) answer, at least in relation to the behaviour of health care users.

The single most important analysis of the effects of different incentives and organizational structures in health care delivery was the RAND Health Insurance Experiment (Newhouse and Insurance Experiment Group 1993). This complex social experiment randomized 2000 families to different insurance plan models that varied the maximum monetary expenditure and the incremental reimbursement per monetary unit spent. A further 3095 people were randomized, either to care from a health maintenance organization or to fee-for-service plans.

The RAND experiment was a monumental and ambitious scheme that attracted considerable attention and was not without its critics (Relman 1983; Welch *et al.* 1987). Although the study is superficially complex, its messages are remarkably simple. If barriers are put in the way of those seeking health care, such as out-of-pocket payments or limitations on services, costs and also volumes of care are reduced.

In the relatively young and healthy population enrolled in RAND, the reduction in the levels of care did not appear to have major consequences, except in groups such as the sick poor (with an effect on predicted mortality rates of about 10 per cent), and changed the likelihood, for example, that a decayed tooth would be filled. Indeed, as Newhouse and Insurance Experiment Group (1993: 180) comment:

... our analyses suggest that cost sharing has a non-specific effect on the use of medical services. In particular, it reduces appropriate and inappropriate services – or highly efficient and relatively inefficacious services – by the same proportion. This is the case for the use of antibiotics, for the medical advantage from being hospitalized, and for particular diagnoses for which medical care should be of substantial and little effect. Cost sharing also reduces the use of preventive services.

The controversial aspect of the RAND Health Insurance Experiment is the interpretation the authors place on these findings, suggesting that the differences in health status between the groups are not of importance or could be dealt with in ways other than less expensive health care to users. Critics have also noted a number of methodological problems, such as difficulties in measuring changes in the health status of the study population (Relman 1983).

Three further quasi-experimental studies, on a much less ambitious scale, have examined the effects of financial disincentives. Soumerai *et al.* (1991, 1994) found that limiting the number of prescriptions that patients could fulfil without payment profoundly affected the utilization of essential drugs in both the frail elderly population and in those with functional mental illness. Co-payments also led to a reduction in the use of both essential and inessential drugs, as also found by Harris and Stergachis (1990).

In summary, it would appear that financial barriers reduce wasteful and efficient practices equally. When there is an excess of waste, such as in a relatively healthy young population, this may not affect health status, at least in the short term. However, when people are receiving essential interventions, financial and organizational barriers appear to be likely to reduce access to these services proportionally. It might be postulated that a careful use of financial barriers, specifically targeting interventions not likely to be beneficial, may be a useful way forward, although most health systems seem a long way from this situation, with the possible exception of Australia in relation to pharmaceuticals.

Important influences on the health care market

The nature of the health care marketplace and its influences may act against the rational application of health care interventions. A number of perverse incentives act on the health care marketplace, including industry and its relationship with those who licence, reimburse and prescribe its products. The purpose of this section is not to criticize the pharmaceutical industry (although some might think that this was reasonable), but simply to consider the rules of engagement within which the industry operates.

The pharmaceutical industry exists almost exclusively to produce and take economic rent from pharmaceutical products. Other related industries, such as devices and diagnostics, may be considered in the same light, although they are of relatively minor importance. A major problem in most industrialized countries is that pricing structures for pharmaceutical products do not reflect their true clinical value in relevant patient groups (Freemantle 1999). Instead, there is considerable separation between the price and the act of prescribing.

The system of licensing and patent protection also tends to act against the interests of patients. For example, newer drugs are promoted heavily, whereas older products, such as beta-blockers, tend to be ignored even when they have considerable benefits and are highly cost-effective in specific patient groups. This is so unless new indications can be found for which patent extensions may be achieved (that is, heart failure for beta-blockers).

The sheer influence of a marketplace for pharmaceuticals should not be underestimated. When industry achieves a true breakthrough product, this clearly benefits both health systems and companies, which should be rewarded appropriately. However, when new drugs have questionable benefit over existing therapies, companies will attempt to achieve a return on their investment in bringing the drug to the marketplace. Not doing so would mean commercial ruin.

A further problem is that separating the value of drugs from their pricing tends to lead to the undervaluing of important new drugs. Occasionally, the pharmaceutical industry does achieve substantial steps forward, but demonstrating the value of their products costs many millions of dollars. A more rational relationship with the industry would suggest a preparedness to pay for that investment and also to share risk. The effect of undertaking the necessary research often indicates that a product has limitations. Currently in the United Kingdom, the Pharmaceutical Pricing Regulatory Scheme rewards companies simply on their investment of historical capital, but the same rewards could be distributed more rationally to reward relevant research investment.

A good example of the power of the pharmaceutical industry to influence practice is provided by an innovative case-control study by Chen and Landefeld (1994), who investigated the link between physicians and pharmaceutical companies. Specifically, they examined the behaviour of 40 physicians in a United States hospital in requesting additions to the practice formulary, compared with a random sample of 80 physicians who did not make such requests.

> Physicians who had requested that drugs be added to the formulary interacted with drug companies more than other physicians: for example, they were more likely to have accepted money from companies to attend or speak at educational symposia or to perform research (odds ratio 5.1; 95% confidence intervals 2.0 to 13.2) . . . This controlled study . . . demonstrated a strong and specific association between . . . behaviour and the physicians' interactions with drug companies, independent of the merits of the companies' products.
>
> (Chen and Landefeld 1994: 686)

In summary, the manner in which health systems value pharmaceuticals and other health technologies does not lead to their rational use in routine clinical practice. Indeed, in many health care systems, such as that of the United Kingdom, the relationship between the health system and the pharmaceutical companies contains perverse incentives that encourage behaviour from the companies and health providers that is not in the best interests of patients.

The hospital setting

Does the hospital as a setting, and the hospital as an employer, offer extra levers in improving clinical performance? Such levers include clinical protocols, peer review and patient audits. There is little evidence on the significance of the setting to inform decision-makers, although it is unlikely that location has no effect. Indeed, in a study of the effect of opinion leaders on unnecessary Caesarean section, Lomas et al. (1991) found a substantial effect in the hospital setting. This finding was not generalized to other studies in a community setting (Thomson O'Brien et al. 2000a), so that it is not possible to determine whether the apparent hospital effect was due to the setting, some other confounding factor or simply the play of chance.

Conclusions

This review of the current state of interventions aimed at promoting optimal clinical practice may be depressing reading for those who find it convincing i whole or in part. Even the availability of good clinical evidence will not. ' own, lead to appropriate changes in clinical practice. Although clinica¹ or guidelines are a necessary part of identifying and setting pr' interventions, their development leaves a good deal to be ' areas are not adequately addressed by guidelines. Ed'' appear to achieve at best only small changes in '

organizational interventions seem blunt tools to achieve change. The latter are as likely to prevent access to efficient interventions as to inefficient ones. Finally, the rules of engagement between industry and health systems produce numerous perverse incentives.

So what can be done to improve the situation? Probably nothing immediately, although some steps may be taken. The increasing availability of well-designed evaluations of the effectiveness and cost-effectiveness of interventions, such as the LIPID trial on pravastatin in over 9000 patients with heart disease (LIPID Study Group 1998), will do much to clarify which are the important interventions. Furthermore, the realization in many health systems that there is a problem will result in progress, through many incremental steps, in ensuring that important interventions become a routine part of clinical practice; witness the overwhelming incorporation of the use of aspirin in patients with acute myocardial infarction. Nevertheless, for those seeking a straightforward answer to the question of how best to optimize clinical performance, it is unfortunate that answering this question currently seems unrealistic.

Acknowledgements

I am grateful to Diane Dawson for comments on an earlier draft and to Anne Burton for assistance in locating relevant references and preparing the manuscript.

References

Bloor, K. and Freemantle, N. (1996) Lessons from international experience in controlling pharmaceutical expenditure II: influencing doctors, *British Medical Journal*, 312: 1525–7.

Chen, M.M. and Landefeld, S. (1994) Physicians' behavior and their interactions with drug companies: a controlled study of physicians who request additions to a hospital formulary, *Journal of the American Medical Association*, 271: 684–9.

Davis, D.A., Thomson, M.A., Oxman, A.D. and Haynes, R.B. (1995) Changing physician performance: a systematic review of the effect of continuing medical education strategies, *Journal of the American Medical Association*, 274: 700–5.

Davis, D., Thomson O'Brien, M.A., Freemantle, N. *et al.* (1999) Impact of formal continuing medical education: do conferences, workshops, rounds and other traditional continuing education activities change physician behavior or health care outcomes?, *Journal of the American Medical Association*, 282: 867–74.

Department of Health (1998) *A First Class Service: Quality in the New NHS*. London: The Stationery Office.

Domenighetti, G., Luraschi, P., Casabianca, A. *et al.* (1988) Effect of information campaign by the mass media on hysterectomy rates, *Lancet*, ii: 1470–3.

Eccles, M., Freemantle, N. and Mason, J.M. (1998a) Evidence based clinical practice guideline: angiotensin converting inhibitors in the primary care management of adults with symptomatic heart failure, *British Medical Journal*, 316: 1369–75.

Eccles, M., Freemantle, N., Mason, J. and North of England Aspirin Guideline Development Group (1998b) Evidence based clinical practice guideline: aspirin for the secondary prophylaxis of vascular disease in primary care, *British Medical Journal*, 316: 1303–9.

Eddy, D.M. (1992) *A Manual for Assessing Health Practices and Designing Practice Policies: The Explicit Approach.* Philadelphia, PA: American College of Physicians.

Freemantle, N. (1996) Are decisions taken by health care professionals rational? A non-systematic review of experimental and quasi-experimental literature, *Health Policy*, 38: 71–81.

Freemantle, N. (1999) Does the UK need a fourth hurdle for pharmaceutical reimbursement to encourage the more cost effective prescribing of pharmaceuticals?, *Health Policy*, 46: 255–65.

Freemantle, N. and Bloor, K. (1996) Lessons from international experience in controlling pharmaceutical expenditure I: influencing patients, *British Medical Journal*, 312: 1469–71.

Freemantle, N., Harvey, E.L., Wolf, F. *et al.* (2000) Printed educational materials: effects on professional practice and health care outcomes, *Cochrane Database of Systematic Reviews*, 2: CD000172.

Harris, B.L. and Stergachis, A. (1990) The effect of drug co-payments on utilization and cost of pharmaceuticals in a health maintenance organization, *Medical Care*, 28: 907–17.

Johnston, M.E., Langton, K.B., Haynes, R.B. and Mathieu, A. (1994) Effects of computer-based clinical decision support systems on clinician performance and patient outcome: A critical appraisal of research, *Annals of Internal Medicine*, 120(2): 135–42.

Ketley, D. and Woods, K.L. (1993) Impact of clinical trials on clinical practice: example of thrombolysis for acute myocardial infarction, *Lancet*, 342: 891–4.

LIPID Study Group (1998) Prevention of cardiovascular events and death with pravastatin in patients with coronary heart disease and a broad range of initial cholesterol levels, *New England Journal of Medicine*, 339: 1349–57.

Lomas, J., Anderson, G.M., Domnick-Pierre, K. *et al.* (1989) Do practice guidelines guide practice? The effect of a consensus statement on the practice of physicians, *New England Journal of Medicine*, 321: 1306–11.

Lomas, J., Enkin, M., Anderson, G.M. *et al.* (1991) Opinion leaders *vs* audit and feedback to implement practice guidelines: delivery after previous cesarean section, *Journal of the American Medical Association*, 265: 2202–7.

Mason, J., Freemantle, N. and Young, P. (1999) The effect of the distribution of Effective Health Care Bulletins on prescribing selective serotonin reuptake inhibitors in primary care: a quasi-experimental study, *Health Trends*, 30: 120–2.

Morgan, S., Smith, H., Simpson, I. *et al.* (1999) Prevalence and characteristics of left ventricular dysfunction among elderly patients in general practice setting: cross-sectional survey, *British Medical Journal*, 318: 368–72.

Newhouse, J.P. and Insurance Experiment Group (1993) *Free for All? Lessons from the RAND Health Insurance Experiment.* Cambridge, MA: Harvard University Press.

NHS Centre for Reviews and Dissemination and Nuffield Institute for Health (1996) Hospital volume and health care outcomes, costs and patient access, *Effective Health Care*, 2(8): 1–16.

O'Connor, G.T., Quinton, H.B., Traven, N.D. *et al.* (1999) Geographic variation in the treatment of acute myocardial infarction: the Cooperative Cardiovascular Project, *Journal of the American Medical Association*, 281: 627–33.

Relman, A.S. (1983) The Rand health insurance study: is cost sharing dangerous to your health?, *New England Journal of Medicine*, 309: 1453.

Soumerai, S.B., Ross-Degnan, D., Avorn, J., McLaughlin, T.J. and Choodnovskiy, I. (1991) Effects of Medicaid drug-payment limits on admission to hospitals and nursing homes, *New England Journal of Medicine*, 325(15): 1072–7.

Soumerai, S.B., McLaughlin, T.J., Ross-Degnan, D., Casteris, C.S. and Bollini, P. (1994) Effects of a limit on Medicaid drug reimbursement benefits in the use of psychotropic agents and acute mental health services by patients with schizophrenia, *New England Journal and Medicine*, 331(10): 650–5.

Thomson O'Brien, M.A., Oxman, A.D., Haynes, R.B. *et al.* (2000a) Local opinion leaders: effects on professional practice and health care outcomes, *Cochrane Database of Systematic Reviews*, 2: CD000125.

Thomson O'Brien, M.A., Oxman, A.D., Davis, D.A. *et al.* (2000b) Audit and feedback: effects on professional practice and health care outcomes, *Cochrane Database of Systematic Reviews*, 2: CD000259.

Thomson O'Brien, M.A., Oxman, A.D., Davis, D.A. *et al.* (2000c) Audit and feedback versus alternative strategies: effects on professional practice and health care outcomes, *Cochrane Database of Systematic Reviews*, 2: CD000260.

Welch, B.L., Hay, J.W., Miller, D.S. *et al.* (1987) The RAND health insurance study: a summary critique, *Medical Care*, 25: 148–56.

Wood, J. and Freemantle, N. (1999) Choosing an appropriate unit of analysis in trials of interventions that attempt to influence practice, *Journal of Health Services Research and Policy*, 1: 44–8.

Yusuf, S., Peto, R., Lewis, J., Collins, R. and Sleight, P. (1985) Beta-blockade during and after myocardial infarction: an overview of the randomized trials, *Progress in Cardiovascular Diseases*, 27(5): 335–71.

chapter fourteen

Hospital organization and culture

Linda Aiken and Douglas Sloane

Introduction

Research on medical effectiveness has grown into a flourishing international enterprise over the past two decades, driven by the search for value, as
industrialized countries have sought to curtail the growth of health care
expenditure (Cochrane 1973; Wennberg and Gittelsohn 1973). Organizational
research has received surprisingly scant attention, however, given the rapid
pace of organizational change in health services (Aiken *et al.* 1997c), and
little is known about the impact on patient outcomes of widespread hospital
reorganization driven by cost containment (Leatt *et al.* 1997; Marmor 1998).
  Curtailing hospital use is a primary focus of national efforts to reduce growth
in health care expenditure (Reinhardt 1996). In the United States, inpatient
days per capita fell by about 40 per cent between 1980 and 1999, resulting in
the lowest per capita rate of inpatient days and the lowest average length
of hospital stay of any comparable country. Additional hospital budgetary
constraints in this period have resulted in widespread initiatives to further
reduce expenditure by redesigning hospital organizations and reducing staffing
(Aiken *et al.* 1997a).
  One cost of hospital reorganization has been professional and public discontent. Nurses in Canada (Driedger 1997), Denmark and Sweden (Bentsen
et al. 1999), the United Kingdom (Royal College of Nursing 1998) and the
United States (Institute of Medicine 1996; Shindul-Rothschild *et al.* 1996;
Davidson *et al.* 1997) have vocally opposed organizational and staffing changes
in hospitals. They cite unsafe professional staffing levels and concern over
eroding quality of care. The public is also discontented with changes in hospitals. A recent international public opinion poll carried out in five countries
(Australia, Canada, New Zealand, the United Kingdom and the United States)
found fewer than one in four respondents reported that their health care

system works well (Donelan *et al.* 1999). The percentage of respondents who ranked their last hospital experience as fair or poor ranged from 18 per cent in the United Kingdom to 27 per cent in Canada. Almost one-third of those polled in a United States national survey reported having less trust in hospitals than they did 5 years before (Hensley 1998).

This chapter is organized into three parts. First, we build a case for greater investment in research on hospital organization that examines the effects of organizational attributes, culture and staffing on patient outcomes. Second, we summarize the relevant research on the determinants of variation in hospital outcomes. Third, we use our research to illustrate the links between hospital organization, culture and outcomes.

Organizational change

The scope and pace of organizational change in hospitals is staggering. Hospital mergers in the United States have increased dramatically since 1994, with roughly 250 mergers per year in the late 1990s. In Canada, hospital regionalization and downsizing of inpatient bed capacity has created controversy among health professionals and consumers (Naylor 1999). The National Health Service in the United Kingdom has experienced two reform efforts in the 1990s, both affecting hospitals (Klein 1998; Le Grand 1999). Yet research on the impact of these organizational changes on patient outcomes has been scarce.

Hospital organizational reform falls into two broad categories. The first is primarily concerned with system changes involving hospitals, and includes multi-hospital alliances and mergers, vertical and horizontal integration of services and the creation of integrated delivery systems, joint purchasing, outsourcing management and similar reforms (Shortell *et al.* 1990). The second is internal hospital restructuring, known as process re-engineering, which can fundamentally alter the design of clinical care and the relationships among care-givers (Blancett and Flarey 1995; Leatt *et al.* 1997). Both forms of reorganization are occurring in the majority of hospitals in the United States and Canada, and increasingly so in hospitals in Europe and elsewhere (Decter 1994; Aiken *et al.* 1997a; Bentsen *et al.* 1999).

Process re-engineering is defined as 'the fundamental rethinking and radical redesign of business practices to achieve dramatic improvements in critical, contemporary measures of performance such as cost, quality, service, and speed' (Hammer and Champy 1993: 32). Re-engineering redesigns job responsibilities and determines who does the work, where the work is located and by what processes or patterns the work will be done. By 1994, almost 70 per cent of the largest corporations in the United States reported having engaged in some form of re-engineering (Champy 1996). Re-engineering became popular in hospitals despite vigorous critiques of its success in other industries (Micklethwait and Wooldridge 1996). Sixty per cent of chief executive officers in hospitals in the United States reported in a national survey that they had implemented hospital re-engineering over the period 1991–96 (Walston *et al.* 2000).

A major purpose of re-engineering is to reduce personnel by increasing productivity and efficiency and to use less costly labour substitutes for professionals where possible. Reductions in nursing staff and skill mix are common targets. In theory, fewer registered nurses are required in this model because the multiskilled team allows nurses to increase the time they spend in direct patient care. However, most re-engineering initiatives also reduce middle-management positions throughout the hospital, leaving clinical nurses at the unit level to supervise the larger, more diverse decentralized labour force. As a practical matter, fewer nursing hours per patient day are often available after re-engineering because nurses' increased supervisory responsibilities more than offset the time saved in delegating non-nursing activities to others.

Team nursing was the dominant form of organizing nurses' work in the 1960s and 1970s. Nurses were dissatisfied with team nursing for a variety of well-chronicled reasons (Brannon 1994). These include their objections to being held accountable for the care provided by relatively untrained personnel, their dislike of managing non-professional workers and their perceptions of an erosion in the nurse–patient relationship resulting from much of the daily care being provided by non-nurses. Nurses in the United States were successful in changing the organization of nursing work to a more professional model, with a significantly higher mix of registered nurses and more direct care delivered by nurses in a model known as primary nursing (Hoffart and Woods 1996). Although little rigorous empirical research links primary nursing to better patient outcomes, primary nursing is a key element of magnet hospitals (Scott *et al.* 1999); that is, institutions that have been shown to have lower mortality than matched hospitals (Aiken *et al.* 1994, 1999). Re-engineering represents a reversal of the trend towards a professional nurse workforce (Brannon 1996). Nurses' dissatisfaction with this element of hospital reorganization has resulted in voluntary resignations and emerging nursing shortages (Baer *et al.* 1996; Davidson *et al.* 1997; Clifford 1998).

The few empirical studies to have evaluated the outcomes of hospital restructuring and re-engineering provide little evidence that structural reforms have achieved their goals of greater efficiency (Leatt *et al.* 1997; Marmor 1998). Recent evaluations of multi-hospital systems (Dranove *et al.* 1996) and vertical integration (Walston *et al.* 1996) suggest that neither strategy has been effective in improving the financial performance and efficiency of hospitals. Walston *et al.* (2000) evaluated the impact of process re-engineering in a national sample of United States hospitals and found that, in most instances, re-engineering adversely affected hospitals' cost positions relative to other hospitals in their local markets. The adverse effect largely resulted from the inability to implement the proposed changes because of widespread opposition, especially from health professionals (Rundall *et al.* 1998). Dissatisfaction among nurses resulting from re-engineering not only potentially increases hospitals' operating costs because of voluntary resignations (Davidson *et al.* 1997); our research indicates that dissatisfaction and burnout among nurses are related to patients' dissatisfaction with the quality of their care.

In summary, hospitals are undergoing dramatic organizational change. Limited research to date suggests that many proposed changes have been met with substantial resistance from care-givers and thus have not been successfully implemented (Rundall *et al.* 1998). In the process, however, the radical nature of the proposed changes has disrupted care, increased dissatisfaction and turn-over among nurses and contributed to shortages of hospital nurses, all of which can adversely affect the quality of patient care.

Review of research on organization and outcomes

Hospitals constitute the health care setting in which patients are the sickest and the rate of adverse events is the highest, and hospital-specific mortality rates and other critical patient outcomes vary substantially. A recent comparison of standardized mortality ratios for Medicare patients discharged from United States hospitals revealed a five-fold difference across hospitals in mortality from myocardial infarction and a ten-fold difference in deaths from congestive heart failure (Rosenthal *et al.* 1997). Hospitals in England differed in overall standardized mortality rates by a factor of two (Jarman *et al.* 1999).

Considerable literature has developed on the determinants of hospital mortality and other adverse patient outcomes (Moses and Mosteller 1968; Kelly and Hellinger 1986; Shortell and Hughes 1988; Chassin *et al.* 1989; Hartz *et al.* 1989; Al-Haider and Wan 1991; Aiken *et al.* 1994; Mitchell and Shortell 1997; van Servellen and Schultz 1999). Much of this literature focuses on how to empirically separate components of outcome variation, caused by severity of illness and other patient characteristics, from manipulable dimensions of hospital organization. Hospital mortality studies focusing on institutional attributes or characteristics usually examine numerous organizational correlates. Most are macro-level structural characteristics such as hospital size, location, teaching status and ownership status (public, private not-for-profit or private for-profit). Resource-related correlates studied commonly include nurse staffing, availability of technology and the qualifications of physicians.

Nurse staffing and patient mortality are consistently inversely related across studies of the determinants of hospital mortality. The higher the number of nurses available per patient-day, the lower the mortality (Shortell and Hughes 1988; Hartz *et al.* 1989; Silber *et al.* 1995; Aiken *et al.* 1999). Similarly, mortality and the skill mix of nursing personnel (registered nurses as a proportion of nursing personnel) are inversely related in the United States (Hartz *et al.* 1989) and in England (Jarman *et al.* 1999).

Nurse staffing and adverse events are also inversely related. Kovner and Gergen (1998) examined the relationship between nurse staffing levels for surgical patients and a set of adverse events in over 500 United States hospitals in ten states. A significant inverse relationship was found between the number of registered nurses per patient-day and urinary tract infections, pneumonia, thrombosis and pulmonary compromise. The researchers estimated that one additional registered nurse hour per surgical patient per patient-day was associated with a 9 per cent decrease in urinary tract infections and an 8 per cent decrease in pneumonia. Similarly, Blegen *et al.* (1998) and Blegen and Vaughn (1998) found that the presence of more registered nurses was associated with lower rates of decubitus, patient complaints and nosocomial infection and that a higher nursing skill mix was associated with significantly lower rates of medication error and patient falls.

No empirical research has documented an optimal nurse-to-patient ratio or nursing skill mix. Mandating specific staffing levels is problematic from a number of perspectives, including that minimum requirements tend to be interpreted over time as sufficient or standard practice (Buerhaus 1997). Nevertheless, because the weight of the evidence shows that nurse staffing and adverse patient outcomes are inversely related, various legislative proposals are pending in the United States mandating minimum nurse-to-patient ratios in certain types of hospital units and restricting the duties performed by unlicensed assisting personnel (Gallagher 1999).

Research on the relationship between physicians and hospital patient outcomes focuses on the experience and specialty of physicians and on communication between nurses and physicians. Generally, this literature finds that patients receiving services from physicians specializing in AIDS have better outcomes (Aiken *et al.* 1999). Higher-volume procedures are associated with better patient outcomes (Flood *et al.* 1984a,b; Thiemann *et al.* 1999), and the better the communication between nurses and physicians, the better the patient outcomes (Knaus *et al.* 1986). In England, the ratio of hospital physicians to beds predicted variation in standardized death rates, as did nursing skill mix (Jarman *et al.* 1999).

The link between hospital organization and outcomes

Flood (1994) provided an informative critique and synthesis of research on the impact of organizational and managerial factors on the quality of health care. She concluded that, too often, studies focus on identifying structural characteristics associated empirically with outcomes rather than on developing models that explain the processes by which structure affects the quality of care and outcomes. Our primary interest has involved whether other factors mediate the effects of nurse staffing on hospital outcomes, and our research has focused on how the relationship between staffing and patient outcomes is influenced by organizational features of hospitals and hospital units that affect what nurses do (Figure 14.1). We have examined these relationships in several large multiple-hospital studies, including a cross-national study involving large numbers of hospitals in Canada, Germany, the United Kingdom and the United States (Sochalski and Aiken 1999).

Our first major attempt to explore the impact of hospital organization on patient outcomes involved a study of three United States hospitals that had been identified by Fellows of the American Academy of Nursing as providing good nursing care (McClure *et al.* 1983). These hospitals had in common a set of organizational characteristics and a culture that valued professional nursing expertise (Kramer and Schmalenberg 1988a,b; Kramer 1990). They were especially successful in attracting and retaining registered nurses, even when hospitals in their local labour market were experiencing shortages of nurses: hence the term 'magnet hospitals'. We were interested in learning whether patient

Figure 14.1 Hospital organization, nurse staffing and patient outcomes

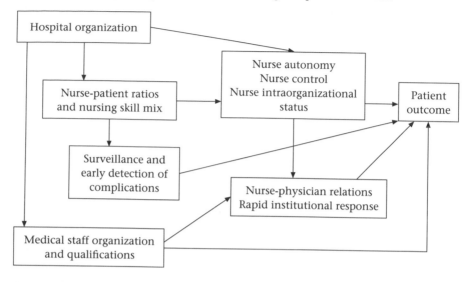

Source: Adapted from Aiken *et al*. (1997b)

outcomes at these hospitals were better than those at comparable hospitals and, if so, why. Using a national database on hospitals, we matched each of the 39 magnet hospitals with five comparison hospitals, yielding a study sample of 234 hospitals. The matching criteria were 12 non-nursing hospital characteristics that previous research had found to be correlated with differences in hospital-related mortality, including type of ownership, teaching status, size, occupancy, proportion of board-certified physicians, technological sophistication, emergency room use and location. We found that case mix-adjusted mortality in the magnet hospitals was significantly lower than in the matched controls (Aiken *et al*. 1994).

We purposely did not match hospitals on nurse staffing so that we could determine analytically whether differences in staffing in magnet hospitals explained their superior outcomes. Magnet hospitals had significantly higher nursing skill mixes and somewhat higher nurse-to-patient ratios. Nevertheless, neither skill mix nor nurse-to-patient ratio significantly affected mortality, nor did they account for any of the differences in mortality across the magnet and control hospitals.

Analysis of organizational data for a subset of 16 of the magnet hospitals revealed that a common set of characteristics in magnet hospitals appeared to be proxies for other variables: greater nurse autonomy, more nurse control over the practice setting and better relationships between physicians and nurses. However, we could not empirically investigate whether these organizational and cultural dimensions unique to magnet hospitals were responsible for their lower mortality, as we lacked such data on the matched control hospitals. Thus, we purposely designed our next study of hospitals to obtain primary data on how organizational context and culture affected clinical nursing care and its outcomes.

Table 14.1 Mean scores on practice environment subscales for 40 organizational units at 20 hospitals throughout the United States according to form of organization

Subscale	Magnet hospitals	Dedicated AIDS units	Conventional scattered-bed units
Nurse autonomy	17.0***	15.1**	14.2
Control over practice setting	22.7***	20.4***	17.4
Nurse–physician relations	6.4***	6.1**	5.8

Significantly different from conventional scattered-bed units: $**P \leq 0.01$; $***P \leq 0.001$

Organizational culture and patient outcomes

The AIDS epidemic in the United States created a natural experiment in hospital reorganization that we exploited to undertake our next study of the impact of organization and culture on patient outcomes (Aiken *et al.* 1997c). Several hospitals in cities with the highest AIDS incidence empowered their nurses to design and manage specialized units for AIDS care (Fox *et al.* 1990). These units appeared at the outset to have many of the organizational attributes and culture of professional nursing observed in magnet hospitals. We designed a study in 40 units in 20 hospitals distributed in all geographical regions of the United States to determine whether the outcomes for people with AIDS varied by the organization of the unit and, if so, whether organizational attributes were responsible for the variation in outcomes. The organizational forms studied included dedicated AIDS units, comparison medical units that provided AIDS care in scattered-bed arrangements and magnet hospitals without dedicated AIDS units (Aiken *et al.* 1997b).

We empirically measured the organization and culture of each unit by using the nurses to report on organizational features that might affect the nature of clinical care at the bedside. Individual-level data derived from surveys were aggregated to the unit level to derive empirical measures of the organizational attributes of greatest theoretical and practical interest (Aiken and Patrician 2000). We created three subscales measuring nurse autonomy, nurse control over the practice setting and relationships between nurses and physicians. Table 14.1 shows the average subscale values on these three features across the three different organizational forms. The mean values on these subscales for magnet hospitals and dedicated AIDS units differed significantly from those of comparison conventional units. Nurse staffing also varied across the models, with magnet hospitals having the highest ratio of registered nurses to patients and conventional units having the lowest ratio.

Having established variation in organization and staffing, we sought to determine whether these settings differed in patient outcomes (such as 30-day mortality after admission and patient satisfaction) and, if so, whether such differences could be explained by variation in organization and staffing. Figure 14.2 shows differences across hospital settings in 30-day mortality for seriously ill patients in our sample. The probability of dying within 30 days was lower in hospitals with specialized units than in conventional scattered-bed units and lower still in magnet hospitals. These differences persisted after

Figure 14.2 Probability of dying among people seriously ill with AIDS within 30 days of admission to 40 organizational units at 20 hospitals throughout the United States according to hospital setting. (The probabilities shown are for more seriously ill patients who require assistance with most activities of daily living or total nursing care.)

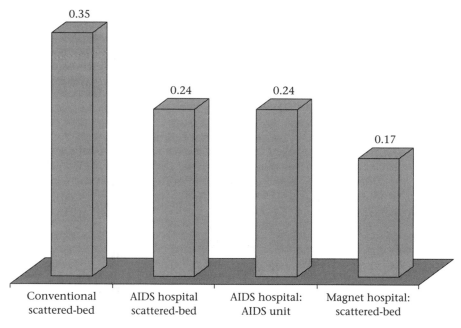

Conventional scattered-bed	AIDS hospital scattered-bed	AIDS hospital: AIDS unit	Magnet hospital: scattered-bed

Source: Aiken *et al.* (1999)

differences across settings in patient characteristics, including illness severity, were controlled. The lower mortality in dedicated AIDS units appeared to be attributable primarily to services from physicians specializing in AIDS and higher nurse-to-patient ratios (Aiken *et al.* 1999). An additional 0.5 nurses per patient-day (or an additional nurse for every six patients on each eight-hour shift) would be expected to reduce the likelihood of dying by roughly one-third. Patients whose physicians were associated with an AIDS specialty service were one-third as likely to die within 30 days of hospital admission. Differences in nurse autonomy, nurse control and physician–nurse relationships did not contribute significantly to explaining variation in mortality after nurse staffing and physician specialty were taken into account, but these organizational attributes were an important explanation for differences in patient satisfaction.

Figure 14.3 shows the differences in average patient satisfaction with the quality of their nursing care between patients in magnet hospital units and dedicated AIDS units relative to patients in conventional scattered-bed units. These results were obtained from regression models before and after adjusting for differences across settings in patient characteristics, nurse staffing and the extent to which nurses control their practice environment (Aiken *et al.* 1999). The large and significant unadjusted difference in patient satisfaction across settings was not accounted for by differences in patient characteristics or, very

Figure 14.3 Unadjusted and adjusted effects of type of unit on the satisfaction of people with AIDS at 40 organizational units at 20 hospitals throughout the United States: ■ magnet hospital unit; □ dedicated AIDS unit

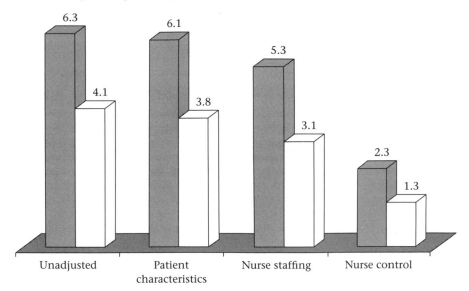

Source: Aiken *et al.* (1999)

substantially, by nurse staffing. The extent to which nurses exercised control over their practice setting, however, accounted for most of that difference.

Our AIDS study data have shown that the organization of hospitals and hospital units affects not only patient outcomes but also nurse outcomes (Aiken and Sloane 1997). We looked at burnout, or emotional exhaustion, among nurses in the same hospital units as the patients in our AIDS study and found that the specialized units and magnet hospitals that tend to exhibit more favourable patient outcomes also have lower levels of nurse burnout. As Table 14.2 shows, differences across hospitals and units were significant and pronounced both before and after controlling for the characteristics of hospitals (such as size, type of ownership and location) and for the nurses who worked in them (such as sex, race, age and experience). Similar to patient satisfaction, the only factor that accounted substantially for the lower levels of burnout in AIDS units and in magnet hospitals was a measure of organizational support, which was a simple composite of items from the nurse autonomy and control scales.

Studying hospitals

Our research on the link between hospital organization and patient outcomes has compiled information from large numbers of nurses and patients and from a variety of sources, but some of the hypotheses of greatest interest have

Table 14.2 Effects of dedicated AIDS units and magnet hospitals in the United States on nurse burnout as measured by the Emotional Exhaustion Scale of the Maslach Burnout Inventory

		Mean difference in nurse burnout[b]	
Model	Factors controlled[a]	AIDS units	Magnet hospitals
1	none	−5.3**	−4.8**
2	H	−5.6**	−5.2**
3	H, N	−4.6**	−4.7**
4	H, N, O	−3.1**	−1.4**

[a] H = hospital effects, or differences between hospitals in burnout. N = nurse characteristics: a block of variables including sex, age, ethnicity, foreign origin, education, experience and sexual preference. O = organizational support, derived from Kramer's Nurse Work Index.
[b] Coefficients indicate mean differences between dedicated AIDS units and magnet hospitals relative to scattered-bed units. Significant effects: $*P \leq 0.05$; $**P \leq 0.01$.

Source: Adapted from Aiken and Sloane (1997)

proven the least amenable to testing. None of our studies on organizational factors have consisted of more than 20 hospitals or, in the case of our AIDS study, twice that number of units. Since the variables we perceive to be the most proximate determinants of favourable patient outcomes are at the hospital and unit level, larger samples of hospitals and units are needed to conclusively answer the questions our research has posed. This is especially true since many of the factors in which we are interested, such as staffing levels, skill mix and nurse control, are related, so that disentangling their effects on patients is difficult.

Our current research has therefore moved from studying specific types of hospitals – that is, magnet hospitals known for good nursing care or hospitals with dedicated AIDS units – to studying representative groups of hospitals. We have determined that our survey methods for obtaining reliable information on hospital organization and culture from nurses employed in hospitals can be implemented at the state, provincial or national level by surveying all registered nurses and aggregating their responses to their hospital of employment. Staffing data are generally available from secondary sources and hospital-specific outcome measures can be calculated from hospital discharge information available through administrative or routine data sources. Thus, we have embarked on a cross-national study of the determinants of variation in hospital outcomes, which will provide us with data from 90,000 nurses and some 700 hospitals (McKee *et al.* 1998; Sochalski and Aiken 1999). This will give us the opportunity to resolve a number of the questions raised in our research over the past decade.

The cross-national study consists of all hospitals in three Canadian provinces (Ontario, Alberta and British Columbia), the state of Pennsylvania (representing hospitals in the United States), Scotland, and selected hospitals in England and Germany. In addition to conventional measures of outcome available from routine data such as mortality rates, the cross-national study seeks to employ a relatively new and promising outcome measure: failure to rescue. The failure-to-rescue rate, defined as the rate of death following complications, is related to hospital resource use, including nurse-to-patient ratios (Silber *et al.* 1995). Preliminary findings show that hospitals within each country vary substantially in organizational context and culture. As expected, major teaching hospitals with a national reputation for providing excellent care also tend to have higher nurse autonomy, more nurse control over the practice setting and better relationships between nurses and physicians. Initial findings from the nurse survey component of the study of 32 National Health Service trusts in England show that the organizational attributes of interest and selected nurse outcomes are significantly correlated. For example, higher nurse autonomy is associated with higher nurse satisfaction, lower nurse burnout and fewer nurses injured by blood-contaminated needles and sharps (Ball 1999). Thus, we expect to make significant progress in understanding the relationship between hospital organization and culture and patient outcomes, including the causal order of relationships, once all the data are available from this very large study.

Conclusions

Abundant research has indicated that nurse staffing and skill mix are important determinants of inpatient mortality and other patient outcomes. Our research has suggested that the organization of nursing care may have an effect on patient outcomes that is independent of, and as important as, staffing and skill levels. Mitchell and Shortell (1997) argue, however, that acute care studies, in general, have been inconsistent in their findings on the effects of organizational characteristics on patient outcomes. This may, as Mitchell and Shortell have noted, be partly caused by the reliance of most studies on mortality and complications to indicate patient outcome or quality of care. Both are strongly associated with patient-level factors, such as the severity of illness, which are difficult to control for. Major challenges for future research on hospital organization and patient outcomes involve determining:

- which outcomes are most affected by hospital organization and culture;
- how organization and culture interact with resource utilization;
- how nurse staffing levels and skill mix affect outcomes; and
- how the effects of these differing hospital characteristics on patient outcomes can be disentangled from the effects of patient characteristics.

Organization and culture are important and insufficiently appreciated factors in explaining variation in hospital outcomes. A better understanding of how these factors influence clinical care and the outcomes of care is key to preserving the aspects of hospitals that favourably influence patient outcomes and reducing resource investment in those that do not.

References

Aiken, L.H. and Patrician, P. (2000) Measuring organizational traits of hospitals: the Revised Nursing Work Index, *Nursing Research*, 49: 149–53.

Aiken, L.H. and Sloane, D.M. (1997) Effects of organizational innovations in AIDS care on burnout among urban hospital nurses, *Work and Occupations*, 24(4): 453–77.

Aiken, L.H., Smith, H.L. and Lake, E.T. (1994) Lower Medicare mortality among a set of hospitals known for good nursing care, *Medical Care*, 32(8): 771–87.

Aiken, L.H., Sochalski, J. and Fagin, C.M. (1997a) Hospital restructuring in the United States, Canada and western Europe: an outcomes research agenda, *Medical Care*, 35 (suppl. 10): S13–25.

Aiken, L.H., Lake, E.T., Sochalski, J. and Sloane, D.M. (1997b) Design of an outcome study of the organization of hospital AIDS care, *Research in the Sociology of Health Care*, 14: 3–26.

Aiken, L.H., Sochalski, J. and Lake, E.T. (1997c) Studying outcomes of organizational change in health services, *Medical Care*, 35(suppl. 11): NS6–18.

Aiken, L.H., Sloane, D.M., Lake, E.T., Sochalski, J. and Weber, A.L. (1999) Organization and outcomes of inpatient AIDS care, *Medical Care*, 37(8): 760–72.

Al-Haider, A.S. and Wan, T.T. (1991) Modelling organizational determinants of hospital mortality, *Health Services Research*, 26(3): 303–23.

Baer, E.D., Fagin, C.M. and Gordon, S. (1996) *Abandonment of the Patient: The Impact of Profit-driven Health Care on the Public*. New York: Springer.

Ball, J. (1999) *Preliminary Nurse Survey Findings in England*. London: International Council of Nurses Meeting.

Bentsen, E.Z., Borum, F., Erlingsdottir, G. and Sahlin-Andersson, K. (eds) (1999) *Når Styringsambitioner Møder Praksis: den Svære Omstilling af Sygehus- og Sundhedsvæsenet i Danmark og Sverige [When Management Ambitions Meet Practice: The Difficult Transformation of the Hospital and Health Care System in Denmark and Sweden]*. Copenhagen: Copenhagen Business School Press.

Blancett, S.S. and Flarey, D.L. (1995) *Reengineering Nursing and Health Care: The Handbook for Organizational Transformation*. Gaithersburg, MD: Aspen.

Blegen, M.A. and Vaughn, T. (1998) A multisite study of nurse staffing and patient outcomes, *Nursing Economics*, 16(4): 196–203.

Blegen, M.A., Goode, C.J. and Reed, L. (1998) Nurse staffing and patient outcomes, *Nursing Research*, 47(1): 43–50.

Brannon, R.L. (1994) *Intensifying Care: The Hospital Industry, Professionalization and the Reorganization of the Nursing Labor Process*. Amityville, NY: Baywood.

Brannon, R.L. (1996) Restructuring hospital nursing: reversing the trend toward a professional work force, *International Journal of Health Services*, 26(4): 643–54.

Buerhaus, P.I. (1997) What is the harm in imposing mandatory hospital nurse staffing regulations?, *Nursing Economics*, 15: 66–72.

Champy, J. (1996) *Reengineering Management: The Mandate for New Leadership*. New York: Harper Business.

Chassin, M.R., Park, R.E., Lohr, K.N., Keesey, J. and Brook, R.H. (1989) Differences among hospitals in Medicare patient mortality, *Health Services Research*, 24(1): 1–31.

Clifford, J.C. (1998) *Restructuring: The Impact of Hospital Organization on Nursing Leadership*. Chicago, IL: AHA Press.

Cochrane, A.L. (1973) *Effectiveness and Efficiency: Random Reflections on Health Services*. London: Nuffield Provincial Hospital Trust.

Davidson, H., Folcarelli, P.H., Crawford, S., Duprat, L.J. and Clifford, J.C. (1997) The effects of health care reforms on job satisfaction and voluntary turnover among hospital-based nurses, *Medical Care*, 35(6): 634–45.

Decter, M. (1994) *Healing Medicare: Managing Health System Change the Canadian Way*. Toronto: McGilligan Books.

Donelan, K., Blendon, R.J., Schoen, C., Davis, K. and Binns, K. (1999) The cost of health system change: public discontent in five nations, *Health Affairs (Millwood)*, 18(3): 206–16.

Dranove, D., Durkac, A. and Shanley, M. (1996) Are multihospital systems more efficient?, *Health Affairs (Millwood)*, 15(1): 100–3.

Driedger, S.D. (1997) The nurses: the front-line caregivers are burned out. Is it any wonder?, *Maclean's*, 110: 24–7.

Flood, A.B. (1994) The impact of organizational and managerial factors on the quality of care in health care organizations, *Medical Care Research and Review*, 51: 381.

Flood, A.B., Scott, W.R. and Ewy, W. (1984a) Does practice make perfect? I: the relation between hospital volume and outcomes for selected diagnostic categories, *Medical Care*, 22(2): 98–114.

Flood, A.B., Scott, W.R. and Ewy, W. (1984b) Does practice make perfect? II: the relation between volume and outcomes and other hospital characteristics, *Medical Care*, 22(2): 115–25.

Fox, R.C., Aiken, L.H. and Messikomer, C.M. (1990) The culture of caring: AIDS and the nursing profession, *The Milbank Quarterly*, 68 (suppl. 2): 226–56.

Gallagher, R.M. (1999) The numbers game, *Nursing Standard*, 13(41): 18–19.

Hammer, M. and Champy, J. (1993) *Reengineering the Corporation: A Manifesto for Business Revolution*. New York: Harper Business.

Hartz, A.J., Krakauer, H., Kuhn, E.M. *et al.* (1989) Hospital characteristics and mortality rates, *New England Journal of Medicine*, 321(25): 1720–5.

Hensley, S. (1998) VHA readies ad campaign: proposed plan would play up local hospitals' strengths, *Modern Healthcare*, 28(4): 2–3.

Hoffart, N. and Woods, C.Q. (1996) Elements of a nursing professional practice model, *Journal of Professional Nursing*, 12(6): 354–64.

Institute of Medicine (1996) *Nursing Staff in Hospitals and Nursing Homes: Is it Adequate?* Washington, DC: National Academy Press.

Jarman, B., Gaults, S., Alves, B. *et al.* (1999) Explaining differences in English hospital death rates using routinely collected data, *British Medical Journal*, 318(7197): 1515–20.

Kelly, J.V. and Hellinger, F.J. (1986) Physician and hospital factors associated with mortality of surgical patients, *Medical Care*, 24(9): 785–800.

Klein, R. (1998) Why Britain is reorganizing its national health service – yet again, *Health Affairs (Millwood)*, 17(4): 111–25.

Knaus, W.A., Draper, E.A., Wagner, D.P. and Zimmerman, J.E. (1986) An evaluation of outcome from intensive care in major medical centers, *Annals of Internal Medicine*, 104(3): 410–18.

Kovner, C. and Gergen, P.J. (1998) Nurse staffing levels and adverse events following surgery in U.S. hospitals, *Image: Journal of Nursing Scholarship*, 30(4): 315–21.

Kramer, M. (1990) The magnet hospitals: excellence revisited, *Journal of Nursing Administration*, 20(9): 35–44.

Kramer, M. and Schmalenberg, C. (1988a) Magnet hospitals I: institutions of excellence, *Journal of Nursing Administration*, 18(1): 13–24.

Kramer, M. and Schmalenberg, C. (1988b) Magnet hospitals II: institutions of excellence, *Journal of Nursing Administration*, 18(2): 11–19.

Le Grand, J. (1999) Competition, cooperation, or control: tales from the British National Health Service, *Health Affairs (Millwood)*, 18(3): 27–39.

Leatt, P., Baker, G.R., Halverson, P.K. and Aird, C. (1997) Downsizing, reengineering and restructuring: long-term implications for healthcare organizations, *Frontiers of Health Services Management*, 13(4): 27–39.

Marmor, T.R. (1998) Hope and hyperbole: the rhetoric and reality of managerial reform in health care, *Journal of Health Services Research and Policy*, 3(1): 62–4.

McClure, M.L., Poulin, M.A., Sovie, M.D. and Wandelt, M.A. (1983) *Magnet Hospitals: Attraction and Retention of Professional Nurses*. Kansas City, MO: American Nurses' Association.

McKee, M., Aiken, L., Rafferty, A.M. and Sochalski, J. (1998) Organizational change and quality of health care: an evolving international agenda, *Quality in Health Care*, 7(1): 37–41.

Micklethwait, J. and Wooldridge, A. (1996) *The Witch Doctors: Making Sense of the Management Gurus*. New York: Times Books.

Mitchell, P.H. and Shortell, S.M. (1997) Adverse outcomes and variations in organization of care delivery, *Medical Care*, 35(11): NS19–32.

Moses, L.E. and Mosteller, F. (1968) Institutional differences in postoperative death rates: commentary on some of the findings of the National Halothane Study, *Journal of the American Medical Association*, 203(7): 492–4.

Naylor, C.D. (1999) Health care in Canada: incrementalism under fiscal duress, *Health Affairs (Millwood)*, 18(3): 9–26.

Reinhardt, U.E. (1996) Spending more through 'cost control': our obsessive quest to gut the hospital, *Health Affairs (Millwood)*, 15(2): 145–54.

Rosenthal, G.E., Harper, D.L., Quinn, L.M. and Cooper, G.S. (1997) Severity-adjusted mortality and length of stay in teaching and nonteaching hospitals: results of a regional study, *Journal of the American Medical Association*, 278(6): 485–90.

Royal College of Nursing (1998) *Evidence to the Review Body for Nursing Staff, Midwives, and Health Visitors: Memorandum*. London: Royal College of Nursing of the United Kingdom.

Rundall, T.G., Starkweather, D.B. and Norrish, B.R. (1998) *After Restructuring: Empowerment Strategies at Work in America's Hospitals*. San Francisco, CA: Jossey-Bass.

Scott, J.G., Sochalski, J. and Aiken, L. (1999) Review of magnet hospital research: findings and implications for professional nursing practice, *Journal of Nursing Administration*, 29(1): 9–19.

Shindul-Rothschild, J., Berry, D. and Long-Middleton, E. (1996) Where have all the nurses gone? Final results of our Patient Care Survey, *American Journal of Nursing*, 96(11): 25–39.

Shortell, S.M. and Hughes, E.F. (1988) The effects of regulation, competition and ownership on mortality rates among hospital inpatients, *New England Journal of Medicine*, 318(17): 1100–7.

Shortell, S.M., Morrison, E.M. and Friedman, B. (1990) *Strategic Choices for America's Hospitals: Managing Change in Turbulent Times*. San Francisco, CA: Jossey-Bass.

Silber, J.H., Rosenbaum, P.R. and Ross, R.N. (1995) Comparing the contributions of groups of predictors: which outcomes vary with hospital rather than patient characteristics?, *Journal of the American Statistical Association*, 90(429): 7–18.

Sochalski, J. and Aiken, L.H. (1999) Accounting for variation in hospital outcomes: a cross-national study, *Health Affairs (Millwood)*, 18(3): 256–9.

Thiemann, D.R., Coresh, J., Oetgen, W.J. and Powe, N.R. (1999) The association between hospital volume and survival after acute myocardial infarction in elderly patients, *New England Journal of Medicine*, 340: 1640–8.

van Servellen, G. and Schultz, M.A. (1999) Demystifying the influence of hospital characteristics on inpatient mortality rates, *Journal of Nursing Administration*, 29(4): 39–47.

Walston, S.L., Kimberley, J.R. and Burns, L.R. (1996) Owned vertical integration and health care: promise and performance, *Health Care Management Review*, 21(1): 83–92.

Walston, S.L., Burns, L.R. and Kimberly, J.R. (2000) Does re-engineering really work? An examination of the context and outcomes of hospital reengineering initiatives, *Health Services Research*, 34(6): 1363–88.

Wennberg, J. and Gittelsohn, S. (1973) Small area variations in health care delivery, *Science*, 182(117): 1102–8.

four

Conclusions

chapter fifteen

Future hospitals

Martin McKee and Judith Healy

The test of whether this book is successful will be whether it encourages a dialogue between those responsible for health care systems and those who manage hospitals. Our aim is to help stimulate a debate that will lead to a fundamental reappraisal of how hospital care is to be provided in Europe in the twenty-first century.

For too long, health policy-makers have treated hospitals as givens. This is hardly surprising. The locations of hospitals, their configurations and the spectrum of activities are typically the result of decisions made so long ago that few can remember how they came about. Today, in making decisions about hospitals, a health policy-maker must involve a range of stakeholders: hospital managers, education authorities, professional regulatory bodies, regional development agencies, private companies and consumer groups. The range and diversity of activities undertaken by the hospital are difficult for any one group to comprehend, with myriad complex interconnections and many unwritten rules. In many countries, professional independence is guarded jealously, with anything seen as external interference rejected as unacceptable. Faced with these circumstances, many policy-makers have adopted the path of least resistance. They have concentrated their attention on how money for the hospital system can be raised and left responsibility for spending it with hospital managers and clinicians, who, it is assumed, know best.

This approach has some merit. The encounter between the patient and the health professional is extremely complex. It is characterized by uncertainty, asymmetry of information and competing and often unspoken values. It does not lend itself to micro-management from afar and, as the experience of the Soviet Union showed, any attempt to do so leads to deprofessionalization and, ultimately, poor quality of service.

Nevertheless, just as 'war is too important to be left to the generals', hospital care is too important to be left to hospital managers and health professionals. Hospitals face enormous pressure to meet the immediate needs of all patients who reach their door, while simultaneously balancing this year's budget. This makes it difficult to look to the long-term needs of the entire population that the hospital is serving, taking account of the services provided by neighbouring hospitals and by health professionals working in non-hospital settings. The immediacy of their patients' health needs distracts the attention of the hospital from the needs of future generations and how to ensure adequate investment in facilities, people and knowledge. The pace of work makes it difficult to stand back and assess whether the care that is being provided is as effective as it might be and whether it is being delivered in a way that responds to the legitimate expectations of patients. The focus on health care may detract from other important functions of the hospital, such as training, research and its broader societal roles. This often involves balancing conflicting incentives and hidden subsidies. Here, policy-makers can do much to ensure that each of these roles is recognized and rewarded. In brief, the creation of a modern, appropriately configured hospital system requires a coordinated effort by those working within the hospital system and those outside it.

One of the pervasive messages in this book is the need to take account of different contexts. Each country has inherited a particular hospital system. Each draws on different levels of resources, not simply financial but also the legacy of long-term investment in facilities, people and knowledge. Countries also face different challenges in the future, with differing patterns of disease and popular expectations. For these reasons, it would be foolish to suggest a blueprint that could be applied in every circumstance. Instead, we have identified and explored a series of issues that we believe will stimulate policy-makers to question why hospital care in their country or region is provided in the way that it is.

One issue policy-makers need to clarify is what, precisely, is meant by the term 'hospital'. As Chapter 1 showed, this word covers many types of institutions, even within a single country. Given the many interpretations and the changing roles of a modern hospital, discussion should focus on the spectrum of services that are provided for a designated population wherever they are delivered, inside or outside the hospital. Thus, rather than looking at the distribution of emergency departments, we should examine the overall trauma management system, including immediate care, evacuation, definitive treatment and rehabilitation. The enormous technical advances in surgical care allow more treatment in free-standing ambulatory surgery facilities. It should also be asked whether long-term nursing care is best provided in large, impersonal institutions or in purpose-built facilities closer to an individual's family.

As Chapter 2 shows, hospitals are a product of history. The arguments that justified their location and layout may or may not continue to apply. What is certain is that these arguments should be reassessed regularly. But even if the current hospitals are configured appropriately, they are unlikely to continue to be so in the future. Chapter 3 sets out a range of issues with enormous implications for hospitals in the future. Populations in many countries are ageing, so policy-makers are very concerned about the implications for health care costs. We argue that these implications may be less than anticipated, at least where social care can substitute for inappropriate and more expensive hospital care. Instead, the main issue for hospitals is that older people will have multiple disorders that require coordinated programmes of care from multidisciplinary teams of professionals with a range of specialist skills.

Population ageing is only one factor behind changing patterns of disease. Changing risk factors, such as smoking and diet, will also influence the diseases that hospitals must deal with. Furthermore, hospitals must also respond to changing public expectations and more demanding consumers.

The tools available to hospitals will also change, opening up new possibilities for diagnosis and treatment. Finally, they will have to work in new policy contexts, which increasingly will reflect European and global developments. Hospitals will have to anticipate and respond to these changes, in the same way that successful manufacturing and service companies monitor and adapt to their environments.

Many of the pressures that hospitals will face will be outside their control, but not all. Throughout history, hospitals have been engaged in an evolutionary struggle with infectious agents. There is a real danger that they will win the battle but lose the war. The unregulated use of antibiotics may offer short-term gains but is ultimately unsustainable.

Policy-makers must also stand back and look at the overall hospital system, since individual hospitals cannot be considered in isolation. Instead, policy-makers should begin from the perspective of a specified population, with defined health needs, and look at the spectrum of health care that is available, whether hospital or community based. As Chapter 6 makes clear, the pattern of hospital services involves balancing geographical access, which calls for dispersed facilities, with the need for a critical mass of interlinked specialties, which requires some concentration. It must also take account of what elements of health care are provided outside hospitals. Advances in technology and changing expectations mean that both the optimal size of a hospital and the interface between the hospital and the rest of the health care system are in a state of flux. For these reasons, the configuration of hospital systems will have to change. Experience from several countries indicates that this is easier when undertaken within a regional planning mechanism. Conversely, devolving a high degree of autonomy to individual hospitals serves to entrench the existing system.

Hospitals can only provide high-quality, responsive care if they have access to a range of external inputs. These include funds for investment in facilities, trained staff and the knowledge needed to provide effective care. Governments, and those acting on their behalf, have a responsibility to ensure that hospitals have access to these inputs and are thus enabled to provide optimal care. However, they also have a responsibility to ensure that hospitals use resources appropriately. This should not involve micro-management of each hospital, but it does require policy-makers, in broad terms, to specify how hospitals should be used and what they should achieve and to monitor the results. This responsibility is referred to as 'stewardship'.

Those responsible for the broader health care system have a range of tools at their disposal. The mixed experiences of hospital reform show that policy-makers should be consistent about what they wish to achieve and ensure that the external incentives that they put in place are aligned with the internal incentives within individual hospitals.

The individual hospital has the primary responsibility for providing quality care. The first step is to provide appropriate facilities. These should be sufficiently flexible to adapt to inevitably changing circumstances. Increasing ambulatory surgery requires fewer beds but more operating theatres, and advances in anaesthesia enable some routine surgery to be removed from the hospital altogether into free-standing ambulatory care facilities. Hospitals should also take account of the vulnerabilities of their patients, many of whom are frightened or confused and have sensory or motor impairments.

Hospitals also need adequately trained staff. They, too, must be able to adapt to changing circumstances. All health care providers must update their skills regularly, and the public increasingly will demand that health professionals demonstrate their continuing competence to practise. Hospitals must ensure that they have systems in place to monitor and enhance the quality of care. This should take into account the evidence summarized in Chapter 13 on the effectiveness of different ways of changing professional behaviour.

Hospital staff require equipment to do their jobs. Again, this needs to be looked at from the perspective of the wider health care system. Decisions must be based on evidence of effectiveness, which requires creating health technology assessment agencies that can develop and disseminate such guidelines. Decisions should also take account of what is available in neighbouring hospitals to avoid duplication or gaps in provision.

All these inputs need to be brought together into a coherent whole. This will be easier if it is within the framework of a supportive hospital culture. Efforts to improve hospital performance are also facilitated by systems that link improvements in quality to control over resources, with managers judged equally on their delivery of high-quality care and achievement of financial targets.

In conclusion, Europe has extremely diverse hospitals, health care systems, values and beliefs. Furthermore, enormous changes are underway in the countries of Europe. Nevertheless, three basic messages apply everywhere. First, hospitals exist to improve the health of the population, a task they fulfil not only by providing health care that responds to the needs and expectations of their patients, but also through teaching and research. Second, hospitals are only one element of a health care system. They cannot be considered in isolation from each other or from the health and social care provided in other settings. Third, improving health and providing responsive and appropriate care are a shared responsibility involving both hospitals and those responsible for the wider health care system. We hope that this book provides the various interest groups with evidence that can guide their shared decision-making.

Index